Epidemiology for Canadian Students

Epidemiology for Canadian Students

Principles, Methods & Critical Appraisal

Scott B. Patten MD, PhD

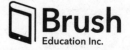

Brush Education Inc.
www.brusheducation.ca
contact@brusheducation.ca

Printed and manufactured in Canada

Cover and interior design: Carol Dragich, Dragich Design. Cover images: ©iStock.com/csheezio—dandelion image; ©iStock.com/urbancow—crowd.

Library and Archives Canada Cataloguing in Publication
Patten, Scott B. (Scott Burton), 1962–, author
Epidemiology for Canadian students : principles, methods and critical appraisal / Scott B. Patten, MD, PhD.
Includes bibliographical references and index.
Issued in print and electronic formats.
ISBN 978-1-55059-572-7 (pbk.).—ISBN 978-1-55059-573-4 (pdf).—
ISBN 978-1-55059-574-1 (mobi).—ISBN 978-1-55059-575-8 (epub)

1. Epidemiology.   I. Title.

RA651.P38 2015   614.4   C2014-908351-3
                                       C2014-908352-1

We also acknowledge the financial support of the Government of Canada through the Canada Book Fund for our publishing activities.

Canadian   Patrimoine
Heritage   canadien

Contents

List of Figures

First principles of epidemiology

1

What is epidemiology?

Objectives
- Define key epidemiological terms.
- Identify the historical roots of epidemiological reasoning.
- Describe the importance of epidemiology to health professionals.

Definition and terms

Epidemiology is the study of the distribution and determinants of disease in populations.

Let's break this down.

Distribution and determinants

The definition of epidemiology uses the terms *distribution* and *determinants*, which describe an important division in the field.

Distribution is the focus of descriptive epidemiology. The ability to describe the distribution of diseases is essential for developing hypotheses about their etiology and for planning health services.

Determinants are the focus of analytical epidemiology. A *determinant* is something that causes a disease (an etiological factor), or that influences the distribution of a disease in a population. For example, a risk factor is a determinant—one that increases the risk of disease. Factors that determine the chances of recovering or dying from a disease are also determinants, because they shape disease patterns in populations.

Descriptive and analytical epidemiology are different, but it's important not to make too much of this distinction. Many epidemiological studies have both descriptive and analytical goals.

Key point: Epidemiology has 2 major branches: descriptive epidemiology and analytical epidemiology.

Population

Epidemiology is a population-based science. Although epidemiology can be concerned with many different kinds of populations, it is always concerned with a population. It focuses on groups of people rather than individuals.

Studies that focus on individual people (case studies or case series) do not usually provide any epidemiological data. Epidemiological studies have the goal of advancing knowledge about populations.

The focus on studying populations does not mean that epidemiology is not relevant for individual people. Much of what we know about the health of individual people derives from epidemiological studies. What makes people sick? What keeps them healthy? What treatments are most likely to return sick people to health? Individual people have a multitude of individual differences. Studies of large groups of people make the effects of such differences cancel out—they bring into focus the health outcomes associated with various exposures in a way that is not possible at the individual level.

For example, defenders of smoking used to say that they knew somebody who smoked heavily and who did not develop any complications. They interpreted this observation as evidence that smoking was not harmful. But an individual case is a poor basis for determining whether smoking is harmful. It would be better to know what happens to large numbers of people who smoke, and to contrast this with the experience of large numbers of nonsmokers. This requires researching groups of people, but the knowledge gained is very relevant for individual decisions. Studying large groups of people can teach us a lot (arguably most of what we know) about determinants of health and disease as they affect individual people.

Key point: Epidemiology emphasizes groups of people rather than individuals, but it can teach us a lot about health risks that are important to individuals.

It is important to keep an open mind about what is meant by the term *population*. In epidemiology, a population can be almost any definable group. The most familiar type of population is defined geographically or politically—for example, the population of Nova Scotia. Epidemiologists are often interested in provincial populations because administration of health care is a provincial responsibility in Canada. Descriptive epidemiological information (e.g., the number of people in different regions of Canada with multiple sclerosis) is necessary for planning and administering services, and for formulating health policy—a point documented in a 2005 study by Beck et al.[1]

However, a population doesn't need to be a geographically defined group. The term *population* could also apply to, for example, recreational skiers, or women, or children with disabilities enrolled in a particular school system.

Epidemiology is a way of answering questions about populations and the term *population* can be used to describe almost any group about which there is a question to be answered.

Key point: A population, in epidemiology, can be almost any identifiable group of people.

Disease

In epidemiology, *disease* is shorthand for almost any type of health outcome, including many that are not normally called a disease—for example, obesity, literacy, and hunger. This is partly because, in the literature, too many terms can lead to complex and cumbersome language.

Just to be clear: it would be perfectly correct to define epidemiology as the study of the distribution and determinants of health-related problems in populations.

Other key terms

Exposure refers to a determinant or potential determinant. For example, a person may be exposed to cigarette smoke, radiation, or psychosocial stress. Often, studies ask whether such factors are health determinants, so it makes sense to call these factors *exposures* until research confirms them as determinants. Investigations of a factor as a potential determinant of disease often reveal that some people have had exposure to the factor and others have not. When collecting data, the presence or absence of the factor can assume different values (in this case exposed or not exposed, yes or no)—in other words, exposure is a variable. The traditional distinction between an independent and dependent variable in experimental science roughly corresponds to exposure and disease, respectively, in epidemiology.

You may see definitions of epidemiology with the term *disease frequency* rather than just *disease* (e.g., "the study of the distribution and determinants of disease frequency in populations"). This wording emphasizes that epidemiological research tends to target groups of people rather than individuals. Other definitions specify "human populations" (e.g., "the study of the distribution and determinants of disease in human populations"). This wording aims to distinguish epidemiology from laboratory sciences, but it creates a problem by excluding veterinary epidemiology—human and animal epidemiologists increasingly work together under a philosophy called "One Health."[2]

Inconsistent terminology is a difficult reality of epidemiology. It can be frustrating: people use terms differently, or use different labels for the same intended meaning. However, since all health science students (and practitioners) need to access and understand the literature, it is best to embrace this diverse terminology, and become familiar with its contradictions, variations, and nuances. In your own work and writing, though, you should aim to use the most specific and applicable term available. This book will offer many suggestions about preferred terminology.

History of epidemiology

The science of epidemiology originated in efforts to address epidemics of infectious disease in the nineteenth century.

John Snow is usually identified as a founder of epidemiology due to his work in public health in London, England. Snow was also an innovator in the field of anesthesiology, but he is now most famous for his investigation of cholera outbreaks. In the 1850s, Snow was able to link cholera deaths to sewage-contaminated drinking water provided by specific utility companies. He also linked a point-source outbreak of cholera to a public water source, the Broad Street pump.[3] He accomplished this not by studying victims in a hospital, morgue, or laboratory, and not by culturing cholera bacilli in a lab— instead, he examined the distribution of cholera deaths in relation to possible determinants. He identified a pattern of distribution consistent with water as the most likely source of infection, which contradicted a theory popular at the time that tainted air—a "miasma"—caused cholera outbreaks. Snow's approach was innovative and represented a major public-health milestone. The London School of Hygiene and Tropical Medicine commemorated his legacy in 2013, the bicentenary of his birth.[4]

The story of John Snow highlights 2 defining characteristics of epidemiology.

First, epidemiology uses probability and statistical reasoning. This broke with scientific conventions at the time, which were more directly aligned with logic and mathematics. During the cholera outbreaks Snow studied, not everyone exposed to sewage-contaminated water developed cholera, and not everyone with cholera was directly exposed to sewage-contaminated water. But people who were exposed had a higher probability of getting cholera—according to Steven Johnson, 6 in 10 drinkers of water from the Broad Street pump developed cholera, compared with only 1 in 10 of nondrinkers.[3] If you look at postulates for linking infectious agents to disease such Koch's postulates (see Table 1), Snow's approach might seem fuzzy and undisciplined, but it has come to dominate health science research—at least research involving human subjects. This is true even within the sphere of medical therapeutics. Today, for example, a drug is "effective" if it produces a desired outcome more often than placebo. If Koch's postulates were used assess the effectiveness of drugs (e.g., "everyone should improve when given the drug, no one should improve without the drug" etc.), it would be almost impossible for therapeutics to advance.

Second, the John Snow story highlights the ability of epidemiology to deliver effective public health strategies before the biology of a disease is clear.

TABLE 1. KOCH'S POSTULATES[5]

1. The infectious agent must be found in abundance in all individuals with the disease, but should not be found at all in healthy individuals.

2. It must be isolated and cultured from a diseased individual.

3. The cultured infectious agent should cause disease in a healthy individual (creating a new case of the disease).

4. The infectious agent must be isolated from the new case and confirmed as identical to the original infectious agent.

The cholera bacillus was not isolated until decades after Snow's work,[6] but his work produced effective public health action. To this day, safe drinking water is the key strategy to controlling diarrheal diseases such as cholera—more effective and more important than treatments targeting the infectious agents themselves (e.g., antibiotics).

Key point: Epidemiological methods originated in studies of infectious diseases, but are key to understanding health and disease in general.

Is epidemiology important to health professionals?

Epidemiology is a foundational health science. A great deal of contemporary health research and the majority of studies conducted with human subjects use epidemiological principles and methods.

The most notable exception is qualitative research, which typically does not draw on epidemiological methods (epidemiology is a decidedly quantitative field). Even qualitative researchers, though, need to read the quantitative literature, which requires knowledge of epidemiology. In addition, researchers often combine qualitative methods with epidemiological approaches in mixed-method studies. For example, Riley et al[7] have recently applied mixed methods to study continuity of care between cardiac rehabilitation services and primary care practices in Ontario.

Key point: Epidemiology is a foundational health science. Understanding the basics of epidemiology enables better understanding of the contemporary health research literature.

The foundational role of epidemiology in health science research makes it an especially important field to study. A solid grasp of epidemiology is also essential for practising health care professionals. Interpretation of diagnostic signs and symptoms, as well as interpretation of test results, depends on concepts from epidemiology. Even the randomized controlled clinical trial—the most important study design for evaluating treatments—is built on epidemiologic foundations.

In a world dominated by technology, it is easy to imagine that a discipline such as epidemiology might become obsolete. After all, how can comparisons between groups of people possibly compete with advanced medical imaging or molecular biology? But consider: How can we gauge the risks and benefits of emerging technologies for health? The answer to this crucial question depends on the foundational concepts and strategies of epidemiology. For example, advances in pharmacology lead to the development of new drugs, but it will all come to nothing—all the investment of time, money, and technology in drug development—if the drugs cannot be shown effective and safe in the real world. This part hinges on epidemiologic data.

Key point: Technological advances create a need for epidemiological research. Epidemiology is a more essential and vibrant discipline now than ever before.

Modern health care systems are driven by data. In Canada, the publicly funded health system has a responsibility to respond to the needs of Canadians, and the administration of this health system means collecting massive quantities of data. Increasingly, these administrative data sets are used to drive health system decisions, to monitor the functioning of the health system, and to track the impact of diseases. Research designed to make the health system better—health services research—is also firmly planted on a foundation provided by epidemiology. In our information age, and with the advances of evidence-based medicine, epidemiology will become increasingly important.

Thinking deeper

Epidemiology in symbols

Epidemiology is the study of the distribution of disease in populations. This is a starting point for expressing epidemiological ideas in symbols, because it implies a division between members of a population that have a disease and members that don't. You can express this as A (for people with a disease) and B (for people without a disease). This expression is complementary because each person either has, or does not have, the disease. The total number of people in the population, then, may be denoted N such that $A + B = N$.

Table 2 embodies the distinction between having a disease or not. This table has 1 row with population values and 2 columns that describe the distinction. It is therefore a 1×2 ("one by two") table.

TABLE 2. 1 × 2 TABLE FOR A POPULATION

Disease	No disease	Total
A	B	N

It is easy to see how a 1 × 2 table can be used to represent the amount of disease in a population. However, epidemiology is concerned with the distribution of disease in populations—so, it is useful to have a table that contains, or represents, a comparison of disease frequency in several groups. A good place to start is with consideration of an exposure. If we divide a population of size N into exposed and not-exposed categories, we can construct a table that depicts the number of people with and without disease in each group. In this case, the cross-tabulation of disease and exposure has something to say about the relationship between exposure and disease. Indeed, examination of this exact contingency (the exposure-disease contingency) is a central paradigm of epidemiologic research. This kind of table is called a 2 × 2 contingency table. A 2 × 2 contingency table has 4 cells based on 2 variables that can each assume 2 values (see Table 3).

In Table 3, note that A and B have different meanings than in Table 2. In Table 2, A included all of the people with the disease. In Table 3, A includes only a portion of those with the disease (those also exposed). The remaining portion (C) includes those who have the disease but are not exposed. Similarly, B now represents only those without disease who are exposed, and D represents those without the disease who are not exposed.

A word of caution about 2 × 2 contingency tables: some books and papers present disease status in the table rows rather than the columns (the reverse of Table 3). This changes the meaning of the symbols A, B, C, and D (assuming that their row and column positions remain the same), and the meaning of row totals ($A + B$ and $C + D$) and column totals ($A + C$ and $B + D$). A subscript to denote exposure and disease status conveys these totals with clarity (see Table 4).

The cells of a 2 × 2 contingency table allow important comparisons. For example, the frequency of disease in the nonexposed component of the population is $C/N_{nonexposed}$. Since diseases do not distribute randomly in populations

TABLE 3. 2 × 2 CONTINGENCY TABLE

	Disease	No disease
Exposed	A	B
Not exposed	C	D

TABLE 4. 2 × 2 CONTINGENCY TABLE WITH ROW AND COLUMN TOTALS

	Disease	No disease	Row totals
Exposed	A	B	$N_{exposed}$
Not exposed	C	D	$N_{nonexposed}$
Column totals	$N_{disease}$	$N_{no\ disease}$	

(they instead distribute in relation to their determinants), it is very interesting to know how $A/N_{exposed}$ compares to $C/N_{nonexposed}$.

Questions

1. In 2006, Bernstein et al[8] applied a case-identification algorithm to administrative data for inflammatory bowel diseases to identify cases of these diseases in 5 Canadian provinces. This allowed estimation of the number of cases in each province.
   a. Administrative data derive partially from physician-billing invoices and hospital-discharge summaries. Do you think this is a good way to identify cases of disease?
   b. Would you classify this study as primarily descriptive or primarily analytical?
   c. Does it concern you that only 5 provinces were included? Why or why not?
   d. Is it important to know how many people have this disease? Why or why not?

2. Maxwell et al[9] studied 2779 clients receiving services from community care access centres in Ontario from 1999 to 2001. Nearly half of these clients had daily pain, but one-fifth received no analgesic treatment. The investigators were concerned that the needs of these clients were not being met.
   a. Is this study "population based"?
   b. Do you think that this study qualifies as an epidemiological study?
   c. Why did the investigators need such a large sample?
   d. What is the descriptive value of their result?
   e. Can you think of a role for this finding in the planning or administration of health services?

3. Tyas et al[10] studied risk factors for Alzheimer disease in Manitoba. They used data from a longitudinal, population-based study of dementia conducted in that province. During 5 years of follow-up, subjects with fewer years of education were found to be at greater risk of Alzheimer disease.
   a. Based on the information provided, would you regard this study as analytical or descriptive?
   b. As you see it, what is the value of this kind of information?

4. Can you identify any similarities between the work of Bernstein, Maxwell, and Tyas, and the work of John Snow?

5. Imagine that you are John Snow and that you are advocating for safer disposal of sewage in nineteenth-century London.
   a. You are accused of failing to appreciate the difference between correlation and causation, and thereby drawing a false conclusion about a causal link. How would you respond?
   b. You are accused of knowing nothing of the etiology of cholera because you have no idea what the infectious agent is. How would you respond?

2

Epidemiological reasoning

Objectives
- State the fundamental assumption of epidemiological research.
- Explain the key concepts of association, proportion, prevalence, and point prevalence.
- Identify the 2 main sources of error in epidemiologic research: random error and systematic error (bias).
- Define critical appraisal.

The fundamental assumption

Epidemiology rests on this fundamental assumption: diseases do not distribute randomly in populations, but rather distribute in relation to their determinants.

Intuitively, this makes a lot of sense. If smokers, for example, are more likely to develop lung cancer, then a pattern of association (or, we could say "contingency") will emerge between smoking and lung cancer. Specifically, you would expect smokers to develop lung cancer more often than nonsmokers. You might also expect people with lung cancer to have been smokers more often than people without the disease. In the language of epidemiology, smoking and lung cancer are associated. If smoking and lung cancer were in fact distributed randomly in the population (if they were independent of each another and therefore not associated), the only value of studying their distribution would be descriptive: to determine how much smoking and lung cancer exists in the population.

Key point: Studying associations between exposures and disease is the "bread and butter" of analytical epidemiology.

Association and causation

Everyone has heard the truism that "correlation is not causation." In other words, an association between 2 variables does not mean that 1 is causing the other. Occasionally, a scientist challenges the value of epidemiological studies because of this—some laboratory scientists, for example, believe only a detailed understanding of the molecular underpinnings of a disease can substantiate causal association.

Certainly, many spurious correlations exist. Did you know, for example, that annual US spending on science, space, and technology correlates strongly (0.99) with the annual number of suicides by hanging, strangulation, and suffocation in the US?[11] This association is not causal—but does that mean no association can be considered causal? Not at all: the reason epidemiology can inform etiology is that, for epidemiologists, questions of cause are related to public health actions, not mechanistic conceptions of cause.

EPIDEMIOLOGY AND SMOKING

The question of whether smoking causes lung cancer is a good illustration. In 1950, Doll and Hill[12] published a study in the *British Medical Journal* called "Smoking and Carcinoma of the Lung: Preliminary Report." They began their study by carefully identifying cases of lung cancer (as well as certain other cancers) from a selection of hospitals in the UK. Doll and Hill interviewed the patients in each case to obtain a detailed record of the patients' smoking history. With this data, they classified the cases into smoking and nonsmoking groups, where exposure (smoking) was defined as anyone who had smoked at least 1 cigarette per day for at least 1 year. They applied the same interview and classification procedure to a comparison (control) group, whose subjects mirrored the lung-cancer group in terms of sex, 5-year age group, and where and when they were hospitalized. This allowed a comparison of the frequency of smoking in the lung-cancer and control groups (an approach that has come to be known as a case-control study). A large majority of the men in their sample were smokers, according to their definition. This included all but 2 (0.3%) of the male cancer patients and all but 27 (4.2%) of the controls. Doll and Hill used an exact statistical test to confirm that a difference this large, or larger, would be very unlikely to emerge by chance (the calculated probability was 0.00000064). They had confirmed an association between smoking and lung cancer.

The discovery of an association between smoking and lung cancer led to public health efforts to decrease the frequency of smoking. These efforts have been partially successful. In men, the frequency of daily or occasional smoking has diminished to 22.1% of males (and 16.5% of females).[13] This, in turn, has resulted in diminishing lung cancer incidence. For example, according to the Canadian Cancer Registry, age standardized (this term will be explained later) carcinoma of the bronchus and lungs declined in men from 74.7 per 100 000 between 1996 and 1998, to 65.0 per 100 000 between 2005 and 2007.[14]

This progress happened even though no mechanism of causation between lung cancer and smoking had been identified. If the world of public health had waited for research to establish the mechanism, imagine the thousands of people who would have died. And waiting may have served no point: understanding the basic physiology may not have assisted in any way with the public health actions necessary for this progress. A strategy document published by Health Canada in 1999[15] listed the following strategic directions: policy and legislation, public education, industry accountability and product control, research, and building capacity for action. None of this depends on molecular biology or even physiology.

Note the parallels between the epidemiology of smoking described in this chapter and the work of John Snow described in chapter 1. The power of epidemiological research to identify etiological connections in the absence of a thorough pathophysiological understanding is clear.

The "acid test" for an epidemiological assertion of cause involves public health action. Will a "cause" in the public health sense (diminishing the frequency of smoking) produce the desired public health effect (a lowering of the incidence of lung cancer)? Had the association between smoking and lung cancer not been causal, public health action would not have been justified and the incidence of lung cancer would not have changed as a result of efforts to discourage smoking. If epidemiological evidence confirms that a public health or clinical action will lead to improved health, then a causal effect has been identified.

Key point: Analytical epidemiologic studies are not often concerned with disease mechanisms (sometimes they are). However, they are often concerned with disease etiology.

EPIDEMIOLOGY AND THERAPEUTIC INTERVENTIONS

A corollary to this way of thinking can also be seen in the literature about the efficacy of treatment and the modern emphasis that is placed on evidence-based medicine. If health professionals are practising evidence-based medicine, they are taking actions that, according to evidence, will lead to the improved health of their patients. These choices do not usually hinge on detailed knowledge of pathophysiology and pharmacology. Health professionals need this knowledge, but this knowledge is not (according to evidence-based medicine) the key deciding factor when selecting among—for example—drug therapies. The key deciding factor comes from observations similar to those made by John Snow, and Doll and Hill—observations that derive ultimately from comparisons of frequencies in different groups of people. Note that, where drug therapies and other therapeutic interventions are concerned, randomized controlled trials are a way of delivering information about frequencies.

Key point: Epidemiological research can identify the causes of disease, but the concept of "cause" is often based on clinical or public health "effects."

Epidemiologic parameters

A parameter, in epidemiology, represents a characteristic of a population. Parameters usually need to be estimated (this is what epidemiologic research does!) and understanding such estimates involves understanding probability.

Proportion

Actions to reduce smoking, and choices about drug therapies, invoke the fundamental assumption of epidemiology and also the idea of comparison. There would be no value in comparing smokers to nonsmokers if the health outcomes at issue were purely random. Similarly, randomized controlled trials comparing different drug therapies would be of little value if treatment outcomes were random. If the results of a diagnostic test were not associated with the disease under evaluation, that test would be useless. The reality that health outcomes are not random makes exploration of those nonrandom elements (associations) valuable.

The fundamental assumption of epidemiology connects progress in health research to statistics—specifically to the link between frequencies (which can be observed in samples or populations) and probabilities, risks, and rates. Gaining the knowledge needed to improve health depends on estimating probabilities, risks, and rates (which must be known) from things like counts and frequencies (which can, at least, be observed).

Epidemiology has a precise term for the concept of frequency: *proportion.* A proportion is a type of ratio, so it consists of 2 numbers, 1 divided by the other. The top number in the ratio is the numerator and the bottom number is the denominator. The special characteristic of a proportion (as opposed to any other ratio) is that the contents of the numerator are contained in the denominator.

Imagine that you have flipped a coin 10 times, and the result is 5 heads and 5 tails. The proportion of the coin flips that are heads is 5/10. The numerator is 5 and the denominator is 10. The 5 heads are included with the 5 tails in the denominator of the ratio. This example, as artificial as it may be, illustrates an important point. If you flip a coin 10 times, you might observe exactly 5 heads. Indeed, this is the expected proportion based on the symmetry of the coin. However, it is also quite likely that you would only observe 3 or 4 heads rather than the expected 5. You would also fairly frequently observe 6 or 7 heads. Nothing about the coin changes, which means the observed proportion of heads in this small series is influenced by chance. Notice that if you had flipped the coin only twice, the vulnerability of this proportion (of heads) to chance is even greater. Based on the symmetry of the coin, we can surmise that 2-flip experiments would produce the following proportions: 0/2 one-quarter of the time, 1/2 one-half of the time, and 2/2 one-quarter of the time (in decimal form, the proportion of heads may be 0, 0.5, or 1). These proportions cover the whole range that a proportion can cover, from 0 to 1. Since the denominator of any proportion includes the contents of the numerator, a proportion can never be more than 1. In the case of our 2-flip example, the entire range of possible values is covered (0, 1, or 2 heads) and the probability of the various outcomes is quite high, suggesting that there is a lot of randomness in what happens when a coin is flipped twice.

THE LAW OF LARGE NUMBERS

There is something magical about proportions. The magic, however, only emerges when the coin is flipped many times, not just twice. If you have the time, try a little experiment: try flipping a coin 100 times, or 1000 times. Or play with an online simulated coin flipper. As the number of flips goes up, the proportion of heads that you observe gets closer and closer to one-half. This is the magic: when you flip a coin once, the proportion you observe will be either 0/1 or 1/1; when you flip it twice, the proportion you observe could be 0/2, 1/2, or 2/2; when you flip it 1000 times, the proportion you observe will predictably be very close to 1/2 (in the language of ratios it will be close to 500/1000, in the language of decimals it will be close to 0.50, and in the language of percentages it will be close to 50%).

The effect you observe as you increase the number of coin flips is an example of the law of large numbers. This law states that when an experiment with a random variable as an outcome is repeated many times, the result becomes closer and closer to an expected value.

To truly understand the power of the law of large numbers, you must reverse this line of reasoning. Imagine that you had a coin that might be a trick coin—let's say that it might have 2 heads or 2 tails—and that you had to flip the coin to figure this out.

If you flip the coin once, you won't be able to tell: you will observe either heads or tails, but because both outcomes are possible for a fair coin and a trick coin, you aren't going to learn very much about the coin.

If you flip the coin twice and observe heads each time, you might begin to think it's a trick coin: you know the probability of this happening is lower. The 2 flips are 2 independent events: if it's a fair coin, we can calculate the probability of seeing heads both times as the product of each event in isolation— 0.5×0.5 or 0.5^2, which is 0.25 or 25%.

What if you flip the coin 10 times and each time it's heads? The probability of this happening is 0.5^{10}, which is an extremely tiny number, approximately 0.001.

The lesson here is that the law of large numbers goes both ways. It allows prediction of long-run probabilities when the expected value of an individual trial is known, but more importantly it allows knowledge to be gained about the probabilities that underlie observed proportions.

Flipping a coin results in heads or tails—a binary outcome. Binary outcomes are at the centre of many health-related questions. A person can have a disease or not, and can be exposed to a risk factor (drinking unsafe water, smoking) or not. A diagnostic test can be positive or negative, right or wrong, and so on.

Key point: A few observations of a binary outcome do not provide very much information about the probabilities associated with that outcome, but observing many independent observations provides a lot of information about those probabilities.

Prevalence

The law of large numbers and properties of coin flipping also apply to prevalence, another key concept in epidemiology.

Prevalence is the proportion of a population with a disease. Prevalence is an example of an epidemiologic parameter. Mathematically, it is a proportion and cannot therefore be less than 0 or more than 1. Epidemiologically, it represents a characteristic of a population: the amount of disease in that population. As with other proportions, prevalence has a numerator and a denominator. The numerator is the number of people with a disease and the denominator includes all members of the population. It should be noted that, occasionally, epidemiologists use the term *prevalence* to refer to the number of people in a population with a disease. However, most commonly, prevalence refers to a proportion as described here.

There are several types of prevalence: the most important is point prevalence, which is the proportion of a population with a disease at a particular point in time. How can knowledge about the prevalence of disease be obtained? Think about flipping a coin again: each flip of the coin is an event that produces either heads or tails. Now imagine this: instead of flipping a coin, you randomly select individual people from a population—say, the population of Canada—and determine whether they have a particular disease. Heads or tails? Disease or no disease? The probability that a member of this population has the disease will reflect the probability that Canadians in general have this disease. If it were possible to examine everybody in Canada and determine whether they had the disease, you could divide the number that have the disease by the total number of Canadians, leading to exact knowledge about the point prevalence of the disease. A sample of 1 person would not add very much to the state of knowledge on this question. As with a coin flip, that person will either have the disease or not, from which you can only conclude that the prevalence is either greater than 0 (if that person has the disease) or less than 100% (if the person does not). But a large sample, which consists of many independent observations, gives more information. The larger the sample—like the more flips of a coin—the stronger the expectation that the observed proportion reflects the underlying point prevalence.

Sources of error

The power of epidemiological research comes from the fundamental assumption of epidemiology and the law of large numbers: epidemiologists can understand disease distribution very clearly if their research studies have large samples. The value of epidemiology for planning services, identifying risk factors, identifying prognostic factors, and interpreting the results of tests follows logically from this. It would seem that the "sky is the limit," and that epidemiology can hardly fail to shed light on the distribution and determinants of any disease.

Unfortunately, it is not quite that simple. Things can go wrong in research.

Systematic error comes from flaws in study design that systematically bias study results. Imperfect measurement is an example of systematic error. In our discussion of coin flipping and random sampling, we assumed we had perfect measurement: that a head could be accurately discerned from a tail, and disease from no disease. Determining whether someone has a disease, however, isn't necessarily a simple matter. If measurement is imperfect, the law of large numbers does not work in the expected way.

Random error comes from chance. For example, it is not always possible to obtain the huge samples that can fully harness the law of large numbers. When sample sizes are too small, as with a small number of coin tosses, the observed disease proportions may fall far from the actual prevalence by chance alone. Random error always becomes smaller as sample size increases.

Extraneous factors can also lead to error—in ways that challenge the fundamental assumption itself. Diseases distribute in populations in relation to determinants, but what if a real determinant just happens to go together with some unimportant factor? It could fool a researcher into thinking that it— the unimportant, extraneous factor—was a cause of the disease. A researcher unaware of this possibility could mistake the extraneous factor for a determinant merely due to its tendency to distribute with a real determinant.

Key point: Epidemiology has a theoretical basis grounded solidly in the law of large numbers. However, in practice there are many potential pitfalls. Students and practitioners of the health sciences and health professionals need to be skilled in identifying vulnerabilities to bias in published epidemiological studies.

The purpose of critical appraisal

When epidemiologists design studies, they need to take deliberate steps to avoid sources of error. If you are training to be an epidemiologist, this will be a big part of your job: to design and conduct good studies.

When you read health research studies, you also need to think deliberately about sources of error. Faced with a study result, you need to ask yourself: What are all the ways that this study result could be wrong? This is called critical appraisal. It means that you don't read a study with the expectation that it is right. Instead, you try to attack it, looking for ways the study's methods make it vulnerable to error. Note that the skills required of an epidemiologist, and those required of a health professional critically appraising a study, are the same: both need to be able to understand all the ways in which research can go wrong.

The principles of critical appraisal shape the health sciences literature. When a researcher submits a study to a journal for publication, the study goes through a process of peer review: experts in the field examine it critically, looking for vulnerability to error. Peer-reviewed journals consider studies for publication only if studies survive this kind of intellectual attack.

Thinking deeper

Expressing prevalence symbolically

The law of large numbers has a focusing effect on the parameter of prevalence. The vulnerability to random differences gets smaller and smaller when estimates of the parameter are based on larger and larger samples. What is going on here? And how can we express this idea symbolically?

In chapter 1, the disease status of a population was depicted using uppercase letters, A and B, in contingency tables. We can extend this symbolic approach to depict the prevalence of disease in a population and produce a formula for calculating this parameter:

$$\text{PREVALENCE} = \frac{A}{A+B}$$

Since $N = A + B$, the formula could also be written as:

$$\text{PREVALENCE} = \frac{A}{N}$$

Note that *prevalence* is uppercase (PREVALENCE): this signifies that we are talking about the prevalence of the disease in an entire population. If a study examined every member of a population and determined, without error, the disease status for each person, the study, if repeated, would produce the same result every time. There is no chance involved. PREVALENCE is therefore not an estimate: it *is* the prevalence. PREVALENCE also functions as a probability: the probability that a randomly selected individual from this population has the disease.

Researchers do not usually have access to information about entire populations. In contingency tables, they may represent this symbolically with lowercase letters to depict disease status (see Table 5). The lowercase letters signal that the counts inside the table derive from a sample rather than from an entire population.

If prevalence is calculated from Table 5, lowercase letters again signal the use of sample-based data:

$$\text{Prevalence} = \frac{a}{a+b}$$

Or, alternatively:

$$\text{Prevalence} = \frac{a}{n}$$

Here, n is the sample size. The probability of selecting any particular member of the population for the study sample is n/N.

RANDOM VARIABILITY, TRUE PREVALENCE, AND SAMPLE-BASED PREVALENCE

Recall that repeating a study to calculate PREVALENCE would result in exactly the same result every time, as long as there was perfect classification of A and B. Chance does not play any role here.

Chance, however, affects calculations of sample-based prevalence. For one thing, not just any a and b people will do for the calculation of sample-based prevalence. You have to assume that the probability of selecting any person from the population does not depend on their disease status. Remember the example of flipping a coin? It was understood that the long-run probability of heads would equal 0.5, because the symmetry of a coin means heads and tails should have equal probability. The same principle suggests that if sample-based prevalence is to tell us something about PREVALENCE, then each member of the population must have an equal probability of being selected. If people with disease (the A people) are more likely to be selected than people without

TABLE 5. 1 × 2 TABLE DEPICTING SAMPLE-BASED DATA

Disease	No disease	Total
a	b	n

disease, you would expect sample-based prevalence to be greater than PREV-ALENCE. If people with disease are less likely to be selected, sample-based prevalence will tend to underestimate PREVALENCE.

However, if each member of a population has an equal probability of selection and if measurement is perfect, the long-run probability that any person we select is an *a* is actually PREVALENCE. For the same reason that flipping a coin thousands of times will almost always result in a proportion of heads near 50%, a study involving thousands of subjects will almost always produce an estimated prevalence very close to PREVALENCE.

CALCULATING STANDARD ERROR

"Almost always" is a key consideration here. Estimated parameters, such as sample-based prevalence, are vulnerable to random variability. An important way to quantify the variability of a parameter is its standard error. The standard error of an estimated proportion (*p*)—such as prevalence—is provided by the following formula:

$$\text{Standard Error} = \sqrt{\frac{p \times (1-p)}{n}}$$

Actually, this is an approximation when it is calculated from a sample, but it is usually good enough. Note that *n* is present within the denominator of the fraction inside of the square root sign. This means that as *n* increases, this fraction will get smaller and smaller. This formula helps to quantify the focusing effect of large samples.

A note about formula and equation formats

This book uses the following formats to present and discuss formulas and equations.
- Formulas and equations that incorporate population-based data (data from an entire population) use uppercase letters for all variables. For example:

$$\text{PREVALENCE} = \frac{A}{A+B}$$

- Formulas and equations that incorporate sample-based data (data from a sample of a population) use lowercase letters, except for spelled-out variables. Spelled out variables use title case. For example:

$$\text{Prevalence} = \frac{a}{a+b}$$

Questions

1. According to data from Statistics Canada,[16] there were 2 363 010 people with asthma in Canada in 2013. Assuming that this figure is correct and that the population of Canada in that year was 35 158 300 at mid-2013, what is the prevalence of asthma in Canada?

2. A study seeking to determine the frequency of delirium (a confusional state due to metabolic dysfunction in the brain) in psychiatric units identified a sample of $n = 401$. From this sample, 9 cases of delirium were identified.[17]
   a. What is the prevalence of delirium in psychiatric units?
   b. What is the estimated standard error of this proportion?

3. In your opinion, is point prevalence a more appropriate parameter for descriptive or analytical studies?

4. Some diseases do not affect entire populations. Prostate cancer, for example, does not occur in women, because women do not have a prostate gland. When calculating the prevalence of this disease, should the entire population be included in the denominator, or only the men?

5. There are various ways to quantify the impact of random variation on epidemiological estimates. Confidence intervals are 1 procedure. These will be described in more detail in a later chapter. In brief, a confidence interval provides a range of plausible values for a population parameter based on observations of a sample. When samples are small, there can be considerable random variation among estimates, and quantification of random error is essential. When samples are large, estimates are likely to be very close to the true value and confidence intervals are less critical. Do you think there is any value in having confidence intervals for estimates that are based on an entire population?

PART II

Fundamental
descriptive parameters

Epidemiology has 2 basic parameter "families"— prevalence and incidence—
that focus on the frequency or rate of single variables.

Prevalence and incidence are also the building blocks of more complex
parameters that capture in more detail the effects of exposure and disease
in populations.

The next 2 chapters look at, first, the basic parameters of prevalence and
incidence, and then at more complex parameters.

3

Basic measures based on frequencies and rates

Objectives
- Distinguish the parameter families of prevalence and incidence.
- Define key parameters within each family.
- Describe the relationship between proportions and odds.
- Describe the relationship between prevalence and incidence.
- Define cumulative incidence and describe how to calculate it.

Parameter families

Epidemiology has 2 basic parameter "families"—prevalence and incidence— that focus on the frequency or rate of single variables. Later chapters describe parameters of more complexity, which compare disease distribution among, for example, exposure groups.

The formulas for calculating prevalence and incidence sometimes look the same—a confusing reality—but prevalence and incidence are entirely different concepts.

The prevalence family

POINT PREVALENCE, PERIOD PREVALENCE, AND LIFETIME PREVALENCE

Chapter 1 noted that epidemiological research has 2 main branches: descriptive epidemiology and analytical epidemiology. In descriptive epidemiology, prevalence is the basic parameter. Note that we are talking here about prevalence as a parameter, not as a sample-based estimate of prevalence, nor as the actual prevalence of a disease in an entire population (PREVALENCE). In most cases, the best, specific term for this parameter is *prevalence proportion*.

(Some people use the term *prevalence rate*, but a rate is different than a proportion, so this counts as sloppy terminology.)

As a parameter, prevalence includes point prevalence, period prevalence, and lifetime prevalence. In some unusual situations, this parameter can also be a count (simply a tally of diseased individuals) rather than a proportion—in these situations, you would call the parameter a *prevalence count*.

Point prevalence quantifies the amount of disease in a population at a point in time. Unless otherwise specified, the term *prevalence* refers to point prevalence.

The Canadian Multicentre Osteoporosis Study[18] produced a point prevalence estimate. This study used a random sample, based on household telephone listings, of 10 061 women and men aged 25 years and older, distributed approximately equally across 9 centres. At the baseline time point, the data were used (among other things) to estimate the point prevalence of osteoporosis in women and men aged 50 years and older (the study used the criteria of the World Health Organization to define osteoporosis). The data showed the point prevalence of osteoporosis among Canadians in this age group was 15.8% for women and 6.6% for men.

The Canadian Study of Health and Aging[19] provides another example of estimating point prevalence. This study was based on a sample of 1835 subjects from a population of 283 510 Canadians who were age 85 and older at the time of the survey. The sampling procedures ensured that the sample represented both household residents in the community and people who were living in institutions. The study estimated the point prevalence of dementia in this age group as 28.5%.

Period prevalence is the proportion of a population that has, or has had, a disease at any time during a defined time interval, such as 1 year or 1 month. Statistics Canada employed period prevalence in the 2002 Canadian Community Health Survey: Mental Health and Well-being.[20] The survey used an interview to assess several conditions, including the 12-month period prevalence of depressive episodes. Investigators asked respondents whether they had experienced various symptoms during the preceding 12 months, and used an algorithm to determine whether respondents' symptoms fulfilled diagnostic criteria for 1 or more major depressive episodes. They estimated that 4.8% of the sample had experienced such an episode.[17] This is an example of a 12-month, or annual, prevalence estimate.

Lifetime prevalence—an unusual type of prevalence—is the count or proportion of people in a population who have had a particular disease at some time in their life. Lifetime prevalence usually applies to diseases that transition in and out of active phases. In Canada, studies of mental illness use this parameter most. People who have had episodes of mental illness remain at risk for future episodes: it is reasonable to think their illness as a lifelong condition subject to recurrence and remission.

For some mental disorders, it is difficult to conceptualize prevalence in any other way than lifetime prevalence. For example, bipolar I disorder is characterized by a lifetime history of 1 or more manic episodes.[21] A manic episode is a discrete period in which a person has elevated mood and increased activity. Usually, people with bipolar I disorder have recurrent episodes of mania and also episodes of depression. However, many people who do not have bipolar disorder develop depression, so depressive episodes indicate a bipolar disorder only if preceded by an episode of mania. The national mental health survey conducted by Statistics Canada in 2002 provides an example of lifetime prevalence.[22] The survey administered a structured diagnostic interview to a sample of more than 35 000 Canadians.[23] It found that 12.2% of the population had had an episode of depression at some time in their life. When it excluded respondents reporting a past manic episode, it estimated the lifetime prevalence of depression as 10.8%.

A troubling characteristic of lifetime prevalence is that it is dependent on age. Whereas period prevalence has a specified interval of observation (e.g., 1 year), the interval of observation for lifetime prevalence depends on the age of the person being assessed. This means that lifetime prevalence does not quantify disease burden as clearly as point prevalence or period prevalence. Also, in practice, lifetime prevalence can be difficult to measure accurately, because it can require subjects to remember long-past signs and symptoms. Some experts argue that these problems make the parameter useless. In a 2010 paper, Dr. David Streiner of the University of Toronto and McMaster University posed the question: "Has lifetime prevalence reached the end of its life?"[24]

Key point: Prevalence is the most common measure of disease burden. While the term encompasses several variants (types of period prevalence and lifetime prevalence), the most common meaning is the proportion of a population with a disease at a point in time (point prevalence).

EXPRESSING PREVALENCE PROPORTION

Except in unusual situations where prevalence is reported as a number (a count), prevalence is expressed as a proportion—for example, as a fraction. In a very small population, such as a group of students in an elementary school class, a fraction provides clear information.

For example, imagine that there are 25 students in a class. During influenza season, 5 of these students become ill with influenza. You could express the period prevalence as 5/25. You could also express it as a decimal (5/25 = 0.20), or as a percentage, which is the decimal form multiplied by

100 (0.20 × 100 = 20%). Many diseases have a much lower prevalence than our classroom example, which makes considering the clearest form of expression important. For example, a systematic review by Pringsheim et al[25] estimated that the prevalence of Huntington disease was 2.71 per 100 000—a form easier to digest than the decimal (0.0000271) or the percentage (0.00271%).

Proportions are intuitive and easy to understand because of their relationship to probabilities. If 5/25 students in a particular class became ill during an influenza outbreak, it is easy to understand that a student in that class had a 20% chance of becoming ill.

Another way to convey the same information uses odds. In our classroom example, this is the number of students who got the disease during the observation interval divided by the number who did not get the disease, or 5/20. The odds of having the disease, expressed as a decimal, are 0.25. As with proportions, you can think of odds as a probability—just like betting odds in horse racing, or when people say "the odds are stacked against you" meaning you have a low probability of success. Clearly, you could use odds rather than proportions to express prevalence, although in practice this is rare. When odds are used to express prevalence, it is especially important to use the most specific language possible: *prevalence odds*.

Key point: Prevalence can be expressed as a count, a proportion, or odds.

The incidence family

THE DIFFERENCE BETWEEN INCIDENCE AND PREVALENCE

The difference between incidence and prevalence is a key distinction in epidemiology. A firm idea of this distinction is the foundation for understanding more complex parameters.

Incidence refers to the new occurrence of a disease. The operative word here is *new*. To be a prevalent case, a person merely needs to have a disease. To be an incident case, a person needs to newly develop the disease. The Canadian Multicentre Osteoporosis Study and the Canadian Study on Health and Aging are examples of studies seeking to estimate both incidence and prevalence. Such studies are an important source of prevalence data because, to estimate incidence, they need to be able to exclude everyone who already has the disease (the prevalent cases).

INCIDENCE PROPORTION, INCIDENCE RATE, AND ATTACK RATE

As a parameter, incidence includes the incidence proportion, incidence rate, and attack rate.

An **incidence proportion** derives from observations over an interval of time. The interval of time—a risk interval—must be specified or the parameter is meaningless. Note the contrast here with point prevalence, which is like a snapshot at a specific point in time. An incidence proportion requires a risk interval: a 5% risk over 1 day is a completely different probability than a 5% risk over 1 hour or 1 year.

To measure an incidence proportion, it is necessary to first identify a population at risk. People who already have a disease at the beginning of a risk interval cannot newly develop the disease during the interval—so measurement involves assessing research subjects at a baseline time point, eliminating those who already have the disease, and assessing the (remaining) at-risk population over a risk interval to see how many develop the disease. The resulting proportion is an incidence proportion, although it would also be possible to measure incidence using odds rather than a proportion.

Key point: Whereas prevalence in its various forms quantifies the amount of disease in a population, incidence proportions represent the risk of newly developing a disease during a specified time interval.

An **incidence rate**, like all rates, describes change in a quantity as a function of time. As an example of a rate, think about velocity. If you drive a car at a velocity (rate) of 60 kilometers per hour, you know you will travel 60 kilometres in 1 hour, 120 kilometres in 2 hours, and 30 kilometres in a half hour. Note that *per hour* could also be written */hour* (e.g., 60 km/hr) or—because the sign of an exponent changes depending on whether it is in the numerator or denominator of a ratio—*hour^{-1}* (e.g., 60 km hour^{-1}). Incidence rates are like velocity: velocity describes the rate at which an object travels, and an incidence rate describes the rate at which people become ill. As with an incidence proportion, an incident rate presupposes that a person is not already ill: it applies to an at-risk population that excludes those who are already ill at the time that observation starts.

Unlike an incidence proportion, which has no time units, an incidence rate has person-time units. These are expressed as time^{-1} (the idea of "being a person" doesn't really need to be specified). The time units associated with incidence rates, while they are always in this form, are themselves arbitrary. Think back to the analogy with velocity: 60 km/hour is the same as 60 km/ 60 minutes or 1 km/minute—the rate does not change, only the units. Similarly, an incidence rate can use any time units—for example, days^{-1}, weeks^{-1}, months^{-1}, or years^{-1}. Epidemiologists aim to select time units that are easy to understand and maximally informative. For example, if the incidence rate for amyotrophic lateral sclerosis in Nova Scotia[26] is expressed as 2.24 per 100 000 person-years (2.24 per 100 000 year^{-1}), a planner can easily imagine the number of new cases likely to arise in at-risk populations in Nova Scotia in a given year. It wouldn't make much sense to report this incidence rate in person-seconds or person-days: this would produce correct, but tiny, numbers of little help to planners.

Key point: Incidence rates are not proportions and not odds: they are rates and expressed in person-time units.

An **attack rate** describes a special type of incidence proportion, where a particular disease corresponds with a particular risk interval.

For example, influenza produces seasonal epidemics in Canada, so the risk interval for influenza is sometimes defined as this seasonal period (November to April). Another example: in some "point source" outbreaks of infectious diseases, the behaviour of the infectious agent can define the risk interval. Say a group of wedding guests is exposed to food contaminated with toxins produced by *Staphylococcus aureus*: they are at risk for developing food poisoning within 6 hours. This 6-hour interval is an obvious choice as the risk interval for calculating the attack rate.

If you are dismayed that anyone would call an incidence proportion a *rate*, you have reason—it is very misleading terminology (reminiscent of the unfortunate *prevalence rate*). Nevertheless, it is a standard terminology.

Severe acute respiratory syndrome (SARS) was an important infectious disease outbreak in Canada[27] where attack rates were reported. The outbreak originated in Guangdong province in China in 2002 and was brought to Canada by travellers infected in Hong Kong in 2003, with the first known case arriving in Canada on February 23, 2003. The initial wave of the outbreak was followed by a second wave consisting of 74 cases reported between April 15 and June 9, 2003. Of these, 29 were health care workers and 28 were people exposed to the virus during hospitalization. Another 17 cases occurred among hospital visitors. Nursing staff at the hospital wards where most of the exposures occurred used a common nursing station, shared a washroom, and ate together in a lounge near the ward. The attack rate among nurses working in an orthopaedic section of the ward was approximately 40% and among those in a gynecology section was approximately 25%. Note that these attack rates are percentages, which are just a type of proportion. The risk interval associated with these estimates is the time period in which the outbreak occurred.

Key point: Attack rates are a type of incidence proportion, and should properly not be called *rates* (but they are).

Basic mortality rates

Mortality rates are a kind of incidence rate. The population at risk for mortality consists of all those who are alive at a point in time. Every time somebody dies, the mortality event is their first (and only) occurrence.

There is a lot of information about mortality in Canada available from Statistics Canada through the Canadian Socio-Economic Information Management System (CANSIM). The information system consists of numerous tables (more than 100 for mortality alone) that users can customize. CANSIM is not limited to examination of mortality, nor even to health statistics, yet there is a wealth of frequently updated health and mortality data there. If you search "Statistics Canada" using an Internet search engine, CANSIM is usually an option that comes up.

Mortality rates are calculated by dividing the number of deaths in a year by the midyear population of that same year. On the surface, this sounds like a proportion, so it is tempting to call this a *mortality proportion*. However, there is a distinction. If you were calculating an annual incidence proportion, you would count the number of deaths that occurred during a year (January 1 to December 31), and divide this by the population at the start of the same year (January 1). A mortality rate uses the midyear population, rather the population on January 1, because the midyear population reflects the occurrence of births and deaths (as well as immigration and emigration) during the year: assuming the population is in a steady state, it describes the person-time in the population. A person born on July 1 provides only half a person-year of time at risk of death, but a person who dies on July 1 also provides only half a person-year of time at risk. In a steady state population, births and deaths are equal and occur throughout the year. For this reason, this kind of mortality statistic can reasonably be called an *annual mortality rate* and is always reported with year^{-1} units.

The relationship between odds and proportions

Converting odds to proportions and vice versa
To report the basic parameters of prevalence and incidence, you can use proportions or odds—these are interchangeable. There is a simple formula for converting proportions to odds:

$$\text{Odds} = \frac{\text{Proportion}}{1 - \text{Proportion}}$$

And there is a simple formula for converting odds to proportions:

$$\text{Proportion} = \frac{\text{Odds}}{1 + \text{Odds}}$$

Odds and proportions have similar values for rare diseases
Here is another interesting characteristic of odds and proportions. When a disease is rare, the prevalence or incidence is quite similar whether expressed

as odds or a proportion. Consider the formulas for a proportion and odds in sample-based data (so, using the a and b notation):

$$\text{Proportion} = \frac{a}{a+b}$$

$$\text{Odds} = \frac{a}{b}$$

When a is small, $a + b$ is very similar to b, and the 2 formulas produce a similar result. So, a disease with a prevalence of 1 in 10 000 (1 person of 10 000 has the disease), the proportion is 0.001 and the odds are almost identical at 0.001001. By contrast, if the proportion is 0.5 then the odds are 1.0, which is not very similar at all.

The relationship between prevalence and incidence

When prevalence and incidence are the same

Let's think about the classroom with 25 students again, where 5 students developed influenza during an outbreak. We could talk about the period prevalence proportion in this situation: the proportion of students with the disease (5/25) during a defined interval (in this case, the period of outbreak).

Could 5/25 also express an incidence proportion?

It could, if all 25 students were free of influenza at the start of the interval. In this case, the interval used to calculate the period prevalence proportion corresponds to the risk interval for calculating the incidence proportion. The 2 proportions are the same. It would also, of course, be correct to describe the incidence proportion as an attack rate in this case.

Prevalence, incidence, and endemic diseases

An endemic disease is defined as a disease whose prevalence has assumed fairly stable levels—a steady state—within a population. There is a very important relationship between prevalence and incidence in endemic disease.

Let's first clearly understand how endemic disease differs from outbreaks, epidemics, or pandemics of infectious disease. In outbreaks, epidemics, and pandemics, disease parameters are unstable. An epidemic occurs when disease exceeds normal, expected levels in a defined community, geographic area, or season. The terms *outbreak* and *epidemic* have similar meanings, but *outbreak* implies an infectious agent and a defined locale. Obesity, for example, currently exceeds expected, historical levels—we often talk about an epidemic of obesity,[28] but never an outbreak of obesity. A pandemic occurs when an infectious disease, such as influenza, sweeps across the globe and creates sequential epidemics in many different populations. In outbreaks, epidemics, and pandemics, the relationship between prevalence, incidence, and mortality is dynamic—there is no steady state. These situations are best understood as departures from a steady state.

The relationship between incidence and prevalence in endemic disease is key to understanding complex parameters in epidemiology. Think of the prevalence proportion as a pool made up of the members of a population with a disease. (Note that this concept of prevalence corresponds to point prevalence, not to period prevalence or lifetime prevalence.) There is an inflow to the prevalence pool (the incidence rate—the rate at which people without disease "flow" into the prevalence pool) and an outflow from the prevalence pool (because of mortality—people dying—or recovery from the disease). The size of the prevalence pool is determined by this inflow and outflow. If more people are getting the disease than are dying or recovering, the prevalence pool increases. If the opposite is true, the prevalence pool shrinks.

In a steady state situation (where inflow and outflow are equal), a simple formula describes the relationship between prevalence and incidence, and it is approximately true most of the time: prevalence is equal to the incidence rate multiplied by the mean duration of illness. More precisely, the prevalence odds are equal to the incidence rate multiplied by the mean duration of disease. The mean duration of illness is influenced by both recovery from the disease (if this is possible) and mortality. For an irreversible disease, the duration is determined only by mortality.

Since the mean duration of illness has time units and the incidence rate has time^{-1} units, these units disappear in the calculation of the prevalence odds.

$$\text{Prevalence Odds} = \text{Incidence Rate}(t^{-1}) \times \text{Duration}(t)$$

Key point: Point prevalence is approximately equal to the product of the incidence rate and the mean duration of illness.

This formula—which expresses the relationship between prevalence and incidence—helps epidemiologists estimate prevalence from information about incidence, and vice versa. For example, the Global Burden of Disease[29,30] study aims to quantify and rank the burden of certain diseases in every country of the world. Burden can be due either to premature mortality or to living with a disease (due to the discomfort and dysfunction that diseases produce). To make these calculations, researchers need information about incidence, prevalence, and mortality, but sometimes do not have adequate data. So, they use mathematical models called DisMod models,[31] which flesh out the basic relationships among incidence, prevalence, and mortality. When information is available for only 2 parameters, the models allow researchers to make an educated guess about the third.

The formula also leads to a qualitative understanding of the relationship between prevalence and incidence, which is particularly valuable. For example, it clarifies the motivations of clinical interventions for public health actions. The formula also shows that reducing incidence through prevention, even in the absence of improved treatment, will diminish the prevalence (and therefore burden) of a disease in a population. It also makes plain the role that the health system plays in population health. Better treatments abbreviate the duration of disease and reduce prevalence, even if incidence does not change. Better treatments may also improve survival (as opposed to curing a disease), which will increase the average duration of disease and, therefore, prevalence in the population.

Cumulative incidence

Cumulative incidence refers to the proportion of cases that accumulate over an interval of observation in an at-risk cohort—a concept very similar to incidence proportion. Indeed, the 2 terms are often used interchangeably. However, there is a subtle distinction: the incidence proportion usually uses the number of people in the at-risk cohort at a baseline time point in its denominator, but cumulative incidence is calculated in ways that take into account the fact that those who become ill during the observation interval are no longer at risk after their illness occurs.

Thinking deeper

Calculating cumulative incidence

Imagine a situation in which the 1-year incidence proportion for an irreversible disease is known to be 0.05. What would the cumulative incidence be after 2, 3, or 5 years?

It seems sensible to simply multiply the 1-year incidence proportion by the number of years—so, the 2-year cumulative incidence would be twice the 1-year proportion ($0.05 \times 2 = 0.1$). However, this wouldn't quite be correct. The reason lies in the basic definition of cumulative incidence.

Imagine that the at-risk population at baseline is $n = 100$. Since the incidence proportion is 0.05, it is reasonable to expect, on average, about 5 people will become ill during the first year. Let's assume that this is exactly what occurs. In the second year, there are no longer 100 people at risk of illness. Five of them have become ill, so now only 95 remain at risk. The number expected to become ill in the second year is now 0.05 of 95 people rather than 0.05 of 100.

The complement of a proportion is 1 minus that proportion. So if the risk of becoming ill during an interval is 0.05, the complement (the risk of not becoming ill) is 0.95. In the calculation of cumulative incidence, it is useful

to think of the proportion of the population becoming ill as the complement
of the number remaining well. Imagine that a 1-year cumulative incidence
is equivalent to the annual incidence proportion. This equivalency could be
written as:

$$\text{Cumulative Incidence}_{1\,\text{year}} = 1 - \left(1 - \text{Annual Incidence Proportion}\right)$$

At first glance, this seems like a silly formula. Why start with the proportion that does not have the disease at baseline and then subtract the complement of the proportion that gets the disease? The value of this expression
becomes clear when there are a series of intervals, which is what cumulative
incidence is all about. At this stage, the expression within the bracket can be
used to represent the probability of staying well through the first year and also
through the second year. Since these are independent probabilities, the joint
probability is their product, such that for year 2:

$$\text{Cumulative Incidence}_{2\,\text{years}} = 1 - \left(1 - \text{Annual Incidence Proportion}\right) \times \left(1 - \text{Annual Incidence Proportion}\right)$$

Or, more simply:

$$\text{Cumulative Incidence}_{2\,\text{years}} = 1 - \left(1 - \text{Annual Incidence Proportion}\right)^2$$

And this leads to a more general way of anticipating cumulative incidence
over a set of risk intervals:

$$\text{Cumulative Incidence}_{n\,\text{years}} = 1 - \left(1 - \text{Annual Incidence Proportion}\right)^n$$

Returning to our hypothetical population in which the annual incidence
proportion was 0.05 and the population size was 100, the last formula tells
us the expected value of the 2-year cumulative incidence: $1 - (1 - 0.05)^2$ or
0.0975.

These formulas deal with only 1 factor that can arise from the relationship
between a series of smaller risk intervals and a bigger risk interval comprising
the smaller intervals: the shrinking of the population at risk as people become
ill from the disease under investigation. These formulas are useful conceptually, but circumstances this simple do not occur often in the real world. For
example, members of the monitored cohort may die, which would diminish
the size of the at-risk population—the formulas do not address this. Similarly,
they do not address reductions of the at-risk population due to other diseases
or circumstances.

EXPECTED CUMULATIVE INCIDENCE: THE EXPONENTIAL EQUATION

The following formula estimates the expected cumulative incidence after a
period of observation (*t*) in a population with a specified incidence rate. This
is called the exponential equation. Like the previous formulas, this formula

only accounts for the diminishing population at risk as incident cases occur (it does not account for other characteristics that could compete with incidence in removing people from the at-risk population). Nevertheless, it is a useful formula.

$$\text{Cumulative Incidence}_t = 1 - e^{-\text{Incidence Rate} \times t}$$

Note that the e in the formula is the base of the natural logarithm, a constant (also an irrational number) that has an approximate value of 2.718. The term after the minus sign in the formula is the inverse logarithm, or exponentiation, of the negative value of the incidence rate multiplied by time.

This formula is not a good substitute for calculating incidence. If the research goal is to estimate a 10-year incidence proportion, then it's best to conduct a 10-year study (as opposed to conducting a 1-year study and using this formula to estimate 10-year cumulative incidence). However, the formula does allow helpful and convenient calculations. Watch out, though, for a common mistake in using this formula: don't forget that a negative sign precedes the incidence rate.

Questions

1. The following table describes the experience of 10 people susceptible to a very dangerous disease. A study of this small population begins on January 1 and observation ends on December 31. Each month, the subjects' health status is assessed and coded as follows: free of disease (grey), ill (black), or dead (white).

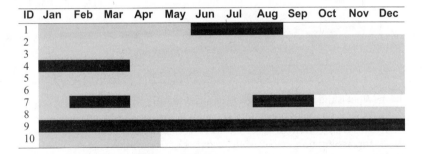

ID	Jan	Feb	Mar	Apr	May	Jun	Jul	Aug	Sep	Oct	Nov	Dec
1												
2												
3												
4												
5												
6												
7												
8												
9												
10												

a. What is the period prevalence of this disease?
b. What is the point prevalence in August?
c. What is the 12-month incidence proportion of this disease?
d. Calculate an annual mortality rate for this population.
e. The experience of subject 7 indicates that this is a recurrent disease. Survivors reenter the population at risk. Under this assumption, calculate an incidence rate for this disease.

2. The following table describes the experience of 10 people susceptible to a rapidly fatal disease. A study of this small population begins on January 1 and

observation ends on December 31. Each month, the subjects' health status is assessed and coded as follows: free of disease (grey), ill (black), or dead (white).

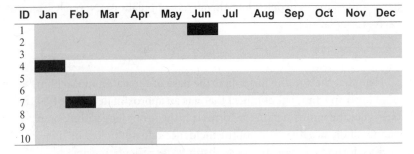

a. What is the period prevalence of this disease?
b. What is the point prevalence in August?
c. What is the 12-month incidence proportion of this disease?
d. Calculate an annual mortality rate for this population.
e. Calculate the incidence rate for this disease.

3. The following table describes the experience of 10 people with a highly recurrent condition. A study of this small population begins on January 1 and observation ends on December 31. Each month, the subjects' health status is assessed and coded as follows: free of disease (grey), ill (black), or dead (white). Assume that each of the episodes is new, including the episode in month 1 in ID = 1.

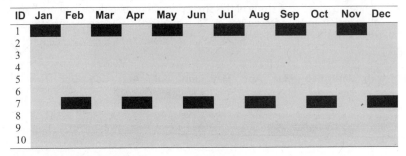

a. What is the period prevalence of this disease?
b. What is the point prevalence?
c. This is a recurrent disease. Survivors reenter the population at risk. Under this assumption, calculate an incidence rate for this disease.
d. What are the prevalence odds? Explain whether you can also calculate the prevalence odds using the following formula: prevalence odds = incidence rate × mean duration.

4. Change the following proportions into odds:
   a. 0.0009
   b. 0.009
   c. 0.09
   d. 0.9

5. Dr. Frederick Banting of the University of Toronto received the Nobel Prize in 1923 for his use of insulin to treat diabetes. Did this accomplishment make insulin-dependent diabetes mellitus more or less common?

Specialized mortality rates and composite measures of disease burden

Objectives
- Define and interpret key specialized measures of mortality: cause-specific mortality rate; age- and sex-specific mortality rate; perinatal mortality rate; infant mortality rate; and case-fatality rate.
- Define and interpret key composite health indicators: QALYs and DALYs.
- Describe the role of these rates and indicators in monitoring population health.

Measures of mortality and disease burden

Chapter 3 introduced the 2 basic parameters of epidemiology—prevalence and incidence—and showed how to calculate these as true values and estimates.

There are situations, however, in which these parameters do not fully capture the burden of disease in a population.

This chapter describes parameters for these more complex situations. These parameters use mortality, prevalence, and incidence as building blocks.

Specialized mortality rates and parameters

Parameters that capture differences in the way diseases affect populations have considerable descriptive value. These include certain specialized parameters calculated from mortality data.

For example, some diseases have a large impact on mortality, such as cancer, cardiovascular disease, and cerebrovascular disease. Some diseases tend to kill young people, such as congenital anomalies, trauma, and suicide. Some, such as stroke, tend to kill elderly people.

In addition, certain mortality rates, especially those for the very young, quantify more than just deaths. The number of children dying around the time of childbirth or in the first year of life is an important way of assessing the general level of social and health system development in a country.

Cause-specific mortality

A statement from the 1955 *United Nations Handbook of Vital Statistics Methods* highlights the importance of cause-specific mortality statistics: "It may truthfully be said that virtually every large-scale problem in preventive medicine has been brought to light—in part at least—by statistics of death, and further that the adequacy of remedial or curative action is, in the last analysis, reflected in these same statistics."[32] Cause-specific death statistics are among the oldest indicators of population health status. In England, "bills of mortality" (weekly mortality statistics) date to the seventeenth century.[33] Abstracts based on bills of mortality produced by William Farr (one of the earliest epidemiologists) were an important data source for John Snow's cholera investigations.[5]

Recall the calculation of a mortality rate (see page 28): the number of deaths in a particular year is counted in the numerator, and the midyear population is taken as an estimate of person-time for the denominator of the rate.

This calculation provides information about the rate at which people are dying, but not about the reasons for their death. Cause-specific mortality statistics address this deficiency. Here, the numerator represents the number of people dying of a specific cause, and the denominator is the midyear population at risk of dying from that cause.

When a cause of death affects only 1 sex (e.g., prostate cancer), the population at risk should only include that sex. For example, the cause-of-death tables published by Statistics Canada[34] report a crude mortality rate for prostate cancer (22.4/100 000 in 2009) for men, but not for women. It would potentially be misleading to report this frequency for the entire population, since prostate cancer is not a health issue for women. Women are not members of the population at risk.

DATA SOURCES ABOUT CAUSE-SPECIFIC MORTALITY

Registration of death is required in all developed countries, making cause-specific mortality statistics among the most widely used health indicators internationally.

A registration of death requires completion of a certificate—usually by a physician, but also by specialized nurses in some provinces[35]—specifying the cause of death. In Canada, where responsibility for health care has been constitutionally assigned to the provinces, relevant vital-statistics legislation varies from province to province. The Vital Statistics Council for Canada works to coordinate and standardize documentation of causes of death (along with other issues, the council is also concerned with certification of births and changes of name). Medical certificates of death are entered into provincial mortality databases and, because of the shared standards, the databases can then be effectively aggregated into a national mortality database. This is called the Canadian Mortality Registry.

Internationally, the World Health Organization compiles international tables of cause-specific mortality for its member states. These international efforts have contributed to effective standardization of procedures for certification of causes of death. The World Health Organization's system for classifying disease, the International Classification of Disease, or ICD, has become the standard classification. It is currently in its tenth edition (ICD-10), with an eleventh edition due by 2017.[36]

A medical certification of death includes demographic information and information from the deceased person's medical history. It identifies an immediate cause of death (the direct cause of death—e.g., respiratory arrest), underlying causes of death (the disease or injury that initiated the sequence of morbid events leading directly or indirectly to death—e.g., carcinoma of the lung), and any antecedent causes of death that are judged to intervene in a sequence of events between the underlying and immediate causes of death. For example, a fall at home could be an underlying cause of death as follows: the fall caused a fracture, which led to surgery and immobility (an antecedent cause), which led to a terminal pneumonia. The last element in the sequence listed on a medical certificate of death should be the immediate cause of death. Death certificates also provide an opportunity to list other associated conditions.

Cause-specific mortality data are made readily available in Canada through Statistics Canada CANSIM tables, which allow users to produce customized output from the national mortality database. The Canadian Institute of Health Information (CIHI) also facilitates access to Canadian mortality data, and carries out analysis and reporting of its findings. The top 10 causes of death in Canada are:

1. malignant neoplasms (cancer)
2. heart disease
3. cerebrovascular diseases (stroke)
4. chronic lower respiratory diseases
5. accidents
6. diabetes
7. Alzheimer disease
8. influenza and pneumonia
9. suicide
10. kidney disease

These top 10 causes of death, which have not changed in their ranking over the past 10 years, amount to 76.4% of deaths in Canada.[37] Some of them have sex-related differences: accidents rank third among leading causes of death in men, but rank sixth for women; suicide ranks seventh for men and thirteenth for women.[37]

When a death appears to be due to unnatural causes (e.g., suicide, accident), or when it is sudden or unexpected, it may trigger an investigation by a coroner's or medical examiner's office. (Note that the use of *coroner* or *medical examiner* depends on the province or territory.) The information collected by these offices can be used as a source of research data. Statistics Canada and the Public Health Agency of Canada have also developed a national database of mortality data from these offices, called the Canadian Coroner and Medical Examiner Database.

Key point: Information about mortality is readily available in most countries, including Canada, and is an important source of epidemiological data.

EPIDEMIOLOGICAL RESEARCH BASED ON CAUSE-SPECIFIC MORTALITY DATA

Many epidemiological studies in Canada have used mortality data.

In a well-known example, Ashmore et al[38] used exposure data from a registry of radiation exposure called the National Dose Registry of Canada to identify a cohort of 206 620 workers who were monitored for radiation exposure. They linked this exposure data to the national mortality database, which allowed them to identify a cohort of more than 5000. They used this cohort to investigate the possible role of radiation exposure in the incidence of cancer and other diseases.

A study by Hwang[39] identified a cohort of homeless men in Toronto in 1995. The Ontario Office of the Registrar General ascertained deaths in this population during 1995 to 1997 using provincial death certificates. Men aged 18 to 24 in this cohort were 8.3 times more likely to die than men in this age group in the general inner-city population. The causes of death were found to depend on age. In younger men, accidents, poisonings, AIDS, and suicide were more common causes of death; in older men, cancer and heart disease were most common, and accidental death was also common.

Aronson and Tough[40] investigated a series of 38 horse-related deaths in Alberta. Since these deaths were "unexpected," the medical examiner's office was a reasonable source of data, and the data were likely representative of accidental deaths related to horses. However, Aronson and Tough noted that only about half the deaths had undergone autopsy, so the exact cause of death may not have been known in all cases. The main finding of this study was that many of these deaths involved head injuries, suggesting that education about the value of helmets was an appropriate preventive strategy.

A study by Boyd et al[41] examined the role of trauma and asphyxia in deaths from avalanches. In collecting data for this study, the investigators reviewed avalanche fatalities that occurred between 1984 and 2005. They searched the database of the Canadian Avalanche Centre, where 220 deaths were recorded. Of those 220 deaths, 204 were also recorded in the databases of the British Columbia Coroners Service or the Chief Medical Examiner of Alberta. Again, about half the deaths ($n = 117$) underwent autopsy. They found asphyxia had caused 154 (or 75%) of the deaths and trauma had caused 48 (24%). Interestingly, they found that the frequency of death due to different causes depended on the nature of activities in which the victims were engaged. Trauma, for example, was the cause of death for 42% of ice climbers and only 9% of snowmobilers.

THE VALUE OF CAUSE-SPECIFIC MORTALITY DATA

For descriptive purposes, mortality data provide a lot of information about what people are dying from. This has obvious value for planning services and for generating hypotheses that analytical studies can evaluate.

However, each record of cause-specific mortality involves the judgement of the professional making the record. Some provinces have produced detailed manuals for completing certifications of death,[42] which may help standardize these judgements. Many Canadian physicians feel inadequately trained in death certification, though, and this may affect the quality of the data.

For example, it might make sense to record suicide as an immediate cause of death (e.g., using an International Classification of Disease code for self-inflicted injury)—but what should be viewed as a contributing cause? In some circumstances, mental disorders (such as depression) that are strongly associated with suicide might be coded as an underlying cause, but such disorders may sometimes be unknown or undocumented.

Other circumstances involve even more difficult, or arbitrary, judgements. A death whose immediate cause was cardiac arrest might have an underlying cause of drug overdose—which might, in turn, have occurred as a possible suicide attempt within the context of a substance use disorder.

Epidemiologists view the causal data contained in registration data with caution.

Key point: Mortality rates are a type of incidence rate. Everyone alive is at risk of death and death is always a new (incident) rather than an ongoing (prevalent) occurrence.

Surveillance

In addition to their value to research, mortality data are a classic source of surveillance data.

Unlike research, surveillance is an ongoing process that provides monitoring through the use of routinely available data sources. In addition, surveillance data must be analyzed, and the information communicated to people who plan and administer health services, or who mobilize public health responses to emerging threats.[43]

Key point: Surveillance differs from research in the'sense that it is an ongoing process, and is inherently coupled with processes of data analysis and communication.

For these reasons, government ministries of health perform most surveillance activities. In Canada, all provincial governments participate in surveillance activities, and the federal government plays a role in the integration and analysis of surveillance data.

Examples of surveillance activities include:

Monitoring of infectious diseases by Canadian provinces: Provinces legislate certain infectious diseases as reportable diseases. Labs, physicians, and other health professionals must then report cases of these diseases to public health authorities. This allows monitoring of the diseases and rapid response to outbreaks. In some cases, rapid response might mean targeting an individual (e.g., prompt treatment for someone with tuberculosis). In other cases, rapid response might mean targeting a population. This kind of surveillance is becoming increasingly important in Canada for certain infectious diseases. For example, falling vaccination rates for diseases such as pertussis (whooping cough) and measles have led to outbreaks requiring rapid implementation of supplementary vaccination programs. Another example: cases of food-borne illness—such as a 2008 listeriosis outbreak linked to a Maple Leaf Foods plant in Toronto, or the staphylococcal intoxication associated with "cronut burgers" at the 2013 Canadian National Exhibition, also in Toronto— have triggered closures of food-serving, -producing and -processing facilities.

National database of notifiable diseases (Public Health Agency of Canada): This database includes information on diseases that all provinces consider notifiable.[44] The Public Health Agency of Canada also provides case definitions for these diseases, an extremely useful resource for communicable disease control in the field.

Chronic Disease Surveillance System (Public Health Agency of Canada): This system synthesizes administrative data collected by the provinces. *Administrative data*—a very common term in Canadian epidemiology— includes information collected during physician billing, drug claims, and other administrative procedures. For example, physicians typically seek payment for their services by submitting "bills" to their provincial health care insurance plan. A bill usually specifies a diagnosis (generally an International Classification of Disease code). In addition, provinces collect data to administer their health care systems. For example, some provinces cover certain drug claims. All of them cover hospital costs in public hospitals (in Canada, almost all hospitals are public hospitals)—so they need to figure out, for example, how much a hospital should get paid for a particular inpatient stay.

National Ambulatory Care Reporting System (Canadian Institute of Health Information): This records emergency department and ambulatory care data.

This is by no means a comprehensive list. National surveillance systems are also in place for blood safety, congenital anomalies, antimicrobial resistance, and many more issues that require monitoring. The website of the Public Health Agency of Canada[45] provides a summary of national surveillance systems, which has links to more detailed information and, in some cases, to reports and data tables.

Key point: Both provincial and territorial as well as federal public health officials participate in health surveillance activities.

Age- and sex-specific mortality rates

It is relatively easy to calculate a mortality rate, but interpreting rates for an entire population can pose challenges.

Here's an important interpretive factor: different causes of death affect people more or less prominently depending on their age, so it is often important to examine mortality rates for particular age groups. This involves identifying the population size within a particular age range and the number of deaths in the population within that age group.

For similar reasons, there may be value in calculating sex-specific rates, or province-specific rates.

In general, such rates are referred to as *specific mortality rates*, although it is always important to label them in ways that clarify what exactly they are being specific about—e.g., age-specific mortality, sex-specific mortality, and so on.

Age and sex are strong determinants of mortality, and they are also classically nonmodifiable determinants. For these reasons, it is very common to make comparisons of mortality within, rather than across, age and sex groups. Due to the importance of these figures, they are routinely tabulated in CANSIM tables available on the Statistics Canada web page. In 2014, for example, number of deaths and mortality rates were available from CANSIM Table 102-0504, which has the title "Deaths and mortality rates, by age group and sex, Canada, provinces and territories, annual." CANSIM has a good directory that can assist users in finding the information they need.[46]

PERINATAL MORTALITY

Several specified rates have wide use because they function as indicators of economic development, general living conditions, social well-being, performance of health systems, and the quality of the environment. These are considered sentinel indicators because they reflect factors relevant to the health of an entire population even if, on the surface, they concern a single age range.

The perinatal mortality rate, also called the perinatal death rate, is a sentinel indicator. In Canada, a perinatal death is defined as the death of a child less than 1 week of age (0 to 6 days) or a stillbirth of 28 or more weeks gestation. Of course, to calculate a perinatal mortality rate, you need both a numerator and a denominator. The denominator here is the number of total births, which consists of live births and late fetal deaths.

A birth counts as a live birth if any sign of life is present after birth (e.g., breathing). To be registered as a stillbirth, there must be no signs of life present, and the fetus must be more than 20 weeks gestation or have a birth weight of at least 500 grams. (A few minor interprovincial differences exist on these points.),

Statistics Canada defines the perinatal death rate as the number of perinatal deaths during a given year per 1000 total births (live births plus late fetal deaths) in the same year, where late fetal deaths are defined as stillbirths of 28 weeks or more gestation. Statistics Canada produces a regularly updated CANSIM table for perinatal mortality.

INFANT MORTALITY

Infant mortality refers to the death of an infant younger than 1 year. It is usually expressed as a frequency, calculated using the infant death count during a given year divided by the live birth count for the same year. Statistics Canada calculates this statistic irrespective of birth weight, but because prematurity and associated birth weight is an important contributor to infant mortality, the infant mortality rate is reported separately (see CANSIM Table 102-0030)[47] for all birth weights and for birth weights over 500 grams.

According to the Conference Board of Canada, Canadian infant mortality rates are shockingly high, even though they have diminished from 27 to 5.1 per 1000 between 1960 and 2007. Of 17 peer nations included in the Organization for Economic Cooperation and Development (OECD), Canada was found to be the second worst (the only nation performing more poorly was the US). However, the rate has continued to drop since 2007: a 2013 update of CANSIM Table 102–0030 reported the rate for 2011 as 4.8 per 1000 live births.[47]

Note that perinatal mortality rates and infant mortality rates are actually frequencies rather than rates, since they are calculated as proportions. They do not need units in the way that a true rate does, and are called *rates* merely for ease of language.

Case-fatality rates

Case-fatality rates are really proportions—another example of using *rate* for ease of language. A preferable term is *case-fatality proportion*, but this is rarely used.

In case-fatality rates, the denominator of the proportion consists of people who have a disease. The numerator consists of those who die while they have this disease. This particular type of mortality measure is unique because the risk interval is not necessarily an interval of time, as is usually the case in the calculation of an incidence proportion or cumulative incidence. Case-fatality rates quantify how many people die when they get sick with a disease, so the fact that they are sick is often more important than any specific time interval.

A 2003 paper published in the *Canadian Medical Association Journal* provides a good example of calculating a case-fatality rate. The paper was written during the outbreak of severe acute respiratory syndrome (SARS) in Toronto. The authors reported that 105 cases of probable SARS had been identified and 13 of these had died, leading to an estimated case-fatality rate of 12.4%.[48,49]

Key point: A case-fatality rate is a special type of incidence proportion in which the risk interval is characterized by an illness state rather than a specified time interval.

Observed survival proportions and relative survival ratios

There is often interest in calculating an index of survival similar to a case-fatality rate, but for a disease that does not have an easily definable duration.

Cancer, for example, may go into remission and then recur. In such instances, case-fatality proportions are calculated over defined time intervals, typically 5 years. The Canadian Cancer Society calls the complement of this type of proportion an *observed survival proportion*.[50]

Consider, however, that people might die from a variety of causes over a 5-year period, particularly since many cancers afflict elderly people. In elderly age groups, mortality related to other causes may not be negligible. (This is different than for SARS, for example, where it may be reasonable to assume that everyone dying during their illness with SARS died of SARS.) For this reason, the Canadian Cancer Society recommends an alternative parameter—the 5-year relative survival ratio, which is the ratio of observed survival in a group of people diagnosed with a cancer to the expected survival in a comparable group of people (free from the specific form of cancer under study) in the general population.[50] A relative survival ratio could be calculated over any duration of observation, but 5 years is typically reported in Canadian cancer statistics.

For all cancers, the relative survival ratio is 63%, meaning that a person diagnosed with cancer has a 63% chance of surviving for at least 5 years, relative to their counterparts in the general population. This ratio is highest for thyroid cancer (98%) and lowest for pancreatic cancer (8%).[50]

Key point: The cancer literature contains some different terminology and addresses the issue of case fatality somewhat differently than the infectious disease literature.

Potential years of life lost (PYLL)

Basic mortality parameters, such as overall (or crude) mortality rates, do not factor for age. Age of death, though, affects the impact of death. Deaths that occur in advanced age disrupt families and society less than deaths that occur earlier in life. For example, a death at age 90 does not deprive society of as many person-years of healthy life and economic productivity as a death at birth or age 20.

The parameter of potential years of life lost (PYLL—also YPLL: years of potential life lost) accounts for the age at which various causes of death occur. PYLL can be reported as years lost or it can be reported as a rate. If it is calculated as a rate, the numerator is the number of years "lost" when people die.

To calculate years of life lost due to a particular cause of death, you need some standard of reference. For example, you could use life expectancy at birth, or some ideal, or hoped for, life expectancy. Or, you could use an age judged to be economically significant, such as the typical age of retirement (before and after which deaths may have a different economic impact). In Canada, PYLL is usually calculated using age 75. In other words, a death at age 70 causes 5 years of lost life, and a death at age 20 causes 55 years of lost life. Note that deaths occurring after age 75 do not count at all.

PYLL can be expressed as a rate using a person-time denominator. When this is done, the person-time in the rate is the midyear population of those under age 75.

Key point: PYLL is a strategy for estimating the impact of various sources of cause-specific mortality. The advantage of PYLL is that it accounts for the different ages at which people die from various causes of death.

Recall that the third highest cause of mortality in Canada in men is cerebrovascular disease.[37] In 1999, the PYLL for cerebrovascular disease in males was 21 353 (here reported as years lost, not as a rate per unit population), whereas it was 150 019 for unintentional injuries and 104 948 for suicide. In women, the PYLL for cerebrovascular disease in 1999 was 18 915, whereas it was 53 780 for unintentional injuries and 25 768 for suicide.[51] In terms of the mortality rate, cerebrovascular disease ranks higher than unintentional injuries or suicide, but with PYLL the opposite is true. This reversal reflects the typical ages at which people die from these different conditions. Accidents and suicides occur across the age range and thereby result in the deaths of a substantial number of young people. Deaths due to cerebrovascular disease are much more common, but most often affect people who are older than 75.

Life expectancy

Life expectancy seeks to produce an estimate of the future survival experience of a contemporary cohort. Unlike basic parameters such as prevalence proportions and incidence proportions (which are real quantities), life expectancy is a projection. It is an artificial parameter.

The most commonly calculated type of life expectancy is life expectancy at birth. Imagine that a large group of babies were born today. Now ask the question: How many years will it be until half of them have died? Stated this way, life expectancy represents the projected median duration of life for a cohort of babies born today.

The challenge is to project the time when half this cohort will be dead. There is no perfect solution to this challenge. The mortality rates experienced by a cohort of babies born today are unknown, since this mortality will occur in the future, much of it in the very distant future. The imperfect solution is to take current age-specific mortality rates and use them to form a best guess about how many will die at any given age. (This is why these calculations are best considered projections rather than parameters.)

Life expectancy offers an intuitively accessible means of summarizing a large number of age-specific mortality rates into a single index that people can relate to. Statistics Canada reports estimates for life expectancy that can be accessed through summary and CANSIM tables.[52] Estimates of life expectancy for various countries are also reported by the World Health Organization and the United Nations. In Canada, life expectancy at birth is approximately 85 years in women and 80 in men.[53] According to Statistics Canada summary tables,[52] from 1920 to 1922, life expectancy was 59 in men and 61 in women.

Health-adjusted life expectancy (HALE) is an indicator of the average number of years that an individual in a population is expected to live in full health, taking into account years lived in a suboptimal state of health. This is an extension of the concepts applied in the calculation of life expectancy. The HALE approach refines life expectancy by adjusting for years of life lived in less than full health. The World Health Organization developed this approach, although its recent burden-of-disease reports use a different measure: disability-adjusted life-years (DALYs).

A 2013 burden of disease study in Ontario[54] used HALE to assess mental illness and addictive disorders. People tend to live for many years with these conditions, so it is not surprising that the impact of mental disorders and addictions on HALE is very large. The study identified 5 mental disorders producing the greatest burden of disease: major depression, bipolar disorder, alcohol use disorders, social phobia, and schizophrenia. The burden of major depression alone was found to be more than the combined burden of Ontario's 4 most common cancers. The Public Health Agency of Canada has also produced a HALE report for Canada.[55]

Composite parameters

In a perfect world, everyone with a disease would receive the best treatment possible. In the real world of limited health care dollars, we have to set priorities. Epidemiological data should guide priority setting, but it means putting different diseases onto a single scale of comparison—a challenging task.

For example, how do you compare the significance of migraine and cancer? According to a 2012 Statistics Canada survey,[56] the prevalence of migraine in the Canadian household population is 8.3% (11.8% in women versus 4.7% in men). The 2-year prevalence of all cancers in Canada[57] is 720.7/100 000, which is less than 1%. Migraine is a long-term recurrent condition that causes pain and disability; cancer is associated with intense treatment needs and high mortality. Comparisons of migraine and cancer must use composite measures capable of quantifying the negative impact of these diseases on individuals' health and duration of life, all on the same scale.

Quality-adjusted life-years (QALYs)

While survival is important, not all survived time is equal. In some cases, disease survivors may have poor quality of life, so a composite parameter of survival time and quality of life during the survival time is useful. (Quality of life refers to a person's self-appraisal of their own health.) This approach is particularly popular in the health economics literature.

It can be challenging, though, to assess quality of life: it involves attaching personal judgements to different health states. A popular approach involves health utilities. Instruments that assess health utility put many different health issues onto a single scale. They do so by assessing the value that people (usually samples of people from population surveys) assign to diverse sets and combinations of health states using specialized techniques (e.g., standard gamble methodologies).

Internationally, the EQ-5D, a 5-item scale developed by the EuroQoL Group,[58] is among the most common health utility instruments. In Canada, the Health Utilities Index (HUI)[59,60] is most popular. The HUI consists of sets of utility weights, meaning that researchers use other instruments to classify a person's health state and then use the HUI to convert the health-state categories into utility scores. The HUI has several versions: recent Canadian studies mostly use the HUI Mark 3.

Some health-utility weighting schemes assign 1 to indicate perfect health and 0 to indicate states comparable to death. These utility scores can be incorporated into the calculation of quality-adjusted life-years (QALYs). This parameter is not widely used in epidemiology, but is widely used in economic evaluations of health outcomes because it allows the calculation of the number of QALYs achievable at a given cost. Since health-utility scales place different illnesses on the same scale of population-based preference, such studies can identify opportunities to improve health at a known unit cost—for example, by comparing the cost effectiveness of different treatments, or by determining whether the costs of a gain in health utility are within an acceptable range. Marra et al[61] applied this approach to a systematic review of a vaccination program for human papillomavirus (HPV).

HPV, which is sexually transmitted, causes cervical cancer in women: vaccination programs targeting HPV prevent this type of cancer, and so prevent the loss of QALYs that would occur in the absence of vaccination. Marra et al reported generally favourable costs per QALY for HPV vaccination. This suggests that HPV vaccination programs would deliver improved health at a rate per unit cost that is usually considered acceptable in the Canadian health system.

> *Key point:* QALYs attempt to quantify the impact of an intervention on quality of life outcomes and are widely used in health economic evaluations.

Disability-adjusted life-years (DALYs)

Disability-adjusted life-years (DALYs) are another composite measure used to quantify the loss of health associated with diseases and injuries. They are the flagship measure of a major international initiative called the Global Burden of Disease Study.

DALYs are often regarded as a measure of disease burden. Disease burden accounts for both premature mortality (years of life lost, which is conceptually equivalent to PYLL) and years lived with disability due to a disease or injury. These 2 aspects of health are melded using a disability weight, such that DALYs are the sum of the following elements:

- years of life lost
- number of years lived with disability multiplied by a disability weight that reflects the extent of health loss experienced due to the disease

Disability weights reflect health state preferences determined by the Global Burden of Disease investigators using survey methods.[62] If a disease has a disability weight of 0.5, living with that disease for 10 years is considered equivalent to dying 5 years prematurely. The Global Burden of Disease Study uses DALYs to rank the burden caused by a comprehensive set of diseases, injuries, and risk factors on population health in different countries[30,63]—information that can assist those countries with setting priorities for population-health initiatives.

DALYs are useful because they deal with an age-old problem in descriptive epidemiology. Death is an easy thing to measure and almost every country measures it. This creates a tendency to see the impact of diseases from that particular perspective. DALYs make sure that the contribution of disabling conditions is recognized in the assessment of disease burden.

According to the Global Burden of Disease Study,[63] the top 10 causes of disease burden in Canada in 2010 were: ischemic heart disease; low back pain; lung cancer; major depressive disorder; musculoskeletal conditions other than low back pain and neck pain; stroke; chronic obstructive pulmonary disease; diabetes; neck pain; and Alzheimer disease. Self-harm ranked next, followed by road injury.[64] This certainly provides a different perspective on health burden than mortality data in isolation.

Key point: Epidemiologists often use rates and proportions to quantify disease impacts and outcomes, but their toolbox also includes composite measures that can provide additional sophistication for capturing the impact of diseases and injuries.

Proportional mortality ratios

Since mortality databases record cause-of-death information when people die, the counts in such databases must normally be linked to population-denominator data (such as a midyear population count) to calculate a cause-specific death rate. A simpler, albeit less informative, way of using mortality data is to calculate a proportional mortality ratio. This is the number of deaths due to a specific cause divided by all deaths during the same interval of time. For example, Sadovnik et al[65] reported that the proportion of deaths due to suicide in a multiple sclerosis cohort was 7.5 times that of the age-matched general population. Unfortunately, this type of ratio does not represent any meaningful risk in the population. As the capacity to link databases has become more advanced, this parameter has been declining in use. However, archived data for proportional mortality can still be found on the Public Health Agency of Canada's webpage.[66]

Thinking deeper

Calculating central tendency

Often, you can describe the behaviour of a variable with statistical parameters that identify the variable's central or typical values: its central tendency. You can combine these measures of central tendency with a measure of dispersion to describe the distribution of that variable. Chapter 2 introduced the standard error of the prevalence proportion, which is a measure of dispersion for prevalence estimates (see page 19).

The 3 most common ways of quantifying central tendency are the mean, the median, and the mode. The mean is the average value of a variable, calculated by adding all the observed values for the variable and dividing this total by the number of observations. The median is the middle value—a value at which one-half of the observations are higher and one-half are lower. The mode is the most-often-occurring value of a variable.

Table 6 presents the ages of 10 people. Let's use this small data set to illustrate how to calculate the mean, median, and mode.

TABLE 6. A DATA SET WITH THE AGES OF 10 PEOPLE

Identification number	Age
1	48
2	35
3	1
4	43
5	31
6	30
7	26
8	46
9	26
10	50

The mean is the sum of each person's age divided by the number of people. The sample size is $n = 10$, and the identification number provides an index that identifies the individual people from the first ($i = 1$) to the last ($i = 10$). In the following formula for mean age, the uppercase Greek letter sigma (Σ) denotes *sum*:

$$\text{Mean Age} = \frac{\sum_1^{10} \text{Age}}{n}$$

This kind of statement is a more efficient way of saying this:

$$\text{Mean Age} = \frac{48 + 35 + 1 + 43 + 31 + 30 + 26 + 46 + 26 + 50}{10}$$

The mean is 336/10 or 33.6.

The median is the value that divides the observations in the sample into 2 parts: the half above the median (in this case, 5 observations) and the half below (the remaining 5). The median is easiest to see if the observations are sorted by age. Table 7 contains the same data as Table 6, but sorts the observations by age.

You can identify the median by counting up to the midpoint (in this case the fifth observation). Here it falls between the values of 31 and 35, and it is traditional to report it as the average of these 2 values, in this case (31 + 35)/2 = 33.

The mode is the value that occurs most often in the data set. In this case, each observed value occurs once with a single exception: 26 occurs twice. Since this is the most-often-occurring value, it is the modal value for age in this data set. The mode is not used very often in epidemiology, but some related terminology is frequently encountered. A distribution with a single central tendency is unimodal, and a distribution with 2 "humps" suggesting 2 central tendencies is bimodal.

TABLE 7. A DATA SET WITH THE AGES OF 10 PEOPLE, SORTED BY AGE

Identification number	Age
3	1
9	26
7	26
6	30
5	31
2	35
4	43
8	46
1	48
10	50

Questions

1. Approximately a quarter of a million people die in Canada each year. Roughly speaking, what is the crude mortality rate in Canada?

2. About 70 Canadians die each year from tuberculosis and about 70 000 die from malignant neoplasms. Roughly speaking, what are the cause-specific mortality rates for these conditions?

3. Calculate the PYLL contributed by the following deaths:
   a. a motor vehicle collision in which 2 people die, aged 20 and 22
   b. a death due to pneumonia in a 95-year-old

4. Identify the 3 main contributors to the following parameters in Canada:
   a. crude mortality
   b. premature mortality
   c. years lived with disability

5. Johansen et al[67] identified first admissions for stroke (people with no admission for stroke within the preceding 5 years) and examined their in-hospital survival in the 28 days following their admission. They reported that 16.7% died during that interval. What type of "rate" is this?

PART III

Vulnerability to error of descriptive studies

Epidemiologic research can go wrong in many ways, but most errors fall into 3 main categories: random error; systematic error leading to bias; and confounding. The next 5 chapters look at these categories of error in the context of descriptive studies and estimates of fundamental descriptive parameters.

5

Random error from sampling

Objectives
- Identify and differentiate the 2 main sources of error in epidemiologic research: random error and systematic error.
- Describe the relationship between sampling and random error.
- Define confidence intervals and how to calculate an approximate confidence interval for a proportion.
- Describe the relationship between sample size and precision in a prevalence study.
- Differentiate estimation and statistical testing.
- Describe statistical testing and define key related concepts: significant versus nonsignificant tests, type I and type II error, and statistical power.
- Explain the influence of sample size on statistical power.

Random error, systematic error, and confounding

Estimates of basic parameters are right or wrong, and they can be wrong because of random (stochastic) error or systematic error—in other words, by chance or because of defects in study design. In addition, if 2 basic parameters are compared, they may mix together (confound) the effects of several different factors.

This chapter focuses on errors due to chance. If you understand the role of chance in epidemiological research, you can take steps in your own research to minimize errors due to chance, and you can stay alert to these errors in the research of others.

Sources of error and critical appraisal

Critical appraisal is about identifying vulnerabilities and weaknesses in research.

It's an important task: research leads to conclusions that affect people's lives.

Assume that the study is wrong
(a "critical" stance)

⇓

Is it wrong because of bias?

⇓ No

Is it wrong because of random error?

⇓ No

Accept that the result may be right

⇓

Interpret the result

FIGURE 1. A SIMPLE SCHEMATIC FOR CRITICAL APPRAISAL

It's also a complicated task. It requires a solid framework for approaching the vast amount of information—in words, methods, and numbers—reported in the typical study. Understanding random error and systematic error is a good place to start. A study can be right or wrong. A critical reader of a study will accept its conclusions only if the study survives critical appraisal—an attack on its design and methods that aims to identify ways in which a study is likely to be wrong.

Two provisos are in order concerning critical appraisal. First, critical appraisal involves attacks of a sort, but not personal attacks. The process of criticism and defence against criticism in science is not a destructive conflict. It is more like a life-giving force in research. It creates a context of rigour and fosters excellence. Researchers usually seek internal reviews of their grant proposals and research papers from colleagues before submitting them to funding agencies and journals. They do this because they understand the value of critical appraisal. Second, in epidemiology at least, the perfect study doesn't exist. If critical appraisal were solely about finding imperfections, it would draw every result into question. Critical appraisal aims to identify potentially important flaws—flaws that threaten the value of the reported information for the goals of clinical practice and public health.

Figure 1 shows that critical appraisal begins with questions about systematic error. There is good reason for tackling systematic error first and random error second. But, a clear definition of systematic error comes from a clear understanding of what is meant by random error—which is why we start with this chapter on random error.

The relationship between random error and sampling

Basic parameters such as prevalence and incidence are real: they actually exist in populations. Random error arises when estimates of these parameters are inaccurate due to chance.

We know population parameters are real for the following reason: if we could count every person in a population, and identify exactly who did and did not have a particular disease, we could determine exactly the true (actual, real) prevalence of the disease. By contrast, an estimate of that parameter is not real in the same way: it is an educated guess about the true population parameter.

Chapter 2 covered ways to represent in symbols the difference between true prevalence and estimated prevalence, where *PREVALENCE* stood for the true parameter, and *prevalence* stood for a sample-based estimate.

$$PREVALENCE = \frac{A}{A+B}$$

where *A* is all the members of a population with disease and *B* is all the members of a population without disease

$$Prevalence = \frac{a}{a+b}$$

where *a* is the members of a population sample with disease and *b* is the members of a population sample without disease

A characteristic of a true population parameter such as PREVALENCE is this: if the parameter were measured multiple times (selecting every member of a population, classifying them with perfect accuracy into diseased and nondiseased groups) the results would always be exactly the same. This lack of variability reflects that a true population parameter is not subject to random error.

To reflect the underlying true parameter, an estimated parameter such as (lowercase) prevalence needs to come from a random sample or, less desirably, some facsimile of a random sample. If not, there is no particular reason to believe the sample-based estimate has any coherent relation to the true parameter. Random samples provide information about true parameters because each observation in the sample is governed by the long-run probabilities that exist in the underlying population through the law of large numbers.

If you were to sample a population several times to repeat the estimate of the parameter, you would likely get a different estimate from each sample. Each sample would almost certainly select a different group of people from the population, and this would deliver different estimates from sample to sample. This variability reflects that estimated parameters are subject to random error: parameters estimated from samples will not always exactly equal the true parameters in a population.

Key point: A parameter (such as prevalence, incidence, etc.) calculated from a population is a real thing with a real definite value, but often such parameters can only be estimated using data collected from samples. The resulting estimates are not real in the same sense. Repeating the process of estimation will lead to different values each time.

Random samples

The samples used to estimate parameters are subsets of larger populations, but they are not just any subsets. The "magic" of the law of large numbers only works if each member of a sample embodies an event (e.g., diseased or not) independent of other events.

The best kind of sample is therefore a random sample—a sample in which the question of who will be selected into the sample cannot be answered. In other words, selection for a random sample is unpredictable. In the sample, each person's disease status is an independent observation that (together with the other observations) reflects the true prevalence in the population.

PROBABILITY SAMPLE, SELECTION PROBABILITY, AND SAMPLING FRAME

A sample for estimating a parameter should also be a probability sample. This means the probability of selecting a person from the population should be known. A simple random sample is the most common and basic form of a probability sample: each member of the population has the same probability of selection.

Imagine that you are conducting a study of the prevalence of smoking in a high school containing $N = 1000$ students. Let's assume your study will have a sample size of $n = 100$. (Note the convention of an uppercase N to represent the number in the population and a lowercase n to represent the number in the sample.) To select your sample, you might list all the students and use some sort of random process to choose 100 from the list. For example, you could assign a number to each student based on the roll of a 10-sided dice, and then choose all the students assigned the number 1 (or any other number up to 10).

This selection process would result in a simple random sample. The sample would also be a probability sample, since the selection probability is known (0.1 or 10%). The list of students would be called a *sampling frame*: a list of population elements that serves as the basis for the selection of a sample.

INFERENCE AND TARGET POPULATION

Inference describes the process of gaining information about a population based on data collected from a sample. Estimation is the most important way of making inferences in epidemiology.

Key point: Probability samples are a type of random sample that serve as the basis for making inferences about populations.

In estimation, the true underlying parameter is called the *target of estimation* and the population to which the estimate applies is called the *target population*.

The process of inference ideally has the following straightforward step at its foundation: a random sample used for inference about a target population must come from the target population. However, very often the target population (e.g., all women of childbearing age) is not suited to enumeration in a sampling frame—which acts against the goal of collecting a probability sample. In this case, a specific population may be identified (e.g., all women of childbearing age in a city or province) as a practical way of representing the larger target population. This produces a conceptual distinction between the target population and the sampled population. These are subtle distinctions. Some studies aim to make inferences of broad significance—for example, "smoking cigarettes during pregnancy causes low birth weight." This kind of statement is intended as fact: there is no reason to believe that it would apply in St. John's and not in Vancouver. Other studies are concerned with more focused inference about a fully specified population—for example, "18% of adult residents of Toronto smoke." So, epidemiological studies can have more-strict and less-strict ways of conceptualizing (and labelling) target populations.

SOURCE POPULATION

When the target population is not fully enumerated in a sampling frame, the population from which the sample is actually drawn may be called a *source population* rather than a *target population*. For example, the target population may be all pregnant women and the source population for a particular study may be all women receiving prenatal care in Halifax at a point in time.

Some researchers refer to the sample drawn from a source population as a *study population*. This is confusing, since the distinction between a sample and a population is critical for epidemiological reasoning. But it's a term you will likely see in the literature—just remember that it's not a population, it's a sample.

Random error

Normally, a researcher would not care very much about the prevalence of a disease in a sample. The estimated prevalence is just a tool to learn about a true population parameter. Data from random samples are necessary for inference, but the data collected from such samples are merely the raw material for making inferences. Researchers calculate parameters from data and use statistics to generate inferences about populations.

Key point: Data from samples are the raw materials from which inferences derive. The tools used to derive and refine those inferences are statistical tools.

Understanding random error requires imagination. Think back to the hypothetical study of smoking in a school with $N = 1000$ students. Suppose you have randomly selected $n = 10$ for inclusion in the study. Here's the part that requires imagination. Imagine that you conduct the same study

100 times, drawing a random sample of $n = 10$ each time. For each sample, you measure how many students smoke (for now, let's assume that you can do this with perfect accuracy) and calculate an estimate of prevalence from the resulting proportion. In Canada, approximately 1 in 10 youths between the ages of 12 and 17 smoke,[68] so for purposes of illustration we will assume that 0.10 is the underlying population prevalence. Figure 2 shows a simulation of what you would expect to see in this scenario. The value for the estimated prevalence peaks at the true value—which in this case is 0.10. So far, so good. But notice that it is possible, if somewhat unlikely, that some of these studies might come up with estimates that are far from the true value, such as 4 times too high.

Of course, in the real world, studies are never repeated many times in this way. Researchers do studies once and they don't know the underlying true parameter. So, in the real world, investigators face the possibility that their estimates may, by chance, fall far from the true parameter. When selection is perfect (as in the simple random sample imagined here) and measurement is perfect, the expected value of a sample-based estimate is exactly the target parameter in the population. But, as Figure 2 shows, chance plays a role in estimation, and an estimate, even from a perfect study, can be wrong. This is the concept of random error (also known as stochastic error and sampling variability).

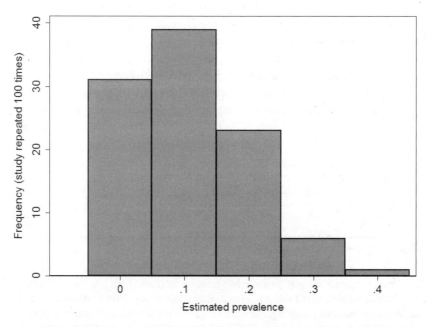

FIGURE 2. SIMULATED DISTRIBUTION OF 100 PREVALENCE ESTIMATES WHERE TRUE PREVALENCE = 0.10 AND N = 10

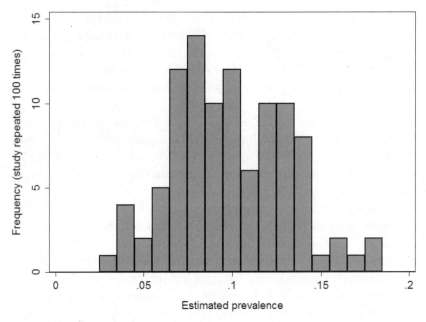

FIGURE 3. SIMULATED DISTRIBUTION OF 100 PREVALENCE ESTIMATES WHERE TRUE PREVALENCE = 0.10 AND N = 100

RANDOM ERROR AND THE LAW OF LARGE NUMBERS

Figure 3 repeats the scenario from Figure 2—so, a study done 100 times in a school with a population of 1000 students—but this time with a sample size of $n = 100$ instead of $n = 10$. The figure shows that a serious error would be less likely. The range of study outcomes is now much narrower.

The distributions of the hypothetical study results presented in Figure 2 and Figure 3 are simulations of sampling distributions, and they show the effect of the law of large numbers on random error: larger samples lower the probability that estimates will differ problematically from target parameters.

Key point: Random error in an estimate of an epidemiological parameter gets smaller as the sample size gets larger.

Pooling estimates to increase sample size

There is a way to salvage studies that have a low sample size (and so have a high probability of random error). This involves pooling estimates from several studies using meta-analysis. In meta-analysis, estimates are only pooled if their differences are small enough to justify pooling. The whole idea of pooling is to find the underlying true value (or, in the case of random-effects meta-analysis, a distribution of values) that the studies are estimating. Pooling study results leads to a more precise estimate.

A good example is a study of depression prevalence in epilepsy conducted by Fiest et al.[69] The literature contained several imprecise estimates of the prevalence of depression in epilepsy. Fiest et al used meta-analysis to combine the results from 9 studies reporting on a total of 29 891 people with epilepsy, leading to an estimated prevalence of "active depression" of 23.1%.

Quantifying random error

Epidemiology has 2 statistical strategies for dealing with random error: confidence intervals and statistical tests.

Confidence intervals

If you are designing a prevalence study, you want a sample size large enough to give you confidence in your estimates. If you are reading a study, you want to know how much confidence you can have in the study's results. Confidence intervals are the preferred statistical method for answering questions about confidence.

Here's a simple way to interpret confidence intervals: when working with sample-based data to generate estimated parameters, confidence intervals define a range of plausible values for true population parameters.

Two numbers called *confidence limits* demarcate confidence intervals: a number at the lower end of an interval's range (the lower confidence limit) and a number at the upper end (the upper confidence limit).

The best types of confidence intervals are exact confidence intervals, which are based on exact probabilities. These are difficult to calculate by hand, but easy to calculate with statistical software packages.

ESTIMATING CONFIDENCE INTERVALS

Many formulas can calculate approximate versions of confidence intervals. Under the assumption that a sampling distribution conforms to a normal distribution—which is a symmetrical bell-shaped distribution (roughly seen in Figure 3)—these formulas often take the following form: the point estimate (the value calculated from the study data) plus or minus the standard error multiplied by a number representing the desired level of confidence for the estimate.

Most investigators seek 95% confidence in their research, which makes the multiplier (based on a normal distribution) 1.96. So, you can approximate a 95% confidence interval (95% CI) as plus or minus 1.96 times the standard error of the parameter being estimated.

A formula for calculating standard error is presented on page 19. For now, let's revisit our hypothetical student-smoking study and assume a standard error of 0.04 for an estimated proportion from a sample of $n = 100$ in which the true population prevalence is 0.10. Multiplying the standard error by 1.96 gives us a value of 0.078, such that an approximate 95% CI is the estimated prevalence (whatever that might be in an individual study—remember that it is not going to be exactly 0.10 very often due to sampling variability) plus or minus 0.078. This provides a range of values within which it is possible to be 95% confident that the true population value lies.

You can also understand confidence intervals as long-run frequencies. For example, you could say that if a study were repeated many times, 95% of the time the confidence interval would include the true value.

PRECISION

The concept of precision is closely related to confidence intervals. Precision refers to the width of a confidence interval. Wide intervals mean low precision and narrow intervals mean high precision.

Precision is inversely related to the risk of random error. It is a key factor to consider in study design, and is directly relevant to critical appraisal of a study's vulnerability to random error. Epidemiological studies need designs that allow them to achieve adequate precision. In practice, this means epidemiological studies must have large sample sizes. Precision-based sample-size calculations estimate the precision achievable in given sample sizes.

Key point: Epidemiological studies must provide adequate precision if their estimates are to be useful. In practice, this means that they must have large sample sizes.

Statistical tests

Epidemiologists use statistical tests less often than confidence intervals. Statistical tests do not have much value in the context of prevalence estimates, so we will use an analytical question to discuss them: whether or not a risk factor (an exposure) is associated with a disease.

Statistical tests begin by formulating a null hypothesis. This amounts to a conjecture that an exposure has no effect on a disease. Of course, in an analytical study, a researcher is likely conducting the study for the opposite reason: because they suspect a particular exposure does, in fact, affect a disease. However, it is much easier to refute a hypothesis than to prove a hypothesis—you only need 1 piece of evidence to refute, but a mountain of evidence to prove (and some say no amount of evidence will entirely prove). So, if a researcher wants to evaluate whether an exposure is associated with a disease, they assume there is no association. In other words, they adopt the null hypothesis for the purpose of trying to disprove it.

Key point: A statistical test can only seek to disprove a hypothesis. These tests cannot directly support a hypothesis.

The next step is to analyze the data collected in the study using an appropriate statistical test. The statistical test assumes the null hypothesis is true, and calculates the probability that what was observed in the data (or something more extreme) would arise given the null hypothesis. This probability is the *P* value associated with the statistical test. If this *P* value is small (5% is the typical critical value against which this determination is made), the null hypothesis is rejected and the alternative hypothesis—that there is an association between exposure and disease—is accepted. If the *P* value is less than 5%, the null hypothesis can be rejected with 95% confidence, and the statistical test is said to be significant.

TYPE I ERROR AND TYPE II ERROR

A statistical test provides a binary outcome. It either rejects, or fails to reject, a null hypothesis, and thereby finds, or fails to find, evidence of an association.

There are 2 ways in which a statistical test can be wrong.

If the null hypothesis really is true, but the results of the statistical test are significant, a type I error has occurred. The probability of type I error is preset by the statistical testing procedure. Since 5% is usually the chosen cut point for assessment of significance, it can be expected that 5% of significant results will be due to chance and therefore represent type I errors.

If the null hypothesis really is false, but a statistical test is not significant, a type II error has occurred. Type II errors are related to the concept of statistical power. Statistical power is the probability of (correctly) rejecting a null hypothesis that is false. The risk of type II error in a study is the complement of power. If the power of a study is 80%, it has an 80% chance of detecting (with a significant test result) that the null hypothesis is false, assuming that the null hypothesis actually is false. Consequently, this level of power signifies a 20% chance that a type II error will occur.

Figure 4 summarizes the types of error associated with statistical tests.

	An association exists in the population (null hypothesis is false)	No association exists in the population (null hypothesis is true)
Statistical test is significant	**No error**	**Type I error**
Statistical test is not significant	**Type II error**	**No error**

FIGURE 4. ERRORS THAT CAN ARISE FROM STATISTICAL TESTS

How can statistical errors be avoided? Type I error is best avoided by limiting the number of tests. If a study evaluates a single hypothesis, the risk of type I error is correctly quantified by the specified critical value, usually 5%. However, if many tests are done, then it is very likely that 1 or more of the significant results will be erroneous. Type II error is best avoided by ensuring an adequate sample size. Sample size is a key determinant of statistical power. Modern statistical software usually includes commands for calculating power according to different assumptions and at different sample sizes. Such calculations are indispensable in the planning of an epidemiological study.

Confidence intervals versus statistical tests
Why are confidence intervals preferred over statistical tests in epidemiology?

One reason is that some of the goals of epidemiology are better accommodated by confidence intervals. Descriptive epidemiologic research often has the goal of estimating a parameter such as prevalence, which has no meaningful null hypothesis to reject. Analytical studies have the explicit goal of evaluating a hypothesis, so in theory statistical testing is a better fit with analytical studies.

However, the goal of evaluating associations is usually done by estimating parameters that embody the comparison of interest (e.g., a comparison between 2 incidence proportions). These parameters have null values built into them. For example, an analytic parameter called *relative risk* is calculated as a ratio: the risk for people exposed to a risk factor (numerator) and the risk for those not exposed to the risk factor (denominator). Under the null hypothesis, the relative risk would be 1.0. As it turns out, if a 95% confidence interval for the null hypothesis fails to include this null value, then a statistical test of the null hypothesis would have been significant at the 5% level of confidence. Therefore, confidence intervals provide all of the information that statistical tests provide, but also much more: they also provide an estimate of the strength of association and identify a range of plausible values for that parameter in the population.

Thinking deeper

Calculating confidence intervals
Chapter 2 presented a formula for estimating the standard error of a proportion:

$$\text{Standard Error} = \sqrt{\frac{p \times (1-p)}{n}}$$

where p is any proportion estimated from a sample of size n

You can use this general formula to calculate an approximate 95% confidence interval (95% CI) in situations where you can reasonably expect a normal distribution for p. You can use the prevalence calculated from a sample to estimate standard error. The following formula gives this general approach, substituting *prevalence* for the unspecified proportion (p):

$$\text{Lower 95\% Confidence Limit} = \text{Prevalence} - 1.96\sqrt{\frac{\text{Prevalence} \times (1 - \text{Prevalence})}{n}}$$

$$\text{Upper 95\% Confidence Limit} = \text{Prevalence} + 1.96\sqrt{\frac{\text{Prevalence} \times (1 - \text{Prevalence})}{n}}$$

Think about our hypothetical student-smoking study again. Table 8 presents data for an iteration of this study where $n = 100$.

This is how you would calculate the approximate 95% confidence interval for the data in Table 8:

$$\text{Lower 95\% Confidence Limit} = \text{Prevalence} - 1.96\sqrt{\frac{0.11 \times (1 - 0.11)}{100}}$$

$$\text{Upper 95\% Confidence Limit} = \text{Prevalence} + 1.96\sqrt{\frac{0.11 \times (1 - 0.11)}{100}}$$

This approximates the 95% CI (rounded to 2 decimal places) as 0.05–0.17, which means you can be close to 95% confident that the true population value is within this range.

Of course, in research, it's better to calculate exact confidence intervals with statistical software, and you should always do exact calculations for work that appears in presentations or publications. For the data in Table 8, statistical software calculates the exact confidence interval as 0.06–0.19, which is fairly close to the formula-derived approximation.

The confidence-interval formula is useful for designing studies that aim to estimate a parameter such as prevalence. Researchers might have a strong idea of the true prevalence—for example, in the case of the hypothetical student-smoking study, we knew 0.10 was likely the true prevalence.[68] They can then estimate the standard error based on the confidence-interval formula, using the expected prevalence and the anticipated sample size. Such a calculation allows prediction about the extent of precision achievable with a particular sample size. If a researcher knows the level of precision required to achieve the objectives of a study, they can evaluate the adequacy of different sample sizes through a series of such calculations. This strategy is called *precision-based sample-size calculation.*

TABLE 8. 1 × 2 TABLE DEPICTING SMOKING STATUS IN A SAMPLE OF N = 100 STUDENTS

Smokes	Does not smoke	Total
11	89	100

Questions

1. What are the key features of critical appraisal? To what extent are these features applied in media reports covering health issues?

2. Describe the defining characteristic of random error in epidemiology.

3. A study by Thege et al[70] reported the prevalence of self-reported sex addiction as 3%, with a standard error of 0.42%. What is an approximate 95% CI for this estimate of the prevalence of sex addiction?

4. The study by Thege et al used a survey conducted over the telephone. Some respondents might have been hesitant to disclose information about their sex lives over the phone. Would this have resulted in random error?

5. Bonaparte et al[26] reported that the age-adjusted incidence rate for amyotrophic lateral sclerosis in Newfoundland in 2003 was 2.13 per 100 000, and reported an associated 95% CI of 0.11–4.15 per 100 000. Provide an interpretation for this confidence interval.

Measurement error that leads to misclassification

Objectives
- Define measurement error, and distinguish it from selection error.
- Distinguish among nominal, ordinal, and cardinal data, and continuous and discrete data.
- Define and explain strategies for describing classification errors: sensitivity and specificity; positive and negative predictive value; Bayes' theorem; likelihood ratios; and reliability.

Measurement error in context
Chapter 5 covered random error in epidemiological research.

Chapters 6, 7, and 8 focus on systematic error. Unlike random error, systematic error does not diminish with larger sample size. It comes from defects in study design that remain unchanged no matter how large the sample. Systematic error leads to bias in epidemiological research—in other words, estimates that systematically over- or underestimate the true values.

For descriptive parameters such as prevalence, there are 2 types of study-design defects that can introduce systematic error: measurement error and selection error.

This chapter and the next look at measurement error: first, at its sources and at ways to quantify its extent; and then, at its effect on parameter estimation.

Chapter 8 looks at selection error and its effects on parameter estimation.

What is measurement error?
Epidemiological estimates are precisely that: estimates of underlying epidemiology, not direct representations. To calculate an epidemiological estimate, you need to assign values to 1 or more variables for all members of the

sample that forms the basis of your estimate. Assigning these values requires measurement.

In a prevalence study, each member of a sample is assigned a variable that can take on different values depending on the member's disease status. Once assigned, these values are recorded as pieces of information collectively referred to as data, and are stored in a data set for analysis.

But, assigning values to variables is not always a perfect process. It is possible that a person with a disease may be incorrectly classified as not having that disease and vice versa.

Epidemiologists are often concerned with classification into categories (especially disease and exposure categories), so errors of classification—misclassification—are a particularly important type of measurement error in epidemiology.

Measurement error compromises the accuracy of epidemiological estimates. It is important to understand how such errors occur so that they can be avoided during study design and, if not, detected during critical appraisal.

Types of data

There are several distinct types of data (all of which provide information). Different types of data require different ways of thinking about measurement. Also, different statistical techniques are appropriate for different types of data. You need to understand data types to do good data analysis, and to understand statistical analyses reported in studies.

Nominal, ordinal, and cardinal data

Nominal data are perhaps the most important data type for epidemiology. As the name suggests, nominal data conform to categories that can be named, such as sex (male and female), marital status (married, unmarried, divorced. widowed), race (Asian, Métis, Caucasian, etc.), and country of origin (Canada, Uganda, Peru, etc.). There is no ordering of these categories. Usually, a diagnosis is a nominal category, as is exposure to a risk factor.

Ordinal data provide information about ranking. Some studies use rating scales to assign numbers to otherwise abstract concepts such as self-esteem, distress, or quality of life. These data have no physical meaning as numbers, and therefore cannot usually be treated as real numbers. For example, many of Statistics Canada's national surveys use the Kessler-6 or K-6 scale (named after its developer, Ron Kessler of Harvard University) to assess nonspecific psychological distress.[71] This scale provides scores on a range of 0 to 24. Because these are numerical scores, it is tempting to give the numbers real meaning—for example, to view a score of 10 as "twice" a score of 5, or to view the difference between scores of 5 and 10 as equivalent to the difference between scores of 15 and 20. However, these scores do not possess mathematical properties.

Here's an example of rating that results in ordinal data. A questionnaire asks, "During the past month, about how often did you feel nervous?" A subject can respond, "all of the time" (which is scored 4), "most of the time" (scored 3), "some of the time" (scored 2), "a little of the time" (scored 1), and "none of the time" (scored 0). The numbers rank narrative statements. Clearly, a score of 4 is greater than a score of 2, but nothing says it's 2 times greater. Normal operations of arithmetic, such as calculating ratios, do not apply to this kind of data.

Cardinal data have real physical meaning, along with all that this implies. Height is an example of cardinal data. A person 2 metres tall is twice as tall as a person 1 metre tall. The difference in their height is exactly the same as the difference in height between people who are 2 and 3 metres tall. Since ratios are meaningful, variables such as height are sometimes said to be measurable on a ratio scale, and since differences are meaningful, this could also be called an interval scale. It is possible for a scale to have interval properties but not ratio properties. For example, the Celsius temperature scale does not allow you to say that 15 degrees is only half as warm as 30 degrees—because 0 on this scale is arbitrary, chosen for convenience (the temperature at which water freezes under specified atmospheric conditions). On the other hand, the Kelvin scale has a real 0 (absolute zero) and therefore is a ratio and an interval scale.

Key point: Three main types of data are: nominal, ordinal, and cardinal.

Categorical versus continuous data

Categorical data have meaningful categories. Nominal and ordinal data, which inherently possess categories, are types of categorical data.

Continuous data can theoretically divide into infinitely smaller categories. Cardinal data, which come from real physical measures such as height or weight, are inherently continuous.

A note about the word data

Epidemiologists, and others, use the word *data* sometimes as a singular term ("the data has a normal distribution") and sometimes as a plural term ("the data have a normal distribution"). This causes a degree of acrimony.

Data derives from Latin: it is a second declension noun of the neuter type. This means that the singular form is *datum* and the plural is *data*. So, by origin, *data* is plural, but its use as a singular term has more and more currency. Some researchers regard the plural usage as a deliberate archaism that serves no purpose.

Other second declension neuter nouns from Latin—those that have not come into common use among the general public—have not evolved in the same way. A good example from epidemiology (and geology) is *stratum* (singular) and *strata* (plural).

This book uses *data* as a plural.

Categorizing continuous variables

In the social sciences, researchers often frown on categorizing continuous variables—variables that are not inherently categorical. Researchers in epidemiology, however, frequently categorize continuous variables. In epidemiology, continuous variables often have meaningful ranges that translate into meaningful categories.

Body mass index, used as an indicator of body composition, is an example. Body mass index is calculated as body weight (in kilograms) divided by height (in metres) squared. This index could theoretically divide into an infinite number of categories—so, it is a continuous variable. However, it is often divided into categories defined by ranges of value, such as underweight, normal weight, overweight, and obese.

Blood pressure is another example. Blood pressure is inherently a continuous variable, but it is often made into a binary variable: normotensive (normal blood pressure) and hypertensive (high blood pressure). Such categorization inevitably results in the loss of some information. For example, if a diastolic blood pressure greater than 90 millimetres of mercury (mmHg) is regarded as hypertensive in a binary categorization, then 89 mmHg will be treated differently than 91 mmHg, even though the actual values are nearly identical. The binary categorization also means that 91 mmHg will be treated the same as 120 mmHg, even though these values are very different.

A lot of categorization occurs in epidemiology despite this obvious loss of information. There is a reason. Epidemiology is a health research discipline, and its methods are closely tied to real-world decision making in professional practice, health service planning, and health policy. Categories often facilitate real-world decisions. They provide guidelines to practitioners about which patients require treatment; they help service planners determine how many people need treatment; and they help policy makers anticipate the preventive value of interventions.

You could say the concept of diagnosis itself imposes categories onto what are sometimes graduated or continuous departures from a physiologic norm. Take blood pressure again. Even though blood pressure is inherently a continuous variable, we know that blood pressure above certain thresholds has impacts on health and requires treatment. In addition, the basic parameters so far discussed in this book (prevalence, incidence) are all based on categorical concepts.

Key point: Artificial categorization is a theoretically problematic manoeuvre, but it often makes sense in epidemiology

---

Quantifying classification errors

As a result of the predominant use of categories in epidemiology, the most important forms of measurement error are those that involve classification into the wrong categories, or misclassification. Fortunately, a set of parameters exists that quantify the likelihood of misclassification and thereby the accuracy of measurement.

Sensitivity and specificity

There are 2 key parameters that quantify the extent of misclassification: sensitivity and specificity.

Both these parameters quantify the performance of a classification method or instrument in relation to a gold standard. A gold standard is a measurement that does not make classification errors. Table 9 shows a way of dividing a group of people according to their true status (the columns, according to a gold standard) and the way in which they are classified by a potentially error-prone test or classification procedure. The table refers to a diagnostic test, so the column titles refer to a gold standard designation of disease status. Note, however, that you could use a table of this type for any type of attribute.

Key point: Determining the performance of a diagnostic test requires comparison to a gold standard.

TABLE 9. 2 × 2 TABLE DESCRIBING THE PERFORMANCE OF A CLASSIFICATION PROCEDURE

	Has the disease	**Does not have the disease**
Test positive	True positive (*tp*)	False positive (*fp*)
Test negative	False negative (*fn*)	True negative (*tn*)

As with many other epidemiological parameters, sensitivity and specificity can be conceptualized as either a frequency or probability. The labels contained in Table 9 (*tp, fp, fn, tn*) offer a means of producing formulas to estimate sensitivity and specificity from a sample:

$$\text{Sensitivity} = \frac{tp}{tp + fn}$$

$$\text{Specificity} = \frac{tn}{tn + fp}$$

Note the use of lowercase letters in these formulas, in keeping with the conventions for sample-based estimates.

VALIDATION STUDIES

The sort of study from which sensitivity and specificity are calculated is called a *validation study*. Validation studies involve a series of steps. First, researchers obtain a sample of people with and without a disease (according to a gold standard assessment instrument). They then administer a test or classification procedure to each member of the sample, which allows them to classify each respondent into one of the 4 groups identified in Table 9: *tp*, *fp*, *fn*, *tn*. From these counts, they can estimate the sensitivity and specificity as a frequency that—if the study is conducted properly and has a large enough sample—provides information about the probabilities of correct and incorrect classification.

Stated in the language of probability, sensitivity is the probability that a person with an attribute is classified correctly by a test (or other classification procedure). Specificity is the probability that a person without the attribute is correctly classified by a test (or classification procedure). Of course, in an epidemiological study, the attribute could be exposure or disease.

Sensitivity and specificity describe test characteristics: they reflect the performance of a test itself, rather than the characteristics of the population in which the tests are used.

Key point: Sensitivity and specificity are characteristics of a test or classification procedure, and do not depend very much on characteristics of the population in which the test is used.

The concept of validity

Sensitivity and specificity quantify the performance of a test or classification procedure in relation to the truth (a gold standard classification). In other words, they provide an assessment of the truthfulness of the results of that test or procedure.

Validity—a term with various uses commonly encountered in the epidemiological literature—refers to the same issue of truthfulness one way or another. So, an epidemiological study is valid if its results provide an accurate reflection of an epidemiologic reality, and a diagnostic test is valid if it accurately identifies the disease status of those who are tested. The term *validity* appears in other contexts as well. It always refers to whether a result is truthful or correct, such as the validity of interpretations or judgements of investigators.

Complements of sensitivity and specificity

Many of the proportions and probabilities encountered in epidemiological studies have complementary proportions and probabilities. The term *complementary* means these probabilities add up to 1. For example, if prevalence is the proportion of a population that has a disease, the complementary proportion consists of those who do not have the disease.

In classification, complementary proportions and probabilities are especially important, and have their own names. The complement of sensitivity is the false-negative rate. (Here, unfortunately, is another questionable use of *rate*. The name for this complement would be better as *false-negative propor-tion*, but this is rarely used.) The false-negative rate is the proportion of those with the disease who are classified incorrectly as not having it.

$$\text{False-Negative Rate} = 1 - \text{Sensitivity}$$

Considering the terminology, it seems perfectly reasonable to call sensitiv-ity the *true-positive proportion*.

The complement of specificity is the false-positive rate (or, preferably, pro-portion). This is the proportion of people without the disease who end up being classified as having it.

$$\text{False-Positive Rate} = 1 - \text{Specificity}$$

Predictive value

Sensitivity and specificity are the most important parameters for quantifying the validity of a testing procedure, but they have a notable limitation. Both parameters are conditional probabilities—necessitating the term *given* in their probability-based definitions. For example, sensitivity is the probability of a positive test given the presence of disease. Specificity is the probability of a negative test given the absence of a disease. However, both probabilities are conditional on a status that is unknown—whether a person has the dis-ease (or other attribute) or not. Obviously, if disease status were known, there would be no need for the test. Because of this limitation, 2 other important classification parameters are needed: positive and negative predictive values.

Positive predictive value is the probability of disease given a positive result on a test or classification procedure. Negative predictive value is the probabil-ity of no disease given a negative test result. The advantage of these param-eters is immediately apparent: they are still conditional probabilities, but they are conditional on something that is known (test status) rather than some-thing that is unknown (disease status). Again, these are frequencies that can be estimated from samples, but which represent probabilities.

A frequency-based formula for positive predictive value, calculated from a sample, is as follows:

$$\text{Positive Predictive Value} = \frac{tp}{tp + fp}$$

Here is a frequency-based formula for negative predictive value, calculated from a sample:

$$\text{Negative Predictive Value} = \frac{tn}{tn + fn}$$

These parameters are very helpful to clinicians who have performed diag-nostic tests and need to interpret the results. They are also very important for screening—where a brief test is administered to populations in an effort to increase early detection of a disease.

Positive predictive value and negative predictive value address a problem with sensitivity and specificity, but these parameters come with their own difficulty—namely, they do not describe test characteristics (unlike sensitivity and specificity). They depend partially on the performance of the test or classification procedure in question, and partially on the frequency of disease in a population. In other words, the same test or classification procedure, with the same sensitivity and specificity, can lead to extremely different predictive values in different populations.

Key point: Predictive values of diagnostic tests and other classification procedures partially reflect the performance of the tests, but partially reflect the characteristics of the population in which the tests are administered.

Bayes' theorem

Bayes' theorem, which is a theorem of conditional probability, provides a formula for understanding the relationship among predictive value, sensitivity, specificity, and the prior probability of disease:

$$\text{Positive Predictive Value} = \frac{Se \times \text{Prior Probability}}{(Se \times \text{Prior Probability}) + [(1 - Sp) \times (1 - \text{Prior Probability})]}$$

where Se is sensitivity and Sp is specificity

Prior probability, sometimes also called *pretest probability*, is the probability that a person being tested has the disease before the test results are known. For example, if testing is performed in a clinic where a known proportion of patients has the disease, this proportion is a tangible baseline frequency—often called a *base rate* in the clinical epidemiology literature (yet another unfortunate use of *rate*). The proportion could also represent a clinician's judgement of the probability of disease in a particular patient, given the patient's signs and symptoms. In the case of a test used for population screening, the prior probability—again, often called the *base rate*—is the prevalence of disease in the population being screened.

Key point: Predictive value can be calculated from characteristics of a test (sensitivity and specificity) and characteristics of the population in which the test is used (e.g., baseline frequency of disease, meaning pretest probability or prevalence).

A similar formula can be used to calculate the negative predictive value of a test:

$$\text{Negative Predictive Value} = \frac{Sp \times (1 - \text{Prior Probability})}{\left[Sp \times (1 - \text{Prior Probability})\right] + \left[(1 - Se) \times (\text{Prior Probability})\right]}.$$

where *Se* is sensitivity and *Sp* is specificity

These formulas may look complicated, but they are similar to the frequency-based formulas presented earlier in this chapter. If you look carefully, you will see the similarities. The numerator of the Bayesian formula for negative predictive value is the product of the frequency of people who do not have the disease (the complement of the frequency of those who do) multiplied by the frequency with which they are correctly classified as not having the disease (specificity). So, the numerator is the expected proportion of true negatives in the sample. The left-hand term in the denominator is identical to the numerator, aligning with the frequency-based definition. The right-hand term in the denominator equates with the expected proportion of false-negative results— given the false-negative rate (1 – sensitivity) associated with the test—multiplied by the frequency of disease. As in the formulas for positive and negative predictive value, the denominator represents both true-negative and false-negative results.

Likelihood ratios

A likelihood ratio is another important way to quantify the meaning of tests or classification procedures. It can be expressed in positive or negative terms, but the positive version—the likelihood ratio positive—is most common. In fact, *likelihood ratio* generally means the likelihood ratio positive.

The parameter can be calculated using the sensitivity and specificity of the test:

$$\text{Likelihood Ratio} = \frac{\text{Sensitivity}}{1 - \text{Specificity}}$$

Conceptually, this is the probability of a positive test when disease is truly present divided by the probability of a positive test when disease is truly absent (or, the true-positive rate divided by the false-positive rate). This likelihood ratio can be used to calculate the impact of a positive test on the best estimate of whether a person has a disease. The relationship is as follows:

$$\text{Posttest Odds} = \text{Pretest Odds} \times \text{Likelihood Ratio}$$

Clearly, this is similar to the Bayesian approach, but it uses odds rather than proportions. The pretest odds are akin to the pretest probability (or a base rate expressed as odds). This is, perhaps, a quicker and more straight-forward way to estimate the likelihood of disease, given a test result, than the Bayesian formula. Odds, however, are less familiar to most people than frequencies and proportions. Fortunately, as noted in chapter 3 (see page 28), it is very easy to calculate odds from proportions and vice versa.

$$\text{Odds} = \frac{\text{Proportion}}{1 - \text{Proportion}}$$

$$\text{Proportion} = \frac{\text{Odds}}{1 + \text{Odds}}$$

Reliability

Interrater and test-retest reliability

Reliability refers to the repeatability of a measure. In epidemiology, there are 2 key types of reliability: interrater reliability and test-retest reliability.

Often, measurement requires a "rater"—for example, a clinician who decides (rates) whether a patient has a disease. If the procedure for diagnosis is reliable, 2 clinicians assessing the same patient should come to the same conclusion. This concept of agreement between different raters is the concept of interrater reliability.

The concept of test-retest reliability applies if a clinician were to assess the same patient more than once—if the procedure for diagnosis is reliable, the clinician should come to the same conclusion each time.

When used in research, these terms do not always apply to assignment of a diagnosis. They may refer to the repeatability of any type of measure of any type of attribute.

Coefficients for quantifying reliability

Where ratings consist of nominal classifications, such as diagnoses, reliability is often quantified with kappa coefficients. Where ratings consist of ordinal or cardinal classifications, reliability is quantified with correlation coefficients.

Correlation coefficients include the Pearson product moment coefficient, the Spearman rank correlation coefficient, and the intraclass correlation coefficient (ICC). The Pearson and Spearman coefficients both compare pairs of measures: the Spearman coefficient uses rankings and is considered more appropriate for ordinal data, whereas the Pearson coefficient is usually more appropriate for continuous data. The ICC compares groups of measures.

Correlation coefficients have a range of values between 1 and −1, where 1 indicates perfect positive linear relationship, −1 indicates perfect negative linear relationship, and 0 indicates no linear relationship. The kappa coefficient has a similar interpretation, although the "linear" part does not apply because the kappa coefficient quantifies agreement between nominal ratings.

Oremus et al[72] published an interesting assessment of reliability statistics. These investigators examined the reliability of scales used to rate the quality of published studies. These quality ratings guide the selection of studies for systematic reviews of the health science literature. The investigators noted that students often do the work of quality rating, so they used student ratings to assess the interrater and test-retest reliability of 2 numeric scales, and of ratings based on categorical indicators (e.g., excellent, mediocre, poor). They used correlation coefficients to assess agreement of the numeric scales and kappa coefficients for the categorical indicators. They found generally poor interrater reliability, but better test-retest reliability. They hypothesized that better training of student raters would enhance the quality of systematic reviews of the literature.

With self-rated measures (e.g., where study subjects rate some aspect of themselves), the concept of interrater reliability does not apply. However, test-retest reliability is still an important characteristic of such measures. For example, Kassam et al developed a scale to measure stigmatizing attitudes about mental illness held by health care professionals. This study was a component of the antistigma work of Mental Health Commission of Canada.[73] Kassam's scale—called the OMS-HC—is a 20-item scale that produces ordinal scores with potential values between 20 and 100. Because this scale produces dimensional ratings rather than nominal ones, kappa coefficients were not appropriate as measures of agreement. Instead, the study used ICCs to quantify test-retest reliability. The study reported an ICC of 0.66, which was interpreted as adequate test-retest reliability.

Thinking deeper

Equivalence of Bayes' theorem and likelihood ratios

Bayes' theorem and likelihood ratios accomplish the same goal: to anticipate the probability of a disease (or other attribute) when a test result is known. They (and other formulas in this chapter) derive from the same 2 × 2 table.

A paper by Joseph et al[74] reported the following 2 × 2 table (Table 10) to test for *Strongyloides* infection in 162 Cambodian refugees arriving in Montreal in the 1980s.

If the serology results are treated as a gold standard in this table (although Joseph et al did not treat them this way), the stool examination is seen to be

TABLE 10. 2 × 2 TABLE FROM JOSEPH ET AL[74]

	Stool exam positive	Stool exam negative	Total
Serology positive	38	87	125
Serology negative	2	35	37
Total	40	122	162

insensitive (38/125 = 30.4%) but highly specific (35/37 = 94.6%). This means that the likelihood ratio positive (sensitivity divided by 1 – specificity) is 5.6.

Imagine you are using the stool examination test in a population with a base rate of 5%. Using Bayes' theorem, the positive predictive value is:

$$\text{Positive Predictive Value} = \frac{0.304 \times 0.05}{[(0.304 \times 0.05) + [(1 - 0.946) \times (1 - 0.05)]}= 0.228 = 22.8\%$$

Note that you can convert a base rate of 0.05 into odds using the formula on page 28 (it becomes a pretest odds of 0.053). The posttest odds of disease can be calculated as the product of the likelihood ratio positive and the pretest odds: 0.053 × 5.6 = 0.296. Converting this back to a proportion (proportion = odds divided by 1 + odds), the result is 0.228 or 22.8%, which is identical to the result attained through the Bayesian calculation.

This example illustrates a general principle: the approach using the likelihood ratio positive and the approach using Bayes' theorem are identical. They are just different ways of looking at the same thing.

Questions

Davidson et al[75] examined the performance of colour Doppler ultrasound in the diagnosis of deep vein thrombosis (DVT) in patients undergoing elective surgeries, with disappointing results. They reported the following 2 × 2 table (see Table 11) showing the results of the ultrasound tests versus the gold standard of venography.

1. What is the sensitivity and specificity of the ultrasound tests versus venography as a gold standard?

2. What are the odds of DVT in the sample? From these odds, calculate the prevalence.

3. What is the likelihood ratio positive for the ultrasound test?

4. Calculate the posttest odds and positive predictive value for those who are ultrasound positive.

5. If the pretest probability is 50% (pretest odds = 1), what is the positive predictive value?

Table 11. Colour Doppler ultrasound versus venography in the diagnosis of DVT[75]

	Venography positive	Venography negative
Colour Doppler ultrasound indicates DVT	8	23
Colour Doppler ultrasound indicates no DVT	13	275

Misclassification bias in descriptive studies

Objectives
- Define misclassification bias as a type of systematic error.
- Describe sources of misclassification bias in terms of sensitivity and specificity.
- Explain the concept of direction of bias in misclassification bias.
- Describe situations in which misclassification bias may result in over- or underestimation of a descriptive parameter.

Misclassification bias in context

Chapter 6 introduced the first of 2 types of systematic error in epidemiological research: measurement error. Specifically, it focused on measurement error that leads to misclassification.

This chapter describes misclassification bias: the effect of misclassification—measurement error—on estimating parameters. (*Bias* means the effect of systematic error.) Since erroneous measurement leads to misclassification, the resulting type of bias could be called *measurement bias*. Another name is *information bias*. However, due to the emphasis of epidemiology on categories and classification, this chapter will use the term *misclassification bias*.

Understanding misclassification bias involves understanding how errors in classification translate into systematic over- or underestimation of parameters such as prevalence and incidence. This chapter will focus on prevalence, but the same principles apply to the estimation of any type of proportion, including incidence proportions.

Sources of misclassification bias

Misclassification bias results from systematic error in measurement—in other words, from flawed disease-detection tests, diagnostic algorithms, classification protocols, and so on. These flaws come from the design of these tests, algorithms, and protocols.

Flawed tests, algorithms, and protocols are like incorrectly calibrated rulers: every time you use them, they give you erroneous measurements. The error they generate does not come from chance (unlike random error), so increasing the number of measurements you make (the sample size) doesn't help. The more things you measure with a flawed ruler, the bigger your pool of erroneous data.

To understand the bias in measurement generated by a flawed ruler, you look at its calibration compared to an accurate ruler. To understand the bias generated by flawed tests, algorithms, and protocols, you look at their sensitivity and specificity.

Low sensitivity

A measurement (e.g., a diagnostic test, a classification protocol) with low sensitivity will not detect disease in all study subjects with disease. Imagine conducting a prevalence study where the measurements (tests, protocols) for identifying the disease are insensitive. You collect the data and classify disease according to the results of the (insensitive) measurements. After data collection, you enter the data into a study database from which prevalence can be calculated. Since only the subjects who tested positive appear in this data set as cases of disease—and since the insensitive measurement did not identify all cases of disease—the numerator of the estimated prevalence proportion will be smaller than it should be. However, all members of the sample, regardless of their disease status or classification, will be present in the denominator. Therefore, low sensitivity (at least when there is perfect specificity) will lead to an underestimation of prevalence.

Key point: Measurements (e.g., tests, protocols) that are insensitive will tend to bias frequency estimates such as prevalence away from the true population parameter in the direction of producing estimates that are too low.

Low specificity

A measurement with low specificity will mistakenly classify some disease-free subjects as diseased. These are false positives. These misclassified subjects will end up in the numerator of the calculated frequency—but again, the denominator of the calculated parameter does not change. This will make the estimated prevalence too high.

Key point: Methods of disease classification that are nonspecific will tend to bias frequency estimates such as prevalence toward values higher than the true population value.

Low sensitivity and specificity

In some situations, a trade-off could exist between sensitivity and specificity, such that the tendency to underestimate due to low sensitivity and the tendency to overestimate due to low specificity would cancel out. This would lead to an unbiased prevalence estimate, but it does not often occur. Most diseases afflict only a small proportion of the population, so prevalence studies contain far fewer people with disease than without. As a result, many more false positives than false negatives tend to occur when sensitivity and specificity are comparable. Specificity needs to be very high in most cases to avoid a substantial overestimation of prevalence.

Describing the direction of misclassification bias

Descriptive parameters such as prevalence and incidence proportion always have values between 0 and 1 because the contents of their numerators are included in their denominators. As a result, the direction of bias can be anticipated given the effect of misclassification on the numerator of the proportion. Misclassification bias can result in an estimate that is too high (positive bias) or too low (negative bias). The idea of using these particular words to describe the direction of bias derives from a formula for relative bias.

This formula depicts bias in relation to the true value of the parameter being estimated. Here is the relative bias formula:

$$\text{Relative Bias} = \frac{e(\text{Prevalence}) - \text{PREVALENCE}}{\text{PREVALENCE}}$$

where *e(Prevalence)* is the expected value of sample-based estimates and *PREVALENCE* is the true parameter

The expected value of the sample-based parameter (the central tendency of the distribution of estimates were the study to be repeated many times)— in the absence of bias—is the same as PREVALENCE. If the distribution of estimates centres around a value that is too low, the formula will produce a negative value. If the distribution of estimates centres around a value that is too high, it will produce a positive value. This demonstrates the value of *positive* and *negative* for describing the direction of misclassification bias. However, while the formula has some conceptual value in understanding the direction of bias, it has little practical value since PREVALENCE is unknown. Indeed, were it known, there would be no need to estimate it.

Other terms for misclassification bias

Unfortunately, the literature uses a variety of terms for misclassification bias.

For example, if diagnosticians are overzealous—counting suspected cases of a disease as disease—the resulting false-positive rate (a lack of specificity)

produces a positive bias and an overestimation of prevalence. *Misclassification bias* would be a good term to describe this, but some epidemiologists call it *diagnostic suspicion bias* or *interviewer bias*. These terms attempt to describe the study defect that is causing bias. However, it is always best to articulate an actual mechanism through which bias might occur, and this usually involves more than just assigning a mechanism.

Compare these statements:

- "This study is vulnerable to diagnostic suspicion bias."
- "Diagnostic suspicion may have lowered the specificity of classification of disease status, leading to an inflation of the numerator of the prevalence proportion with false positives, causing misclassification bias and leading to an overestimation of prevalence."

The first statement is less wordy, but the second statement is much more informative and precise.

Key point: There are many terms to describe different forms or mechanisms of bias that might occur in specific studies, but it is not necessary to know these terms.

The relationship between bias and random error

What should be considered first, random error or bias? This is an important question in study design and in critical appraisal.

You can make a case for considering bias first. In the absence of bias, a study's results remain vulnerable to random error. In the presence of bias, however, it is difficult to say what random error means. In unbiased studies, confidence intervals quantify the extent of vulnerability to random error. However, if an estimate is systematically biased, it is difficult to say what the confidence intervals are quantifying.

If you calculate a conventional confidence interval for a biased estimate, the interval will centre on the biased estimate rather than the true population value. As the sample size increases, the width of those confidence intervals will become narrower, but still centre on the wrong thing. With increasing sample sizes, confidence intervals for a biased estimate will actually be less likely to incorporate the true parameter value. Any interpretation of those confidence intervals (such as a statement of confidence that the true population value lies within the range specified by the 2 confidence limits) is untrue.

Bias results from study-design flaws: careful study design can usually avoid them. Where misclassification bias is concerned, this means making sure that study variables are measured accurately. In reviewing a study with serious design flaws, such as inaccurate measurement, a thoughtful critical appraiser will not pay much attention to the statistics (knowing these to be wrong) and will instead focus on the effects of systematic error.

Thinking deeper

Exploring the magnitude of misclassification bias

An estimate of prevalence is based on a 1 × 2 table (see Table 12). You can generate this kind of table if you have classified a sample into diseased and nondiseased groups.

On page 18, we described the calculation of prevalence from a table such as Table 12 in a way that did not acknowledge classification errors: the formula for prevalence was simply $a/(a + b)$ or equivalently a/n. If, however, a study is vulnerable to misclassification bias, the numbers in the table do not actually represent people with or without the disease. Instead, they partially represent a flawed way in which the study has classified its subjects as having or not having disease.

To anticipate the effect of misclassification, you can break down each of the columns in this table. You can divide subjects identified as having the disease—denoted a in the table—into 2 groups: those correctly classified as having the disease (the true positives, tp) and those incorrectly classified as having the disease (false positives, fp). You can similarly divide those identified without the disease (denoted b) as correctly classified (true negatives, tn) and incorrectly classified (false negatives, fn). This is a sobering thought. The law of large numbers is the driving force behind epidemiological research and of course it is still operating—but, where misclassification bias enters in, the law no longer operates in the service of valid estimation. A prevalence estimate is calculated as:

$$\text{Prevalence} = \frac{a}{a+b} = \frac{a}{n}$$

This is actually estimating an entity expressed in the next formula (below). Note that, because the denominator of a prevalence proportion contains the entire sample regardless of how classified, the possibility of misclassification does not affect the denominator and it can therefore be written simply as n rather than $tp + fp + fn + tn$.

$$\text{Prevalence} = \frac{tp + fp}{n}$$

The expected number of true positives is the proportion of those who actually have the disease and are classified correctly (sensitivity × a), and the

TABLE 12. 1 × 2 TABLE WITH SAMPLE-BASED DATA FROM A PREVALENCE STUDY

Disease	No disease	Total
a	b	n

expected number of false positives is the number without the disease multiplied by the false-positive rate: $(1 - \text{specificity}) \times b$. Pulling it all together, the result is a strange looking formula:

$$e(\text{Prevalence}) = \frac{(\text{Sensitivity} \times a) + \left[(1 - \text{Specificity}) \times b\right]}{n}$$

where $e(Prevalence)$ is the expected value of the estimated prevalence

Note that if sensitivity and specificity are both perfect (having values of 1), this equation reduces to the following form (a way of saying that measurement is perfect and that the estimated prevalence is not subject to misclassification bias):

$$\text{Prevalence} = \frac{a}{n}$$

Let's return to our formula for $e(Prevalence)$:

$$e(\text{Prevalence}) = \frac{(\text{Sensitivity} \times a) + \left[(1 - \text{Specificity}) \times b\right]}{n}$$

Consider what would happen to estimated prevalence if sensitivity or specificity were less than perfect. Suppose that specificity is perfect and sensitivity is less than 1. In this instance, the formula reduces to the following (since specificity is 1, the right-hand term in the numerator disappears):

$$e(\text{Prevalence}) = \frac{\text{Sensitivity} \times a}{n}$$

So, if there is perfect specificity, imperfect sensitivity will always lead to an underestimation of prevalence.

What happens when sensitivity is perfect and specificity is less than 1? In this circumstance, the equation reduces to:

$$e(\text{Prevalence}) = \frac{a + \left[(1 - \text{Specificity}) \times b\right]}{n}$$

Whenever specificity is less than 1, the numerator of the prevalence equation will be inflated by false positives, and the expected value of the sampling distribution for this parameter will be systematically higher than that of the true population value.

You can use these formulas to anticipate the direction of bias—and also the magnitude of bias. You could, for example, consider the impact of a sensitivity or specificity of 0.5 versus 0.9 on the expected value of the estimated prevalence by replacing sensitivity and specificity with these values and calculating the expected value of the estimate.

Questions

1. The Canadian Longitudinal Study on Aging (CLSA) is a 20-year prospective study. The study includes measurement of a set of chronic medical conditions. The scope of the CSLA (which has a sample size of 50 000) is too large to have each participant assessed by a clinical diagnostician, so it uses self-reported diagnoses. Because self-reported diagnoses may be inaccurate, the investigators sought to develop algorithms based on self-report data. They calculated the sensitivity and specificity of proposed algorithms in relation to high-quality clinical assessments, which served as a gold standard.[76] There were 20 people with 1 of several chronic conditions included in the algorithm-study sample.

   a. One assessment involved an algorithm for symptoms of Parkinson disease (parkinsonism). The algorithm had excellent sensitivity and specificity: both were 100%. Does this mean that studies using the algorithm (especially the CLSA) would be free of misclassification bias?

   b. One of the algorithms for diabetes was 100% sensitive but only 70% specific. Do you think that application of the algorithm would lead to over- or under-estimation of the population prevalence of diabetes?

2. Foebel et al[77] investigated the validity of a rating instrument called interRAI to diagnose neurological conditions. InterRAI was intended for use in people receiving home care, long-term care, and mental-health care. The investigators compared the data they collected through interRAI with data from—presumably accurate—patient records. They reported excellent specificity but variable sensitivity, depending on the diagnosis. For example, for traumatic brain injury the specificity was 99% and the sensitivity was 22%.

   a. Would you anticipate bias in a prevalence estimate of traumatic brain injury?

   b. If so, in what direction?

3. Kassam et al[73] developed a scale to assess mental-illness-related stigma in health professionals. Several studies have used this scale to assess the level of stigma held by members of various health professions and their trainees.

   a. People who hold negative beliefs (stigma) toward people with mental illness may not admit to their beliefs. Do you think this could make studies estimating the mean level of stigma vulnerable to bias?

   b. If so, in what direction?

4. Mothers whose newborn babies have malformations often think hard about possible causes of those malformations. Drugs and medications are often suspected of increasing the risk of fetal malformations.

   a. Would a tendency of mothers whose babies have malformations to think hard about drugs or medications they may have taken during pregnancy introduce bias into an estimate of the frequency of use of those drugs and medications?

   b. What would be the best way to control such bias?

5. A major source of data for epidemiological research in Canada is administrative data. These data are collected during the process of administering the health system during tasks such as reimbursing hospitals for the care they provide or paying fees to physicians for services that they perform. Marrie et al[78] have developed algorithms for the detection of comorbidity in neurological patients using linked administrative databases in Manitoba. As a validation standard, they conducted chart reviews, allowing calculation of sensitivity and specificity for alternative algorithms. Do you agree that a chart review can be used as a gold standard?

8

Selection error and selection bias in descriptive studies

Objectives
- Define selection bias as a type of systematic error arising from participation or nonparticipation in a study.
- Identify sources of selection bias: selection itself, nonconsent, attrition, and (in some cases) missing data.
- Describe the mechanism by which defective selection can introduce bias into an estimated frequency such as prevalence.
- Describe the direction of bias in a defective prevalence study in which selection depends on disease status.

Selection bias in context

So far, we have covered random error (chapter 5), and 1 of 2 types of systematic error and bias in epidemiology: measurement error leading to misclassification (chapter 6) and misclassification bias (chapter 7).

This chapter covers the second type of systematic error and bias in epidemiology: selection error and bias.

For clarity, the breakdown that follows compares: random error; misclassification error and bias; and selection error and bias.

Type of error	Sources of error	Type of bias
Random error	Chance	N/A
Systematic error		
• Measurement error	Flaws in study design (flawed measurement leading to misclassification)	Misclassification bias
• Selection error	Flaws in study design (flawed sampling procedures that choose participants)	Selection bias
	Other factors related to participation (e.g., subjects withdrawing from a study)	

In selection error, all sources of error are related to participation, so some researchers call the bias that results *participation bias*. Note that only 1 of the sources of error in selection error really counts as a defect in selection (in the strictest use of the word): flawed sampling procedures, which determine who researchers choose as study participants. We use *selection error* as shorthand for other factors related to participation, even if sampling procedures are not flawed, because they all lead to bias through a similar mechanism. These factors include, for example, decisions by subjects not to participate in a study, or not to participate fully.

Key point: Selection bias is a type of systematic error that results from study-design defects, and other factors, that affect who participates in an epidemiologic study.

Selection error from sampling procedures

To understand flawed sampling procedures, you need to understand ideal sampling procedures. Ideal sampling procedures deliver probability samples, where the probability of selection for each member of the sample is known.

Ideal sampling: probability samples

Chapter 5 discussed the concept of random sampling (see page 55). In simple random sampling, each member of a population has the same chance of being selected into a sample. In other words, the selection probability for each member of the population is the same. With random sampling (assuming perfect measurement), the law of large numbers ensures that the proportions observed in samples closely reflect the true population values, at least when samples are large.

Simple random sampling belongs to a broader category of sampling procedures called *probability sampling*.

In probability sampling, there is a known probability of selection for each member of the population, but each member doesn't necessarily have the same probability of selection. Stratified sampling—another type of probability sampling—involves differing (but known) probabilities of selection for members of a population. Researchers use stratified sampling to make estimates within population subgroups. To limit the imprecision of these estimates, they ensure adequate numbers of subjects from target subgroups in their study samples.

For example, national surveys conducted by Statistics Canada, such as the Canadian Community Health Survey,[79] use stratified sampling. Because these surveys are federal initiatives, they are designed to provide useful estimates to all the provinces. However, some provinces are much larger than others. A simple random sample of the Canadian population would lead to small sample sizes in small provinces such as Prince Edward Island—which would make estimates made for this province imprecise. As a result, the design of the study ensures that selection probabilities for small provinces are larger than they would be in a simple random sample.

Stratified sampling also played a role in a mental health survey conducted in New Zealand: the probability of selection for Maori people was doubled, and for Pacific people quadrupled, to allow estimation in these subgroups.[80]

Most studies using stratified sampling have overall estimates as a goal, in addition to estimates for subgroups. For example, the surveys conducted by Statistics Canada aim for national estimates as well as provincial estimates. In making national estimates, researchers offset the unequal selection probabilities with sampling weights. These ensure that national estimates do not overrepresent subgroups.

In stratified sampling, researchers deliberately alter selection probabilities to make them unequal in known ways, and use sampling weights to prevent these unequal probabilities from introducing bias in overall estimates.

By contrast, unequal selection probabilities due to defective study design introduce bias in ways that cannot be corrected after the fact.

The real world of imperfect sampling

Even if researchers intend to obtain a probability sample, in reality they may not achieve equal probability of selection for all study subjects, or they may not know the exact probability of each subject's selection. Either of these problems can lead to selection bias, and they can occur at different steps of the sample-selection process.

The first step in sampling is to identify a sampling frame (chapter 5 also discusses sampling frames—see page 55). This is sometimes easy. For example, if you want to study the population of students at a particular university, a list of all registered students would provide a logical and straightforward sampling frame. But what if you want to make inferences about the population of a city or town? In this case, a list of residents may not exist. The only list, in theory, would be a census. Census lists do exist, but they are not usually accessible to researchers for reasons of privacy—in Canada, federal census data are protected by the Statistics Act.

The next step is selecting a sample from the sampling frame. If a real sampling frame is available (i.e., a list of all people in a population of interest), you can obtain a true probability sample fairly easily. For example, if you want a 10% simple random sample from a list of university registrants, you could enter the list into a spreadsheet or database, and then randomly generate an integer in the range of 0 to 9 (all with equal probability) for each entry. You could then choose all of the entries with a specific value as a means of randomly selecting 1 in 10.

When a list of an entire population is not available, though, probability sampling is not possible

STRATEGIES FOR REPRESENTATIVE SAMPLING

Without a real sampling frame, the best you can do is to collect a representative sample—a sample, in other words, that you believe represents the real population.

Many studies use area frames and telephone frames as the basis for representative sampling.

Key point: While probability sampling is always the preferred procedure, researchers must often devise other ways to obtain representative samples.

AREA FRAMES

Area frames define populations geographically. To obtain a representative sample from an area frame, you would typically do the following: first use maps to define geographical areas, then identify households within those areas, and finally select individuals from those households. Statistics Canada uses area frames for a variety of national surveys, including the Labour Force Survey.

TELEPHONE FRAMES

Telephone frames come from lists of telephone numbers, such as Internet telephone directories or old-fashioned paper telephone directories. Telephone directories, however, have never provided reliable sampling frames because people can choose to keep their numbers unlisted. Historically, this problem was addressed by random digit dialing (RDD), which involves randomly manipulating telephone numbers to equalize the probability of reaching listed versus unlisted numbers. Random dialing often uses single digit substitution: you select a telephone number from a list of telephone numbers and substitute 1 of its digits (usually the final digit) with a randomly generated number between 0 and 9. Presumably, using the random-digit phone number makes the chance of reaching an unlisted number or a listed number the same.

Telephone frames usually involve phone numbers that connect to households, not to individuals. If a research team reaches a household through telephone sampling, they must typically select 1 person from that household to participate in their survey. This is not a trivial matter. The most common procedure is to select 1 person randomly, or to use a nonrandom procedure, such as selecting the person with the most recent birthday.[81] Random selection in a household with 2 people results in a 50% chance of each person being selected; in a household with 10 people, it results in a 10% chance. The number of phone lines coming into a household also changes selection probabilities (the more phone lines to a household, the higher the selection probability for members of that household). Sampling weights can be used to offset these problems.[82]

Some problems, though, limit the usefulness of telephone surveys in less manageable ways.

Telephone surveys worked quite well before the 1990s, at which point their usefulness began to decline. In general, they show a trend toward declining response rates. Telephone fraud and telemarketing may have contributed to this trend: people are more cautious about providing personal information over the phone, and they use call-blocking and call-screening technologies— all of which can affect response rates to RDD surveys. A recent RDD survey conducted in Alberta had to call 36 068 telephone numbers to obtain a sample of 3304 participants.[83]

An even greater threat to telephone sampling comes from the rise of mobile phones over landlines. Mobile phones are not usually listed in directories, so you can't use them to produce a representative sample through digit substitution. You could try calling large numbers of randomly generated phone numbers, but many of these numbers would be nonworking, or would reach businesses or fax machines: you might call hundreds of them before connecting to a potential participant.

Finally, not everybody owns a telephone. If the target population is a community population, investigators want an equal chance of reaching each person—something that cannot happen by phone if not everybody has a phone.

Key point: Telephone survey methods are of declining importance in epidemiology due to difficulties in obtaining a representative sample in this way.

OTHER SAMPLE FRAMES

Mail surveys were once a mainstay of epidemiological research, but they are also becoming less and less useful.[84] People are using mail less and show an increasing tendency not to respond to mailed survey requests. Furthermore, stamps are very expensive.

The decline in telephone and mail strategies for sampling has generated a lot of interest in Internet-based sampling. However, the Internet does not provide a good foundation for representative samples: there is no enumeration of people with Internet access or any way to systematically enumerate a sampling frame consisting of those people.

TRENDS IN SAMPLE FRAMES

Major data collection platforms have increasingly become the foundation for epidemiological research. These platforms include registries of disease. For example, cancer registries are very important sampling vehicles in cancer epidemiology.[50] Registered diseases are growing in number, and registries now exist for neurology,[85] muscular dystrophy,[86] and trauma.[87,88] The establishment of a cerebral palsy registry at McGill University has made Canada a leader in this area.[89] In addition, provinces have registries of persons insured for health care—and since Canada has universal health care, these can prove useful for sampling.

National surveys conducted by Statistics Canada are another important source of data for epidemiological research. The most important health survey is the Canadian Community Health Survey, which collects data from approximately 65 000 Canadians every year on a continuous data-collection cycle. These surveys collect extensive and far-reaching data using high-quality sampling based primarily on an area frame. Statistics Canada has procedures in place for epidemiologists to access these data, with safeguards to ensure compliance with the Statistics Act. The procedures require research to take place inside regional data centres—a set of secure data-analysis facilities with locations at many of Canada's major universities. Statistics Canada calculates sophisticated sampling weights for these data, which it also makes available to researchers.

Selection error from other factors: consent, attrition, and missing data

Obtaining a sample is obviously a very challenging aspect of selection in epidemiology, but the challenges don't stop there. Just because a person has been selected for participation in a study doesn't mean they will participate.

Unlike the national census, people are not legally obliged to participate in research. To participate, people must provide consent for participation. Rather than a legal principle, consent reflects an ethical principle called the *respect for persons* principle. This principle means that people should decide for themselves whether they wish to participate in a research study. To make such a decision, people must know the implications of their participation (what it would mean to agree to participate) and they must be free of coercion so that their choices about participation are fully autonomous.

People hold different opinions about health related topics, and some have more trust than others in health research and health researchers. Some people selected into a study sample decline to participate. Others may agree to participate, but may refuse to answer certain questions—this results in missing data, which in turn may result in selection bias. In longitudinal studies, participants may lose interest and drop out, resulting in sample attrition. Attrition can also occur because participants move out of the study area, or because researchers fail to track changes in participant contact information, and for many other reasons.

Key point: Any factor affecting participation in a study that is related to the condition being studied has the potential to introduce selection bias.

The mechanism of selection bias in prevalence estimates

Suppose that a study's sampling procedure is flawed in the sense that people with disease are more likely to be selected into the study than people without disease. This means that the numerator in the prevalence calculation (denoted *a*) will be too large.

$$\text{Prevalence} = \frac{a}{a+b}$$

Let's assume prevalence is estimated from a simple random sample and classification has been free of error. The observed proportion of people with disease has an expected value—*e(prevalence)*—related to the proportion of people in the population that have the disease (the true population value). The expected value of the count represented by *a* is the population value (*A*) multiplied by the selection probability $p_{selection}$.

$$\text{e(Prevalence)} = \frac{A \times p_{selection}}{\left(A \times p_{selection}\right) + \left(B \times p_{selection}\right)}$$

Clearly, if there is only 1 selection probability ($p_{selection}$), which is the case for a simple random sample, there will be no bias since the expected value of the estimate will be the population prevalence. So, $p_{selection}$ cancels out and the equation reduces as follows:

$$\text{e(Prevalence)} = \frac{A}{A+B} = \text{PREVALENCE}$$

However, if there were 2 different selection probabilities—1 for people with the disease and 1 for people without the disease—then systematic error will result. The expected value of the estimated parameter would not be the true value of the population. If people with the disease had a higher probability of selection, the numerator of the prevalence equation would be too large and prevalence would be overestimated. If people without the disease had a higher probability of selection, the denominator would be too large and the prevalence would be underestimated. The same principles apply to other barriers to participation, such as nonconsent, attrition, and failure to provide necessary data. If these barriers correlate with disease status, they will systematically skew prevalence estimates from true values.

Ethics in epidemiological research

Canada's 3 main research-funding agencies have mapped out a framework for ethical research. This framework is called TCPS2—the *Tri-Council Policy Statement: Ethical Conduct for Research Involving Humans,* now in its second edition.[90] TCPS2 requires ethical decisions to be made at the local level by ethics review boards, which are officially constituted to bring the right mix of perspectives and expertise to ethical deliberations.

Key point: Health research in Canada is guided by a national tri-council policy statement, but administered at a regional or institutional level through duly constituted ethics review boards.

Many principles are involved in health research ethics. These principles form part of complex decisions to allow or disallow studies—decisions that also engage different priorities, perceptions, and beliefs. Ethical principles important to epidemiological research include:

Respect for persons: Researchers must respect the autonomy of research subjects.

Beneficence: Research must aim to do good rather than harm.

Nonmaleficence: Research should avoid doing harm wherever possible. Of course, there is almost always some potential for harm and some potential for benefit in research.

Utilitarian principle: The possibility of good should outweigh the possibility of harm.

Confidentiality: Research must have safeguards in place to ensure personal information does not fall into the wrong hands—for example, safe data storage and strict protection of information collected during research.

Privacy: Research must respect people's inherent right to keep their personal information to themselves. Research almost always involves collecting personal information of some type and therefore always entails a degree of invasion of privacy. This negative aspect of research must be minimized by appropriate limits (only collecting information that is needed by the study) and by the hope that this harm will be offset by useful results that lead to positive changes in health.

Justice: Research should benefit those who bear the harms of research. It is unjust to exploit a group—for example: students, prisoners, or the socioeconomically disadvantaged—to obtain knowledge that does not directly benefit the group. In the past, some health researchers coerced participation from vulnerable groups such as psychiatric patients[91] and vulnerable members of Canada's First Nations.[92] Such activities transgress the ethical principle of justice.

Thinking deeper

Selection bias in symbols

The rules governing the occurrence and direction of selection bias are intuitive:

- If people with the attribute whose frequency is being estimated are more likely to participate, the estimated frequency will be biased upwards (positive bias).
- If people with the attribute are less likely to participate, the estimate will be biased downwards (negative bias).

Note that each scenario represents a departure from the ideal of a simple random sample (where every person in the population has the same probability of selection into a study). To understand how this type of bias unfolds, a new concept is required: conditional selection probability.

Recall the 1 × 2 table—restated below as Table 13—from which prevalence for a target population could be calculated assuming that we had complete data on each person in that population (and also assuming perfect measurement):

TABLE 13. 1 × 2 TABLE FOR A POPULATION

Disease	No disease	Total
A	B	N

To calculate an estimated prevalence for this population, some members of the population will be selected. Table 14 restates the 1 × 2 table for calculating estimated prevalence from a sample population (denoted as usual with lowercase letters):

TABLE 14. 1 × 2 TABLE FOR A SAMPLE

Disease	No disease	Total
a	b	n

Recall the concept of selection probability ($p_{selection}$). Selection probability is the probability that a member of the target population is selected into the sample.

In a simple random sample, there is a single selection probability that applies to each member of the population. In a sample influenced by selection errors, however, the selection probability for those having the disease differs from the selection probability of those who do not have the disease—so, 2 probabilities are at work. To think through the precise mechanism of selection bias in a prevalence study, it is necessary to define these 2 probabilities.

The conditional nature of these probabilities is depicted by a vertical line that can be read as "given." The probability of selection given disease is $p_{\text{selection|disease}}$ and that for nondisease is $p_{\text{selection|nondisease}}$.

The expected value for the number of people with disease in a study sample is the number of people in the target population with the disease (A) multiplied by the probability of selection given that they have the disease. Depicting this as an expected value using the letter e:

$$e(a) = A \times p_{\text{selection|disease}}$$

And the expected value for the number of people without the disease is similarly:

$$e(b) = B \times p_{\text{selection|nondisease}}$$

This allows an expanded version of the formula for an estimated prevalence that incorporates the idea of a selection probability:

$$e(\text{Prevalence}) = \frac{A \times p_{\text{selection|disease}}}{\left(A \times p_{\text{selection|disease}}\right) + \left(B \times p_{\text{selection|nondisease}}\right)}$$

Imagine that each selection probability is 0.1 (in other words, that 1 in 10 members of the population are selected into the study—a simple random sample). In this case:

$$e(\text{Prevalence}) = \frac{A \times 0.1}{(A \times 0.1) + (B \times 0.1)}$$

Factoring out the selection probability in the denominator:

$$e(\text{Prevalence}) = \frac{A \times 0.1}{0.1 \times (A + B)}$$

Or:

$$e(\text{Prevalence}) = \frac{A}{A + B}$$

This is another way of saying that, for any simple random sample, the expected value of the prevalence will be the true population prevalence—in other words, it will not be biased.

If the selection probabilities for diseased and nondiseased subjects are unequal, the expanded equation makes clear that bias will result. It also makes clear that, in this event, increasing the sample size (which essentially means increasing the selection probabilities) will not fix this problem.

As with all types of bias, selection bias casts a shadow over all statistical analyses based on the biased samples.

Questions

1. The Canadian Community Health Survey is a large-scale initiative that includes both general health surveys and surveys that have more specialized content. In 2012, a mental-health-focused survey was conducted.[93] This survey used a combination of an area frame and a random digit dialed (RDD) telephone frame. The survey collected data by interviewing some subjects face to face, and some subjects via telephone. Alcohol and drug dependence (among other disorders) were assessed in the survey. The greater social distance associated with telephone interviewing means that respondents were more willing to disclose their use of alcohol and drugs, thereby leading to a higher estimated prevalence of alcohol and drug dependence.

    a. Do you think that this could be an important cause of selection bias?
    b. Mental disorders tend to be stigmatized conditions. Stigmatization consists of negative attitudes and behaviours. Could fear of stigma result in selection bias in a study of this type? How?
    c. The response rate in this survey was about 70%. If the response rate had been 100% instead of 70%, could selection bias occur?

2. Another feature of the Canadian Community Health Survey (CCHS) is that its target population consists of household residents. People with severe dementia tend to live in institutions, rather than at home. People with dementia are therefore less likely to be selected into the CCHS than people without dementia. Will this cause selection bias in an estimate of dementia prevalence?

3. A study used physician-billing claims and hospitalization data (a type of administrative data) to estimate the prevalence of autoimmune inflammatory myopathy in the province of Alberta, both in the general population and in aboriginal populations.[94] To be coded as having this condition, it was necessary to see a physician or be admitted to hospital. Could this have caused selection bias?

4. Several iterations of the CCHS have sought to measure schizophrenia prevalence using self-report items included in an interview.[95] People with schizophrenia, when they are ill, can develop delusions that cause them to feel that they are in danger (a persecutory delusion). Conceivably, some people with this illness, if they were ill at the time of the interview, might have refused to participate.

    a. Could a lower response rate among people with schizophrenia lead to selection bias in an estimate of schizophrenia prevalence?
    b. If so, in what direction?

5. A longitudinal study followed a community sample of 3304 for 3 months to assess their risk of depression.[83] Those who were not depressed at baseline were tracked prospectively with telephone interviews every 2 weeks to estimate their incidence of depression. Those who became depressed may have felt tired or hopeless, which may have increased their rate of attrition from the study. Would this have resulted in a biased incidence estimate?

Confounding in descriptive studies

Objectives
- Define confounding.
- Define and describe strategies to adjust for confounding in descriptive studies: stratification, direct standardization, and indirect standardization.
- Describe the concept of weighting.

Confounding in context

So far, this book has discussed 2 categories of error in epidemiological research: random error, and defective study design leading to misclassification bias and selection bias. We have explored these in the context of descriptive studies and basic parameters, particularly the parameter of prevalence.

This chapter looks at the third key category of error: confounding. In descriptive studies, confounding results in a failure to accurately assess important (useful, actionable) variables from a variety of variables at play in a population.

The problem of confounding: intermixing of effects

If a determinant cannot be changed, it is of little interest. Classic examples of nonmodifiable determinants are age and sex. They contribute strongly to the risk of many conditions, yet they cannot be changed. Populations often differ in terms of such nonmodifiable determinants. Descriptive epidemiologic comparisons of different populations are therefore complicated by the fact that potentially interesting differences might merely reflect underlying differences in nonmodifiable determinants. For this reason, there is a lot of interest in determining whether health outcomes differ among populations apart from the effects of certain nonmodifiable determinants. If differences remain after adjustment for nonmodifiable determinants, those differences are more interesting and more likely to result from modifiable factors.

Key point: Modifiable determinants of health outcomes are much more important than nonmodifiable determinants. Only modifiable determinants can lead to effective preventive interventions.

The intermixing of more and less interesting effects when populations are compared is called *confounding*. In descriptive epidemiology, the main procedures to handle confounding involve standardization. Procedures for standardization adjust for the nonmodifiable, and therefore less interesting, effects of (most commonly) age and sex in 2 populations. This allows unconfounded comparisons. While standardization for age and sex is commonplace, the same procedures can be used, in principle, to adjust for almost any variable that might confound more interesting comparisons.

After such adjustments, persistence of a difference between 2 populations poses the question of why that difference exists. A persistent difference most likely arises from the effects of modifiable risk factors. At this stage, the focus of epidemiological inquiry shifts from description to analysis—from descriptive studies to analytical studies. Descriptive studies tend to generate hypotheses about etiology, whereas analytical studies often address specific hypotheses about disease etiology.

A note about terminology

Terminology for variables that influence health status can take a variety of forms. A cause of a disease, in epidemiology, is usually referred to as a *risk factor*. A variable associated with increased risk in a way that is not due to a cause-effect relationship may be called a *risk marker* or *risk indicator*. Because most diseases have multiple contributing causes, questions of causation often assume a nuanced meaning in epidemiology—a meaning not adequately captured by a simplistic single-cause-leading-to-single-effect logic. As a result, some epidemiologists prefer to regard risk factors as component causes.

An example of a nonstandardized difference in mortality

Standardization procedures most often apply to the interpretation of mortality data, which is a form of incidence data.

Unadjusted mortality rates reveal large differences between Canada's provinces and its northern territories. Another note about terminology: *crude mortality* is another name for an unadjusted mortality rate.

Key point: In epidemiology, rates and frequencies can be presented as adjusted or unadjusted (crude) parameters.

Chapter 4 discussed the reports of mortality in Canada's provinces and territories that Statistics Canada regularly updates and publishes (see page 37). Let's look at that data again.

To find mortality data on the Statistics Canada website, it's best to browse by subject, starting from the main page, and follow the links to what you need. (Don't run a search from the main page using a nonspecific search term such as "mortality.") For example, you can browse to the subject "health," which has a link to the subject "life expectancy and deaths," which leads to a list of resources that include both summary tables and detailed CANSIM tables for mortality.

A look at the summary table for deaths in 2011 indicates that the territory of Nunavut had 166 deaths in 2011 and Ontario had 89 195 deaths.[96] These mortality counts are, of course, difficult to interpret because the populations of Nunavut and Ontario are different. It would be helpful to turn these into rates by dividing the number of deaths by the midyear populations of Nunavut and Ontario.

Population counts and projections are also easy to find on the Statistics Canada website through browsing by subject. Under "health," follow the link for "population and demography." In this case, rather than using a summary table, it's best to go to the relevant CANSIM table, which allows manipulation by the user. Most summary tables on the Statistics Canada website reference their source CANSIM table in a footnote: in this case, the source is Table 051-0001.[97] Here, by selecting the tab "add/remove data," you can select the territory of Nunavut, and see that the total population at midyear in 2011 was 34 196. For Ontario, it was 13 263 544. The crude mortality rate in Nunavut is therefore 166/34 196 or 4.85 per 1000 years^{-1}. For Ontario, the crude mortality rate is 6.72 per 1000 years^{-1}.

On the surface, this would appear to be an important descriptive epidemiologic finding. Why are the rates higher in Ontario? Might there be significant environmental differences or perhaps psychosocial factors accounting for this difference? In keeping with the general role of epidemiology in public health, the finding might motivate a search for such causes in the hope that modifiable determinants might be identified, leading to public health interventions capable of preventing the apparent excess mortality in Ontario.

However, many factors differ between Nunavut and Ontario, which could account for the difference in mortality rates, and some of these factors are more interesting than others. These factors are not evident in a simple consideration of mortality rates—indeed, they are intermixed in these crude rates. Two of these factors are age and sex. If the apparent difference in mortality rates were due exclusively to differences in age or sex, then the difference in mortality rates would not be useful for identifying preventive opportunities, because age and sex cannot be changed.

A proviso, of course, is that the difference in crude mortality does say something. A greater proportion of Ontario residents die each year than Nunavut residents. This may be important information for some purposes, such as planning health services for end-of-life care. To identify opportunities for prevention, however, you would want to know whether the difference in mortality is due to something more than differences in age or sex.

Strategies to adjust for confounding in descriptive studies

Stratification

Stratification is the simplest type of adjustment to unconfound variables.

If a difference in a mortality rate is due to sex or age, or both, then those differences will not be apparent within sex or age strata. A difference that is due to sex cannot explain a difference between women in 2 populations, for example. Similarly, a difference between 2 populations that is due to age cannot explain a difference seen within the same age groups when the 2 populations are compared.

The Statistics Canada website has links to CANSIM tables that report age- and sex-specific mortality rates. Table 15 shows the mortality rates by sex for Nunavut and Ontario in 2011 from CANSIM.[98] As opposed to crude mortality, these estimates reflect sex-specific mortality rates in each locality. They can also be referred to as *sex-stratified mortality rates*. The CANSIM system makes it particularly easy to extract data from its national tables and create customized tables like Table 15. After customizing a table, you click the "download" tab at the top of the title (be sure to download the data "as displayed," not the entire table). This provides the customized table as a comma-delimited data file, which you can import into almost any spreadsheet, database, or statistical software.

Table 15 shows that mortality rates are higher in men than women in each location. The sex-specific mortality rates continue to be higher in Ontario than Nunavut. Table 16 presents the same data, stratified this time by age group.

This age-stratified data presents a very different picture from the crude mortality rates and sex-specific mortality rates, which showed higher rates in Ontario. Almost all of the age-specific mortality rates are higher in Nunavut. There is also a typical pattern of age-specific mortality: fairly high mortality in the first year of life (something almost always seen in age-specific mortality

TABLE 15. SEX-STRATIFIED MORTALITY RATES PER 1000 YEAR^{-1} FOR ONTARIO AND NUNAVUT[98]

	Ontario	Nunavut
Male	6.7	5.6
Female	6.6	4.2

TABLE 16. AGE-STRATIFIED MORTALITY RATES PER 1000 YEAR[-1] IN ONTARIO AND NUNAVUT[98]

	Ontario	Nunavut
under 1 year	4.6	26.3
1 to 4 years	0.1	0.3
5 to 9 years	0.1	0.9
10 to 14 years	0.1	0.3
15 to 19 years	0.3	3.1
20 to 24 years	0.4	2.9
25 to 29 years	0.4	1.4
30 to 34 years	0.5	1.5
35 to 39 years	0.7	2.8
40 to 44 years	1.1	3.1
45 to 49 years	1.8	5.3
50 to 54 years	3.0	5.2
55 to 59 years	4.7	5.5
60 to 64 years	7.3	14.1
65 to 69 years	11.5	25.7
70 to 74 years	18.2	73.9
75 to 79 years	30.4	65.9
80 to 84 years	52.1	84.3
85 to 89 years	89.5	290.3
90 years and over	173.1	125

data), low mortality until middle age, and rapidly increasing mortality with increasing age.

The pattern in the age-stratified data indicates that the crude mortality rates were misleading. Nunavut appears to have a higher rate of mortality, once the effect of age is accounted for. The suggestion from the crude data (apparently lower mortality in Nunavut) is not valid within any age category. A possible exception is the 90+ age group, which shows higher age-specific mortality in Ontario. However, the idea that age-specific mortality in Nunavut would drop in the 90+ age group is not plausible, so this aberration must represent a chance effect (random error) due to a small number of observed deaths in Nunavut. The misleading impression provided by the crude mortality rate must have come from confounding by age. Since age is a strong determinant of mortality, a differing age distribution in Ontario versus Nunavut has created a misleading set of crude mortality estimates.

Confounding can invalidate epidemiological estimates, just like errors of classification and selection. However, as a threat to validity, confounding falls into a slightly different category than misclassification and selection bias. With misclassification and selection bias, study-design defects lead to systematic error, false data, and, as a result, invalid results. The crude mortality estimates from Nunavut and Ontario are not invalid in the same sense. Crude mortality in a particular case is a valid estimate of the true crude mortality rate in the population. It is not wrong—it is just misleading. An adjusted estimate, such as an age-stratified rate, is no longer misleading because it disentangles the characteristics of Nunavut from the age of the people who live in Nunavut.

Key point: Stratified rates are a form of adjusted rates. Stratification is 1 procedure for adjustment.

Table 17 shows the same data as Table 16 with simultaneous stratification for age and sex. This table begins to show some of the weaknesses of

TABLE 17. AGE- AND SEX-STRATIFIED MORTALITY RATES PER 1000 YEAR^{-1} IN ONTARIO AND NUNAVUT[98]

	Male		Female	
	Ontario	Nunavut	Ontario	Nunavut
Under 1 year	5.1	35.8	4.1	15.4
1 to 4 years	0.2	0	0.1	0.6
5 to 9 years	0.1	0	0.1	1.8
10 to 14 years	0.1	0.6	0.1	0
15 to 19 years	0.4	5.0	0.2	1.2
20 to 24 years	0.6	4.8	0.2	0.7
25 to 29 years	0.5	0.7	0.3	2.1
30 to 34 years	0.7	1.5	0.4	1.6
35 to 39 years	0.9	3.4	0.5	2.0
40 to 44 years	1.3	5.6	0.8	0.9
45 to 49 years	2.1	5.0	1.5	5.7
50 to 54 years	3.6	6.3	2.5	3.8
55 to 59 years	5.8	7.1	3.6	3.5
60 to 64 years	9.1	20.8	5.5	7.6
65 to 69 years	14.0	28.2	9.1	23.3
70 to 74 years	22.4	87.6	14.4	58.3
75 to 79 years	37.1	32.3	25.0	108.1
80 to 84 years	62.4	31.3	44.7	117.6
85 to 89 years	108	214.3	79.2	352.9
90 years and over	186.5	90.9	167.8	153.8

stratification as an adjustment technique. While the same general trends are evident, the division of the fairly small Nunavut population into age and sex strata makes the numbers sufficiently small that patterns become more difficult to see.

Direct standardization

Stratification is a perfectly good way to adjust for potential confounding variables, but it has drawbacks. It requires you to look through a data table row by row. Also, stratification magnifies errors of chance. Since small samples lead to more random error, dividing a large data set into smaller strata increases the random variation typically seen in stratum-specific estimates.

When stratum-specific rates are available, direct standardization is a common way to simplify comparisons between rates. In direct standardization, you choose a standardizing population and use it as a bridge between the 2 rates.

Direct standardization takes a set of stratum-specific rates and weights them by the stratum-specific structure of the chosen standardizing population. In the Nunavut-Ontario mortality-rates comparison, the procedure asks: If both of these populations had the same age and sex distribution (that of the standardizing population), what would their expected mortality rate be?

The choice of a standardizing population is somewhat arbitrary. In the Nunavut-Ontario comparison, it would be possible to use the age and sex distribution of either Nunavut or Ontario. A common choice, however, is to use the age and sex distribution of the national population. A standardizing population should be roughly similar to the populations being standardized.

In direct standardization, the standardizing population is divided proportionally, and the proportion of the population falling into each age and sex group becomes a means of weighting the stratum-specific estimates. The stratum-specific estimates are multiplied by these weights, and then all the weighted rates are added to produce the standardized rates. Tables 18 and 19 provide an example of standardization for the Nunavut-Ontario comparison for age in males and females, respectively. In each case, the stratum-specific values from Table 17 are presented (with the under-1-year and the 1-to-4 year categories combined), along with the proportion of the national population in each age-sex stratum according to 2011 population estimates.[97]

The age-standardized rates from Table 18 and Table 19 show that Nunavut has a higher mortality rate than Ontario once the effect of age is addressed.

Statistics Canada has recently produced a CANSIM table for cause-specific mortality that has age-standardized mortality as an output option. In the CANSIM table, the age-standardized mortality is expressed per 100 000 years[-1], and simultaneously adjusts for age and sex rather than adjusting for age separately in males and females. The results are consistent with the

TABLE 18. DIRECT STANDARDIZATION FOR AGE OF ONTARIO AND NUNAVUT MORTALITY DATA FOR MALES[97,98]

| Age at time of death | Male mortality rates | | Weights* | Weighted rates (Ontario) | Weighted rates (Nunavut) |
	Ontario/ 1000 year^{-1}	Nunavut/ 1000 year^{-1}			
0–4 years	1.1	7.6	0.057171	0.07	0.43
5 to 9 years	0.1	0	0.054552	0.01	0.00
10 to 14 years	0.1	0.6	0.057993	0.01	0.03
15 to 19 years	0.4	5	0.067383	0.03	0.34
20 to 24 years	0.6	4.8	0.070139	0.04	0.34
25 to 29 years	0.5	0.7	0.069862	0.03	0.05
30 to 34 years	0.7	1.5	0.068227	0.05	0.10
35 to 39 years	0.9	3.4	0.066666	0.06	0.23
40 to 44 years	1.3	5.6	0.070251	0.09	0.39
45 to 49 years	2.1	5	0.080488	0.17	0.40
50 to 54 years	3.6	6.3	0.079347	0.29	0.50
55 to 59 years	5.8	7.1	0.068969	0.40	0.49
60 to 64 years	9.1	20.8	0.05958	0.54	1.24
65 to 69 years	14	28.2	0.04378	0.61	1.23
70 to 74 years	22.4	87.6	0.031903	0.71	2.79
75 to 79 years	37.1	32.3	0.024435	0.91	0.79
80 to 84 years	62.4	31.3	0.017079	1.07	0.53
85 to 89 years	108	214.3	0.008778	0.95	1.88
90 years and over	186.5	90.9	0.003397	0.63	0.31
Directly standardized rate/1000 population				6.66	12.09

*proportion of the national male population in each age category

directly age-standardized rates presented in Table 18 and Table 19. They show higher standardized mortality in Nunavut (470 and 1124 per 100 000 years^{-1} in Ontario and Nunavut, respectively).[99]

The most important thing to remember about directly standardized rates is that they are imaginary. Conceptually, a directly standardized mortality rate represents a mortality rate that is expected to occur in the imaginary scenario where both Nunavut and Ontario have exactly the same age distribution as the national population. Neither of them does. Because it is an imaginary rate, the standardized rate should not be assigned any particular significance other than its intended purpose, which is to facilitate comparisons. Looking at Table 18 and Table 19, the key point is that for both men and women, the Nunavut rate is higher. It would be wrong to compare the sex-specific rates in this case, because the male and female tables use different

TABLE 19. DIRECT STANDARDIZATION FOR AGE OF ONTARIO AND NUNAVUT MORTALITY DATA FOR FEMALES[97,98]

	Female mortality rates			Weighted rates (Ontario)	Weighted rates (Nunavut)
	Ontario/ 1000 year^{-1}	Nunavut/ 1000 year^{-1}	Weights*		
0–4 years	0.9	3.4	0.053458	0.05	0.18
5 to 9 years	0.1	1.8	0.050914	0.01	0.09
10 to 14 years	0.1	0	0.053752	0.01	0.00
15 to 19 years	0.2	1.2	0.063045	0.01	0.08
20 to 24 years	0.2	0.7	0.066999	0.01	0.05
25 to 29 years	0.3	2.1	0.068165	0.02	0.14
30 to 34 years	0.4	1.6	0.067353	0.03	0.11
35 to 39 years	0.5	2	0.065719	0.03	0.13
40 to 44 years	0.8	0.9	0.06871	0.05	0.06
45 to 49 years	1.5	5.7	0.077932	0.12	0.44
50 to 54 years	2.5	3.8	0.0774	0.19	0.29
55 to 59 years	3.6	3.5	0.068075	0.25	0.24
60 to 64 years	5.5	7.6	0.059828	0.33	0.45
65 to 69 years	9.1	23.3	0.045478	0.41	1.06
70 to 74 years	14.4	58.3	0.035261	0.51	2.06
75 to 79 years	25	108.1	0.029062	0.73	3.14
80 to 84 years	44.7	117.6	0.023693	1.06	2.79
85 to 89 years	79.2	352.9	0.016008	1.27	5.65
90 years and over	167.8	153.8	0.00915	1.54	1.41
Directly standardized rate/1000 population				6.61	18.37

*proportion of the national female population in each age category

standardizing weights. (In Table 18, the weights are the proportions of men within the national population in each age group. In Table 19, the weights are the proportions of women within the national population in each age group.) In addition, it would be inappropriate to compare these directly standardized rates to those of other countries.

Note that Table 18 and Table 19 present separate age-standardized rates for men and women, but standardization commonly adjusts simultaneously for age and sex.

Indirect standardization
Indirect standardization is another strategy for increasing the comparability of 2 populations.

A typical scenario involves concern that an occupational group may have an elevated risk of an adverse health outcome. You could address this question by comparing the crude mortality rate in the targeted workers (or some other group, which for ease of language will be called the *exposed group* here) with that of other occupations or the general population. The outcome of interest is usually mortality, but it can be another outcome. In the discussion that follows, *mortality* will be used to designate outcome to simplify the language. Unfortunately, a simple comparison between an exposed occupational cohort and the general population, due to the possibility of confounding, would probably not be a valid comparison. Often, age- and sex-specific incidence or mortality rates are available for the general population, but not for the occupational (or other) cohort in question, so you can't use direct standardization to address this confounding. Another approach—indirect standardization—is necessary.

As with direct standardization, indirect standardization uses a standardizing population. In indirect standardization, stratum-specific (usually age- and sex-specific) rates from the standardizing population are multiplied by (you could say *weighted by*) the proportion of the exposed cohort falling into each of those age-sex categories. This multiplication predicts the expected deaths (or other outcome) in the exposed cohort, under the null hypothesis that the cohort has the same age- and sex-specific mortality rates as the standardizing population.

The next step is to divide these expected deaths by the actually observed deaths, creating a parameter called the *standardized mortality ratio* (SMR). If the expected and observed deaths have very similar values, the SMR will be close to 1. This means that the exposed group does not have an elevated risk of death. On the other hand, if the group has an elevated risk of mortality, the SMR is greater than 1.

$$\text{SMR} = \frac{\text{Observed}}{\text{Expected}}$$

where *observed* means the actual number of deaths that have occurred in the exposed cohort and *expected* is the sum of the expected number of deaths in a series of age- and sex-specific strata

---

Key point: Indirect standardization involves the calculation of an SMR, a parameter that embodies a comparison of an exposed cohort to a general population rate.

The abbreviation *SMR* can also stand for *standardized morbidity ratio* if the outcome of concern is not mortality. The same principles apply. Also, the same procedure can be used to standardize incidence rather than mortality. In this case, the resulting parameter is called the *standardized incidence ratio* (SIR).

Here's an interesting feature of the SMR for exposed occupational groups: intuition suggests that a value of 1 should indicate a lack of effect of the exposure on mortality or morbidity, but an SMR of 1.0 is actually a cause for concern. The reason is an effect called the *healthy worker effect*. People working at a job are expected to be healthier than people who are not working, so when an SMR is calculated for an occupational cohort using the general population as the standardizing population, expectation is that the SMR should be less than 1.

Another point about the SMR is that this parameter is often expressed as a percentage:

$$SMR(\%) = \left[\frac{Observed}{Expected} \right] \times 100$$

We'll use the comparison of all-cause mortality in Nunavut and Ontario in 2011 to demonstrate calculating an SMR. Table 20 shows the population

TABLE 20. STANDARDIZED MORTALITY RATIO FOR NUNAVUT: INDIRECT STANDARDIZATION FOR AGE USING THE NATIONAL POPULATION AS THE STANDARDIZING POPULATION[96-98]

	National age-specific mortality rates (/1000 year^{-1})	National age-specific mortality rates (year^{-1})	Nunavut population	Expected deaths
Under 1 year	4.8	0.0048	791	3.7968
1 to 4 years	0.2	0.0002	3386	0.6772
5 to 9 years	0.1	0.0001	3410	0.341
10 to 14 years	0.1	0.0001	3178	0.3178
15 to 19 years	0.4	0.0004	3368	1.3472
20 to 24 years	0.5	0.0005	3200	1.6
25 to 29 years	0.5	0.0005	2920	1.46
30 to 34 years	0.6	0.0006	2777	1.6662
35 to 39 years	0.8	0.0008	2120	1.696
40 to 44 years	1.2	0.0012	2211	2.6532
45 to 49 years	1.9	0.0019	2002	3.8038
50 to 54 years	3.1	0.0031	1629	5.0499
55 to 59 years	4.8	0.0048	1186	5.6928
60 to 64 years	7.5	0.0075	936	7.02
65 to 69 years	11.8	0.0118	483	5.6994
70 to 74 years	19.1	0.0191	292	5.5772
75 to 79 years	31.4	0.0314	190	5.966
80 to 84 years	53.7	0.0537	77	4.1349
85 to 89 years	92.7	0.0927	26	2.4102
90 years and over	178.3	0.1783	11	1.9613
Total deaths expected				62.8709
Observed				166
SMR				2.64
SMR (%)				264%

of Nunavut in 5-year age strata[97] and age-specific mortality rates for the overall Canadian population.[98] Multiplying the counts in the Nunavut age strata by the national age-specific mortality rates (which are converted to decimal values here to simplify the units, and presented in addition to the 1000 years[-1] rates recorded in CANSIM) leads to an expected number of deaths in each age stratum. As with direct standardization, these are imaginary estimates that represent the number of deaths that would be expected to occur within each stratum in Nunavut under the assumption that Nunavut residents have the same mortality rates as the national population. Finally, the actual number of deaths in 2011,[96] which in this case is 166, is used to produce the SMR.

The elevated SMR leads to the same conclusion as the results of direct standardization: age standardized mortality is elevated in Nunavut.

Thinking deeper

The concept of weighting
This chapter has described 2 procedures for comparing populations in the presence of possible confounding variables. These procedures, especially direct standardization, provide an introduction to the concept of weighting.

Direct standardization uses the proportion of the standardizing population in a particular age and sex stratum to weight age- and sex-specific rates or frequencies in 2 populations. This facilitates more meaningful comparisons between the populations.

Population surveys often use a similar weighting procedure to approximate simple random sampling (which produces ideal samples).

Imagine some of the national surveys that Statistics Canada conducts. These surveys use multiple-stage selection procedures, because obtaining a simple random sample for Canada's large and dispersed population poses many obstacles. A random sample would first require a list of every survey-eligible person in the country (e.g., a list of all household residents who are not members of the armed forces and do not live on reservations or in institutions)—a very long list, and difficult to compile. After selecting a random subset of subjects from this list, researchers would need to contact the subjects—and possibly travel across the country to interview them, which would be prohibitively expensive.

However, by selecting a particular geographical area for a survey, a researcher can travel to that area, obtain a list of households within it, contact those households, and randomly select 1 or more participants from among the residents of each household. This multiple-stage approach is much more efficient than simple random sampling in large-scale population surveys.

A multiple-stage approach to sampling means that different members of the sample have different selection probabilities. For example, imagine the step in a multiple-stage sampling procedure where a researcher randomly selects 1 person from a household into a study: if that household has 2 members, the probability of either of them being selected is 0.5, which is one-half the selection probability associated with a 1-person household. The same problem would emerge with selection of households from areas that contain different numbers of households.

SAMPLING WEIGHTS

The problem of different selection probabilities is addressed by the calculation of sampling weights. A common type of weighting uses the inverse (in other words, the reciprocal) of the sampling probability. If each observation from 2-person households is multiplied by a probability weight (the inverse of the 0.5 sampling probability, $1/0.5 = 2$), and the resulting weight is used in the calculation of an estimate, this corrects the problem of unequal selection probability, and the weighted prevalence estimate will again reflect what would have been seen in a simple random sample.

The calculation of sampling weights is usually more complicated than our example: multiple-stage sampling procedures can have many steps, and studies using them build in stratified sampling as well. Each step may alter the probability of selection, which complicates the calculation of sampling weights.

The calculation of sampling weights can also attempt to address the possibility of selection bias that results from refusal, nonconsent, attrition, and so on. If such "drop-outs" have characteristics in common, sampling weights can adjust for them. These are called *nonresponse weights* or (since they usually amount to an adjustment to another weight calculated to account for broader study-design issues) *nonresponse adjustment to sampling weights*. Think back to the discussion of selection bias in a chapter 8: selection bias occurs when the probability of selection is influenced by disease status. Disease status, of course, is not known when a person drops out or refuses to participate in a study. Adjustments for nonresponse, therefore, must incorporate some guesswork. They must try to make adjustments based on characteristics of those who do not participate, but not on the key characteristic (i.e., whether their participation depended on disease status). For this reason, adjustments for nonresponse are no substitute for the best way to avoid such bias: making sure that the rate of participation is high.

UNEQUAL SELECTION PROBABILITIES, CLUSTERING, AND WEIGHTING

A sampling procedure that results in unequal selection probabilities is an example of a design effect. Design effects result from the ways in which a study was deliberately designed. An example is the effect of a sampling procedure that results in unequal selection probabilities. This design effect can be corrected using sampling weights. Attrition and nonconsent are not design effects since they are not a planned component of the study. These are study-design defects: they represent problems in the way a study was conducted. Design effects are more predictable than the problems that arise from study-design defects and can more easily be corrected using data analysis procedures such as weighting.

Multiple stages of selection produce design effects. In these situations, the members of the sample fall into clusters, such as geographical areas. The problem with clustering is that members of a cluster are likely more similar to each other than randomly selected people in the general population. Failure to account for this design effect results in underestimation of standard error if conventional statistical analyses are used, and, consequently, unrealistically narrow confidence intervals for estimated parameters. Survey-analysis software has special procedures to correct for this design effect and generate accurate confidence intervals.

WEIGHTING IN STATISTICS CANADA DATA

The national surveys conducted by Statistics Canada provide several options for properly addressing the issues of unequal selection probabilities and clustering.

When Statistics Canada conducts a survey, it typically produces 2 data sets, including a public use microdata file, or PUMF. (PUMFs are available for download by researchers and students at major Canadian universities.) PUMFs place continuous variables in categories and remove certain variables as safeguards to protect against the identification of individual survey respondents.

Each survey respondent in a PUMF file has an associated weight. This is a frequency weight and is somewhat different than the type of sampling weight described above (where the weight represents the inverse of the selection probability). A frequency weight specifies the number of people in a population represented by each individual respondent. Statistical software can use this weight to produce valid estimates.

Statistics Canada also has an approximate method for dealing with clustering in PUMF data, based on tables of approximate coefficients of variation. These tables are provided for each PUMF, and allow you essentially to look up an approximately correct standard error for an estimate. This does not allow you to conduct complex analyses, but does allow the calculation of confidence intervals for estimates using PUMF data.

Statistics Canada's regional data centres, located at most major Canadian universities, house full Statistics Canada data sets. These large and complex data sets allow detailed analysis. Statistics Canada produces replicate bootstrap weights that allow calculation of valid estimates, with accurate confidence intervals.

The regional data centres in Canada are an underused resource. Most university-based researchers in Canada are eligible for access to these data sets. Those who check into them are often surprised to find the centres have collected and stored important data related to their areas of interest.[100]

Statistics Canada describes the content and study-design characteristics of the various data sets on its website.

Questions

1. Zablotska et al[101] studied the long-term mortality and cancer incidence experienced by uranium workers and mill workers employed in Port Radium, NWT, and Beaverlodge, Saskatchewan, and at a radium and uranium refining and processing plant in Port Hope, Ontario. They linked the workers' records to the Canadian Mortality Database (CMDB) and the Canadian Cancer Database to ascertain cancer-related mortality to 1999. They observed 42 cases of deaths due to non-Hodgkins lymphoma in their cohort, compared to 46.28 expected deaths determined using statistics from the general population.

   a. What type of standardization is this?
   b. What is the SMR for mortality due to non-Hodgkins lymphoma?
   c. Provide an interpretation of the result.

2. As a component of the Vancouver Injection Drug Users Study (VIDUS), Spittal et al[102] monitored 520 female intravenous drug users, 68 of whom died during follow-up. Using the female population of British Columbia as a standardizing population, they calculated an SMR for this group of 47.3.

   a. What does this SMR mean?
   b. What are some possible explanations for an SMR of this magnitude?

3. Karmanis et al[103] used Swedish health data to evaluate whether women treated for anorexia nervosa might have a lower cancer incidence. Their rationale was that caloric restriction lowers cancer incidence in some animal models. Using the general population as a standardizing population, they reported an SMR of 2.5 for lung cancer mortality. Can you think of a possible explanation for this finding?

4. Callaghan et al[104] followed a cohort of patients discharged from California hospitals after admissions for alcohol- and drug-related diagnoses. The patients were followed for 16 years, after which the investigators calculated age-, sex-, and race-adjusted SMRs for deaths due to motor vehicle accidents. These SMRs ranged from 2.3 for cannabis to 3.8 for cocaine. The SMR for alcohol was 4.5. In your opinion, what are the implications of these SMRs?

5. Nijjar et al[105] wanted to investigate whether different ethnic groups have different risk of acute myocardial infarction (AMI) in the province of British Columbia.

Using hospital administrative data, they attempted to identify all patients with incident AMI in BC during a defined time interval. Ethnicity was determined by analyzing surnames. The investigators used direct age standardization to support comparisons of incidence among 3 groups. Among men, those of South Asian ethnicity had the highest age standardized incidence rate (SIR), followed by those of Caucasian and Chinese ethnicity. The investigators found a similar ranking in women. These investigators were not studying mortality, which is the most common use of direct standardization. In your opinion, is it appropriate to use direct standardization in an incidence analysis like this?

PART IV

Study designs and their vulnerability to error

So far, we have covered the fundamentals of epidemiology by discussing descriptive studies. Most epidemiological studies, however, are analytical, or at least have some analytical goals.

Descriptive studies measure the distribution and prevalence of disease. By contrast, analytical studies measure association between exposure and disease, and make inferences about causation.

Analytical studies are vulnerable to the same kinds of error as descriptive studies, but sometimes with added complications that require different strategies.

10

Cross-sectional studies

Objectives

- Define cross-sectional studies.
- Differentiate between the potential descriptive and analytical goals of cross-sectional studies.
- Describe the following measures of association: prevalence differences, prevalence ratios, prevalence odds ratios, and specific types of linear equations.
- Explain how to interpret measures of association calculated from cross-sectional data.
- List strengths and weaknesses of cross-sectional studies.

Critical appraisal and classification of study designs

The ability to correctly classify study designs is a useful skill.

Classifying the design of a study facilitates communication: a single label (e.g., "cross-sectional study") conveys information about the study's methodology.

Study-design classification also helps with critical appraisal, because particular methodological vulnerabilities are typically associated with different designs. In addition, the process of classifying a study's design requires close attention to key aspects of its methodology, which helps to bring a conceptual structure to the process of critical appraisal.

Study-design classification resembles aspects of clinical assessment, such as taking a history from a patient or conducting a physical examination. It involves an organized series of steps and questions that collect key information. Classification of a study design probes the way in which a study was conducted. As you read a study, you look for evidence. This makes reading a study into a procedure for evaluating that study.

Key point: Critical appraisal is more than just reading a study and intuitively identifying problems with it. Critical appraisal involves asking and answering a series of key questions. It is a more formal way of looking at studies, and seeks clear conclusions about the value of studies. Classification of study design is an early step in critical appraisal.

Approaches to study-design classification

The best approach to study-design classification is to determine the key features studies actually possess.

A common approach, however, is to categorize studies presumptively as either descriptive (concerned with the distribution or prevalence of disease) or analytical (concerned with causal connections between exposure and disease).

This presumptive descriptive-analytic division emphasizes the goals and motivations generally associated with particular study designs. For example, the cross-sectional study design is often considered descriptive, because it cannot usually allow causal inference. Cross-sectional studies measure exposure and disease at a single point in time, so they cannot meet a basic criterion for causal judgement: that causes must temporally precede effects. Therefore, causal inference is usually not possible from a cross-sectional study.

However, there are some instances where exposures can reasonably be interpreted as preceding the onset of disease, even in cross-sectional data. For example, if the exposure is a birth-related event or a gene, and the disease has its onset well after birth—say, in adulthood—cross-sectional data may be sufficient to clarify temporality.

So, cross-sectional studies can be analytic, which makes the descriptive-analytic distinction a risky starting point for classifying study design.

The distinction is also risky because the goals of investigators are not always clearly evident. An investigator may have analytic aims, but may deliver data that are descriptive only. Or, they may have descriptive aims, but nevertheless interpret some of their findings as having causal significance. Because of these ambiguities, it is better to classify study designs on more defensible grounds than the presumptive descriptive-analytic distinction.

Key point: Accurate classification of a study's design should start with documented features of the study, not with the stated or assumed descriptive-versus-analytical motivations of the investigators.

What is a cross-sectional study?

Epidemiological studies fall into 3 main categories: cross-sectional studies, case-control studies, and prospective-cohort studies.

Cross-sectional studies are studies in which all data are collected at a single point in time. A study designed to estimate point prevalence (called a *prevalence study*, see page 15) is an example of a cross-sectional study. A prevalence study provides a snapshot of disease status in a population at a point in time. Prevalence studies are generally descriptive in their goals, but they can also have analytical goals involving hypotheses about disease-exposure associations. Most often, such goals involve determining the existence of a disease-exposure association, or generating etiological hypotheses, rather than evaluating etiological hypotheses. In such instances, the key characteristic of a cross-sectional study is that both the disease and exposure variables are measured at a single point in time.

It's important, however, to stay flexible about what is meant by "a single point in time." Obviously, no study can occur in an instant. A prevalence study may take months or even years to conduct. Conceptually, however, these studies take place at a point in time: they neither look back into the past (retrospectively), nor forward into the future (prospectively).

Examples of cross-sectional studies

CANADIAN COMMUNITY HEALTH SURVEY

The Canadian Community Health Survey (CCHS) is an ongoing program of cross-sectional surveys carried out by Statistics Canada.

The CCHS survey program has several goals:[79]

- support health surveillance programs by providing health data at the national, provincial, and intraprovincial levels
- provide a single data source for health research on small populations and rare characteristics
- provide timely release of information and easy accessibility to a diverse community of users
- create a flexible survey instrument that includes a rapid response option to address emerging issues related to the health of the population

Data collection for the general health component of the CCHS is continuous, occurring throughout the year, but the data are aggregated into annual and 2-year data sets that describe the health of the Canadian household population at what can be considered points in time. The CCHS collects data on the prevalence of various chronic health conditions, and the prevalence of important risk-factor exposures such as smoking. It also measures certain health status characteristics (e.g., distress) using validated instruments and describes the use of health care resources.

CHILD ABUSE AND ADULT MENTAL HEALTH STATUS: AFIFI ET AL

Not all cross-sectional studies are exclusively concerned with estimating parameters such as prevalence. Some seek to quantify associations between exposures (such as risk factors or other determinants) and disease outcomes.

The parameters estimated by these studies seek to embody a comparison between 2 groups—typically an exposed group and nonexposed group. Like all cross-sectional studies, these studies measure disease and exposure at the. same point in time.

For example, in 2014, Afifi et al[106] published a study of the association between child abuse and adult mental health status. The objective of the study was to establish an association between events from the past and health outcomes many years later. Information about both exposure and disease were collected at a single point in time (through data collection in the Canadian Community Health Survey).

BREAST FEEDING AND OBESITY: VON KRIES ET AL

A study from Germany in 1999 investigated the possible association of breast-feeding with obesity.[107] Obesity was assessed in children undergoing routine assessment at the time of school entry. A questionnaire recording breast-feeding practices was completed by the parents of a subset of the children. Even though exposure (to breast-feeding) was retrospectively assessed in this study, the data collected were cross-sectional because both exposure (breast-feeding history) and disease (obesity prevalence) were measured at a single point in time.

EFFECTS OF DRUGS TO TREAT PARKINSON DISEASE: WEINTRAUB ET AL

In 2010, Weintraub et al[108] used a cross-sectional study to quantify a possible association between drugs for treating Parkinson disease and impulse-control disorders.

Parkinson disease is a progressive neurological disease characterized by tremor, rigidity, slowed movement, and gait problems, as well as cognitive and behavioural changes. These symptoms are believed come from the death of dopamine-producing cells in the brain. Treatment of Parkinson disease often includes drugs—dopamine agonists—that act on the same brain receptors as dopamine. However, due to one of dopamine's other roles in the brain (e.g., neurotransmission in the reward centres of the brain), dopamine agonists are associated with an increased frequency of impulse-control disorders. When taking dopaminergic medications, people with Parkinson disease may anticipate greater rewards from potentially risky activities such as gambling or sexual activity. To study this association, Weintraub et al conducted a cross-sectional study. They identified dual goals for their study: to estimate the "point frequency" (prevalence) of impulse-control disorders in people with Parkinson disease, and to assess the association of these disorders with dopamine-replacement therapies (a category that includes dopamine agonists and also levodopa, which is converted to dopamine in the brain). The investigators, exemplifying the intermixture of descriptive and analytical motivations that underlie many epidemiological studies, hypothesized that patients treated with dopamine agonists would have a higher prevalence of impulse-control disorders than those not treated with dopamine agonists. Study subjects with Parkinson disease were recruited from movement-disorder centres in the United States and Canada. Their use of medication was recorded, and an assessment with validated instruments was used to identify 4 impulse-control disorders: problem gambling, compulsive sexual behaviour, compulsive buying, and binge eating.

The final study sample included 3090 participants. Dopamine agonists were used in about two-thirds of the sample. An impulse-control disorder was identified in 13.6% of the sample. Those treated with a dopamine agonist had a higher prevalence of 1 or more impulse-control disorders (17.1%) than those not treated with dopamine agonists (6.9%). This translated into an odds ratio of 2.72, which was reported with an associated 95% CI of 2.08–3.54. The authors concluded that these medications were associated with an elevated prevalence of impulse-control disorders in this population.

How cross-sectional studies look at association

Many cross-sectional studies go beyond estimation of prevalence to include an assessment of risk factors. In this situation, the data can be represented by a 2 × 2 table—a version of the table encountered in chapter 6 (see Table 9, page 69). Rather than quantifying the contingency between a test and a gold standard, this 2 × 2 table depicts the association between an exposure and a disease.

The fundamental dichotomy between population and sample are just as important as always. Therefore, it is best to present 2 2 × 2 tables: Table 21 displays the exposure-disease contingencies in a population (using the convention of uppercase letters) and Table 22 displays contingencies as observed in a sample drawn from that population (using the convention of lowercase letters).

TABLE 21. 2 × 2 TABLE FOR DATA FROM A CROSS-SECTIONAL STUDY OF AN ENTIRE POPULATION

	Disease	No disease
Exposed	A	B
Nonexposed	C	D

TABLE 22. 2 × 2 TABLE FOR DATA FROM A CROSS-SECTIONAL STUDY OF A SAMPLE

	Disease	No disease
Exposed	a	b
Nonexposed	c	d

Tables 21 and 22, in themselves, are not particularly effective in communicating the contingency. The question of interest in such a cross-sectional study is whether the prevalence of disease differs between the exposed group and the nonexposed group. You can use the tables to calculate a prevalence estimate for each group and then compare the 2 prevalence estimates. Considering the sample data, this reduces 4 numbers to 2 proportions, facilitating comparison:

$$\text{Prevalence}(\text{exposed}) = \frac{a}{a+b}$$

$$\text{Prevalence}(\text{nonexposed}) = \frac{c}{c+d}$$

It would be even better to examine the association with a single number. There are a variety of ways to do this, such as subtracting 1 prevalence from the other (a prevalence difference), or making a ratio of the 2 prevalences (a prevalence ratio), or calculating the prevalence as odds and making a ratio of odds in the exposed group and nonexposed group (a prevalence odds ratio). Such parameters embody a comparison of the 2 prevalences, and are therefore measures of association.

Prevalence differences

Here's how to calculate a prevalence difference for a population:

$$\text{PREVALENCE Difference} = \frac{A}{A+B} - \frac{C}{C+D}$$

For a sample, it is:

$$\text{Prevalence Difference} = \frac{a}{a+b} - \frac{c}{c+d}$$

Differentiating the second equation from the first serves as a reminder that a sample-based estimate is subject to random or stochastic error. If you repeated this study many times, and calculated the prevalence difference many times, a distribution of prevalence differences would emerge. If the sample sizes from these repeated studies were small, this distribution would be broad. By contrast, if the repeated studies had large sample sizes, this distribution would be narrower. If procedures for measurement and selection were perfect, the law of large numbers provides a reason to believe that the distribution will centre around the population value. The estimates arising from such "perfect" studies may sometimes differ quite a bit from the population value, but if the study is sufficiently large, significant differences are unlikely.

We say "perfect" as a reminder that imperfect measurement and selection can lead to systematically erroneous prevalence estimates. Measures of association based on prevalence estimates are, like the prevalence estimates themselves, vulnerable to study-design defects that lead to misclassification bias and selection bias.

Key point: A prevalence difference is a measure of association because it embodies a comparison between 2 simpler parameters, which are prevalences in exposed and nonexposed groups.

Prevalence ratios

To calculate a prevalence ratio, you divide the 2 prevalences:

$$\text{PREVALENCE Ratio} = \frac{\dfrac{A}{A+B}}{\dfrac{C}{C+D}}$$

Or, for a sample:

$$\text{Prevalence Ratio} = \frac{\dfrac{a}{a+b}}{\dfrac{c}{c+d}}$$

Note that a ratio is simply 1 number divided by another, which means the prevalence proportion itself is technically a ratio—and sometimes also called a *prevalence ratio.*

Odds ratios

Odds ratios are commonly encountered, and use odds rather than prevalence proportions. (Differences in odds, however, are not used.)

An odds ratio can refer to any ratio of odds. Therefore, when calculating an odds ratio from a cross-sectional study, it is best to explicitly label that parameter as a prevalence odds ratio.

$$\text{PREVALENCE Odds Ratio} = \frac{\dfrac{A}{B}}{\dfrac{C}{D}} = \frac{AD}{BC}$$

Or, for a sample:

$$\text{Prevalence Odds Ratio} = \frac{\dfrac{a}{b}}{\dfrac{c}{d}} = \frac{ad}{bc}$$

> *Key point:* An epidemiological association between exposure and disease can be expressed as the ratio of prevalence in nonexposed and exposed groups (including prevalence odds).

Linear equations

The formulas for prevalence difference, prevalence ratio, and prevalence odds ratio all derive from the classic 2 × 2 contingency tables depicting an exposure-disease relationship, such as Table 21 and Table 22.

The same goal of comparing 2 prevalence estimates can also be accomplished by a linear equation—a simple equation that describes a line using an intercept and slope term.

To see how this works, we can form such an equation using 3 symbols: alpha (α), beta (β) and X_e. Here, α is the intercept term and β is the slope term for the linear equation. X_e is a variable that represents exposure to a risk factor. Suppose that—in addition to being part of the equation for a line—α represents prevalence in the nonexposed group and β represents the risk difference. To make this type of equation work, we also need the indicator variable (X_e) representing exposure. An indicator variable for exposure assumes a value of 0 (meaning not exposed) or 1 (meaning exposed). This leads to a simple form of a linear equation:

$$\text{Prevalence} = \alpha + \beta X_e$$

Note that in its simplest form, as above, this equation doesn't actually describe a line, merely 2 prevalence estimates: a prevalence for the exposed group and a prevalence for the nonexposed group. X_e can have 2 values: 0 to represent nonexposure and 1 to represent exposure. For the group that is not exposed, where the value of X_e is 0, the term to the right of the plus sign disappears: prevalence equals α. For the exposed group, where X_e is 1, the prevalence equals $\alpha + \beta$, which makes sense because this is the baseline prevalence in the nonexposed group plus the amount of extra prevalence (the prevalence difference) that goes along with exposure.

> *Key point:* The same information provided by a 2 × 2 contingency table for disease and exposure can be represented using an equation that has a linear form.

The value of expressing 2 prevalence estimates using a single equation of the type shown above may not be obvious at this stage. The equation doesn't add any information beyond presenting the 2 frequencies themselves. However, equations of this form are important tools for addressing confounding and effect modification, issues of importance in analytic studies. The relationship described above is a starting point for the use of linear models for epidemiological analysis.

LOG-TRANSFORMED PREVALENCE

There is another interesting relationship that emerges from the general idea of depicting prevalence data for exposed and nonexposed groups using an equation of linear form. This relationship unfolds when the equation describes the natural logarithm (here abbreviated *log*) of the prevalence. Consider the following equation:

$$\text{Log Prevalence} = \alpha + \beta X_e$$

Here, the log prevalence in the exposed group is $\alpha + \beta$, and the log prevalence in the nonexposed group is α. In this case, β is the difference in the log prevalence associated with exposure. The log prevalence in the exposed group minus the log prevalence in the nonexposed group is β, so taken together with the rule for subtraction of logarithms ($\log a - \log b = \log a/b$), you can see that β in this type of model is actually a log prevalence ratio. Again, the value of this type of equation may not be obvious at this stage, but it is a foundation for important analysis strategies.

LOG-TRANSFORMED PREVALENCE ODDS

Epidemiological studies often use odds (in our current discussion of cross-sectional studies, these would be prevalence odds) to describe association. The study of effects associated with drugs to treat Parkinson disease by Weintraub et al[108] is an example (see page 115).

The use of odds to describe association leads to an equation of linear form in which the β coefficient is a log odds ratio, or—more specifically for the purposes of this chapter—a log prevalence odds ratio. This type of equation is the basis of another approach to statistical modelling that is widely used in epidemiology: logistic regression analysis.

$$\text{Log Odds} = \alpha + \beta X_e$$

Key point: Log-transformed models based on linear equations are the basis of several approaches to epidemiological analysis. The coefficients in such models represent the log of ratio-based measures of association.

Strengths and weaknesses of cross-sectional studies

Strengths

Valuable snapshots of disease: Cross-sectional studies provide accurate snapshots of the amount of disease in a population at a point in time. This is very useful for descriptive purposes. Planners and administrators of health services use this kind of information to anticipate the level of services required to meet the needs of populations. Since cross-sectional studies often use probability sampling, they can provide very good estimates of population parameters.

Description of disease occurrence across multiple variables: Cross-sectional studies can describe the occurrence of disease in relation to multiple exposure and disease variables. The Canadian Community Health Survey is an example of a study that measures many exposure and disease variables. It's important to remember, though, that cross-sectional associations (as quantified by prevalence differences, prevalence ratios, or prevalence odds ratios) do not provide comparisons of risk. Prevalence is determined by incidence (a concept closely aligned with risk) and also by duration. Duration, in turn, is influenced by mortality and other aspects of prognosis. This means that cross-sectional associations may (or may not) reflect an impact of exposure on disease etiology, mortality, or prognosis. Nevertheless, such estimates can be informative: they can help specify groups with a high burden of illness and may generate hypotheses for future studies.

Cost efficiency: Cross-sectional studies can be less expensive to conduct than other types of studies because they do not track participants over time, something that usually costs a lot of money.

Invulnerability to attrition: Attrition (loss of participants) is a vulnerability of studies that follow subjects over long periods of time, and can result in selection bias. Attrition does not affect cross-sectional studies, because these studies collect data at a single point in time.

Weaknesses

Lack of causal inference: Cross-sectional studies rarely directly contribute to understanding causation. This is largely because they measure disease and exposure at a point in time, which often precludes determination of the temporal relationship between exposure and disease. Since a cause must logically precede an effect, the point-in-time data of cross-sectional studies is a strong impediment to causal reasoning.

No determination of risk: Cross-sectional studies cannot determine risk. An exposure that increases the incidence of disease will increase prevalence, other things being equal, but an exposure that leads to more rapid death will decrease prevalence by shortening the duration of disease. An exposure that affects the rate of recovery from a disease can increase or decrease the prevalence depending on whether it decreases or increases the rate of recovery.

Inefficiency for rare diseases: Cross-sectional studies can be an inefficient way to study rare diseases or associations with rare exposures. A cross-sectional study might end up collecting a lot of data only to have a small number of respondents in some of the cells of the 2 × 2 table arising from the data. This will usually lead to wide confidence intervals.

Insensitivity to time-dependent frequency changes: Cross-sectional studies can be misleading when disease frequency changes over time. For example, diseases that occur more often in winter—say, seasonal affective disorders or seasonal influenza—will have different prevalences depending on the season when they are measured.

Key point: Like all study designs, the cross-sectional design is associated with strengths and weaknesses. It is the best design for some purposes and not for others.

Thinking deeper

Confidence intervals for odds ratios

This chapter has made a distinction between sample-based and population-based analyses. Sample-based analyses are subject to random error, so confidence intervals for such estimates are needed. Confidence intervals help to quantify the vulnerability of an estimate to random error. Formulas to calculate confidence intervals are available for all the parameters discussed in this chapter, but the formulas are not always accurate. It is usually better to use statistical software to calculate exact confidence intervals for such parameters.

With this proviso in mind, there is a formula for calculating confidence intervals for an odds ratio that usually works quite well. It is worth understanding this formula for at least 2 reasons. First, it allows such calculations to be made quickly—e.g., while reading a study in which confidence intervals are not reported. Second, practicing this sort of calculation can help to solidify your understanding of confidence intervals. The trick to this particular formula is that instead of being based on the odds ratio itself, which tends not to be normally distributed, the formula is based on the log odds ratio.

Table 23 shows a 2 × 2 table from the Weintrub et al study.

TABLE 23. 2 × 2 TABLE FOR DATA FROM A CROSS-SECTIONAL STUDY[108(p592)]

	Impulse-control disorder	No impulse-control disorder
Exposed to dopamine agonists	348	1692
Nonexposed to dopamine agonists	72	978

The odds ratio from Table 23 is:

$$\text{Prevalence Odds Ratio} = \frac{\dfrac{a}{b}}{\dfrac{c}{d}} = \frac{ad}{bc} = \frac{348 \times 978}{72 \times 1692} = 2.8$$

Note that this odds ratio is slightly different from what the study reported. In the study, the data were stratified by country (US versus Canada) and a more complex type of odds ratio, the Mantel-Haenszel odds ratio, was used for the calculation while accounting for this stratification.

Odds ratios are not normally distributed, so it is difficult to calculate approximate confidence intervals. However, the log of the odds ratio is approximately normally distributed. So, you can convert the odds ratio to a log odds ratio, calculate 95% CIs for the log odds ratio using a normal approximation, and then convert the log odds ratio's confidence limits back to the original scale using the inverse log function. The calculation can also be done in a spreadsheet. The natural log of the odds ratio is log(2.8), or 1.03. An approximate formula for the standard error of this log odds ratio is:

$$\text{Standard Error of the Log Odds Ratio} = \sqrt{\frac{1}{a} + \frac{1}{b} + \frac{1}{c} + \frac{1}{d}}$$

In this case, it is:

$$\text{Standard Error of the Log Odds Ratio} = \sqrt{\frac{1}{348} + \frac{1}{1692} + \frac{1}{72} + \frac{1}{978}} = 0.136$$

As usual, the confidence limits are the point estimate (remember that this is the log odds ratio) plus or minus an appropriate z value multiplied by the standard error. If the goal is a 95% CI, the appropriate z value is 1.96. So the confidence limits in this case are 1.03 plus or minus 1.96 × 0.136, which is 0.761 and 1.29. To convert the confidence interval back to the regular scale, the inverse log of these limits should be calculated, which leads to a 95% CI of 2.14–3.64.

Questions

1. List 4 advantages and 4 disadvantages of cross-sectional studies.

2. Do you agree with the following statement? "It is impossible to make causal inference from cross-sectional data." Why or why not?

3. Using the data from Table 23:
   a. What is the prevalence of impulse-control disorders in this population?
   b. Calculate an approximate 95% CI for this proportion.

4. Using the data from Table 23, calculate a prevalence difference for the use of a dopamine agonist.

5. Using the data from Table 23:
   a. Calculate the log odds of having an impulse-control disorder for the exposed and nonexposed subjects.
   b. With the help of an indicator variable assuming values of 0 for the nonexposed group and 1 for the exposed group, formulate an equation of the linear form $y = \alpha + \beta X_e$ that can represent the 2 log odds of impulse-control disorder.
   c. Calculate the inverse log of your β coefficient from part b of this question. What does this represent?

Case-control studies

Objectives
- Define case-control studies.
- Explain how to interpret measures of association calculated from case-control data.
- Describe recall bias.
- Describe the rare disease assumption.
- Distinguish between induction and latency periods for disease, and describe the dynamic of component causes of disease.
- Define primary, secondary, and tertiary prevention.
- List strengths and weaknesses of case-control studies.

What is a case-control study?
Case-control studies usually have analytic goals: they usually aim to evaluate hypotheses about disease etiology (what causes disease). Some case-control studies have descriptive aims: to generate hypotheses rather than testing them.

Case-control studies differ from cross-sectional studies in their selection of research participants. In a case-control study, participants are selected based on their disease status. This is a radical departure from the typical cross-sectional study, which aims for simple random samples (where each person in the population has an equal probability of selection) or probability samples (where each person has a known probability of selection). Case-control studies really have 2 processes of selection, because they select 2 groups: a group of cases and a group of controls.

Since selection is based on disease status, these studies cannot estimate the frequency of disease. Instead, they focus on estimating associations between risk factors and disease.

> *Key point:* Case-control studies aim to estimate associations between risk factors and disease, and are therefore usually analytical in their orientation.

Design of case-control studies

Case-control studies involve identifying a set of cases (people who have a disease under investigation) and a set of controls (people who do not). Their goal is to assess exposure in both groups, and so disease etiology.

Assessment of exposure in case-control studies is, by necessity, retrospective, because people in the "case" group already have the disease under investigation. This means that case-control studies literally look back in time. They select cases and controls in the "here and now," and then assess past exposure (retrospectively) in each group.

Some investigators used to call case-control studies *retrospective studies*, but this term is now considered obsolete. Although case-control studies are almost always retrospective, other study designs also look back in time.

Figure 5 presents a schematic of the case-control study design.

> *Key point:* Case-control studies have 2 key characteristics: they select participants based on disease status (cases and controls), and they assess exposure retrospectively.

Association in case-control studies

A 2 × 2 contingency table, like Table 24, is a good starting point for understanding how case-control studies can estimate risk-factor associations. This table has some familiar features and a few new wrinkles.

The use of lowercase letters shows that this table represents sample data. Because the cases and controls are differentiated based on their disease status, the column headings now reflect this terminology: they refer to cases and controls, rather than disease and nondisease. Also, because the design of the study affects the proportion of participants selected as cases and controls, the table has a new row for the total in each group.

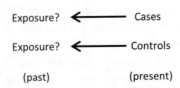

FIGURE 5. SCHEMATIC OF THE CASE-CONTROL STUDY DESIGN

TABLE 24. 2 × 2 TABLE FOR DATA FROM A CASE-CONTROL STUDY

	Cases	Controls
Exposed	a	b
Nonexposed	c	d
Total	n_{cases}	$n_{controls}$

Think back to the features of cross-sectional studies based on simple random samples: because the selection probabilities are equal for each member of the population sampled, the expected values falling into each contingency cell (a, b, c, d) reflect those same contingencies in the population. At least this is true in the absence of study-design defects involving participation and classification. In case-control studies, the situation is different: the investigator decides how many cases and how many controls will be in the study. For this reason, unlike cross-sectional studies based on simple random samples, case-control studies have no expectation that the proportion of cases provides an estimate of the population prevalence:

$$e(\text{Prevalence}) \neq \frac{a+c}{a+b+c+d}$$

In a cross-sectional study, if the selection probabilities are higher for those with a disease, it follows that prevalence will be overestimated due to selection bias. If the selection probabilities for those with a disease are lower than for those without a disease, a prevalence estimate will underestimate the population prevalence.

In a case-control study, the unequal selection probabilities are not a study-design defect leading to bias, but a deliberate study-design feature. The selection probability for cases is always much higher than for controls, but this does not preclude estimating the association. These studies are designed to produce valid estimates of disease-exposure associations, not estimates of prevalence.

Key point: In a case-control study, the selection probabilities for cases are typically much higher than those of controls.

THE IMPACT OF DIFFERENT SELECTION PROBABILITIES FOR CASES AND CONTROLS

In fact, far from representing a study-design defect, the ability to have different selection probabilities for cases and controls is a major advantage of the case-control design and a key reason for its enduring popularity. It allows investigators to selectively recruit cases, even of rare diseases, into a study.

This possibility can be exploited to an extreme degree in case-control studies. Imagine a rare disease for which all of the cases in a health region or province are treated at a single clinic. In this situation, you could conduct a case-control study with a selection probability for cases of 1.0 (100%), meaning that the study would include every single case. However, it would be very inefficient to attempt to have the same selection probability for controls. The value of the case-control design is its ability to use a subset of potentially eligible controls in the population as a referent against which to compare the cases.

The selection of cases is only a part of subject selection in case-control studies. It is usually the easier part. The most difficult challenges involve the selection of controls. The selection of controls must occur in a way that supports valid estimation. The rationale of this study design is that differences in exposure between cases and controls should reflect etiology of the disease, so selection must not depend on exposure in any way that differs between the cases and controls. Otherwise, differences observed may partially or wholly represent methods of selection rather than a disease-exposure association. Here's an example of a tricky problem in control selection. Suppose that a case-control study of a rare disease selects its cases from a specialized clinic. Various exposures might have affected the probability of a case attending that clinic. For example, people with other illnesses, or with worrisome lifestyle characteristics such as smoking or alcohol consumption, may have a higher likelihood of being referred to such a clinic. If exposures of interest to a case-control study have an influence on the selection of cases, a control group with exactly the same influence of exposure on selection would need to be found.

To understand the impact of different selection probabilities on estimating exposure-disease associations in case-control studies, let's revisit the familiar 2×2 table for sample-based data, as presented in Table 24. Because the 2×2 data no longer reflect the prevalence of disease, a prevalence ratio or prevalence difference is no longer a suitable measure of association. The best measure of association is the odds ratio. Another look at the formula for an odds ratio helps to explain why:

$$\text{Odds Ratio} = \frac{\dfrac{a}{c}}{\dfrac{b}{d}} = \frac{ad}{bc}$$

Higher selection probabilities for cases (a and c) and lower selection probabilities for controls (b and d) will not necessarily introduce bias into the estimated odds ratio, because the odds ratio is not dependent on the counts in the different cells. Instead, the odds ratio depends on the odds of exposure in cases relative to controls. For this reason, even if the selection probabilities for cases and controls are very different (they always are), a case-control study can still produce valid estimates of the underlying population odds ratio.

Key point: If properly conducted, case-control studies can provide valid estimates of the odds ratio for an epidemiologic association.

The efficiency of case-control studies

You may reasonably ask: So what? After all, a simple random sample can also produce unbiased estimates of the odds ratio. Indeed, a simple random sample seems more straightforward, since the contingency table for the sample will then directly represent the population contingencies.

The value of the case-control study, however, lies in its efficiency. Efficiency is the extent of precision (width of the confidence intervals) that a given investment of resources in a study can obtain. In a case-control study, you can obtain cases from places such as cancer registries or health care settings. This is extremely efficient compared to simple random sampling, especially for rare diseases. A simple random sample would result in a small number of cases (especially for a rare disease)—so even if the sample size were very large, it would likely generate imprecise estimates. Essentially, the case-control design allows for the more efficient use of a smaller subset of population members than a simple random sample, leading to gains in efficiency.

Key point: The main advantage of the case-control design is its efficiency. The design is efficient because selection of cases can be accomplished flexibly and the control group is usually only a small subset of the analogous group in the general population.

The organization of the Canadian health system can add to the efficiency of case-control studies. The Canadian health system operates largely on a single-payer model, so it often pursues population-based clinical services to reduce duplication of services. If the population served is geographically defined (e.g., a health region or province), it is referred to as a *catchment area* for that clinical service. Catchment areas are ideal for conducting case-control studies. If a clinic serves all members of the catchment area population with a specific disease, selection cannot depend on exposure in the cases. Similarly, any noncase (potential control) in the catchment area would have been a case had they developed the disease, regardless of exposure. Other types of health system organization can also interface very well with the case-control design. For example, many case-control studies use hospital-based cases: some select all patients presenting to a particular hospital for a particular disease during a defined period.

An example of a case-control study

Hackam et al[109] conducted a case-control study in Ontario to assess the potentially protective role of angiotensin-converting enzyme inhibitors (ACE inhibitors) in preventing rupture of aortic aneurisms. This study used linked administrative data to identify patients admitted to hospital with ruptured aneurisms. This was the case group. Patients admitted to hospital with unruptured aneurisms were the control group. The investigators observed a significant protective effect of ACE inhibitors: the odds ratio was 0.82, with a 95% CI of 0.74–0.90. The odds ratio, as with other ratio-based measures of association, has a null value of 1.0: values less than 1.0 are interpreted as being protective. In the study by Hackam et al, the upper limit of the confidence interval does not reach this null value, which is the basis for the investigators' assertion that ACE inhibitors have a significant effect. In situations where a 95% CI for a measure of association does not include the null value, the result will be significant at the 5% level of confidence. The confidence limits clarify that the protective effect may be as strong as odds ratio = 0.74, or as weak as odds ratio = 0.90.

Selection bias in case-control studies

The efficiencies of the case-control design come at the cost of 2 main vulnerabilities: selection bias and misclassification bias.

Selection bias is not necessarily a point of vulnerability for every case-control study. In general, however, the case-control design is vulnerable to selection bias.

The concept of selection bias is more complicated for case-control studies than for simple parameters such as prevalence.

For simple parameters, there is a single outcome, usually a disease. If the presence of the disease affects the probability of selection, bias results. In other words, if the selection probability for those with the disease differs from the selection probability for those without the disease, this defect produces bias. This is a fairly simple rule to follow.

More complex rules are needed to assess whether selection bias has affected the estimated odds ratio in a case-control study. To grasp these complex rules, it is best to view the odds ratio as an actual ratio of odds and not as a cross product. In other words, it is best to think of the odds ratio as this:

$$\text{Odds Ratio} = \frac{\dfrac{a}{c}}{\dfrac{b}{d}}$$

Rather than this:

$$\text{Odds Ratio} = \frac{ad}{bc}$$

Also, it's useful to approach the more complex rules in terms of the simple rule—as the simple rule applied twice, once for the numerator and once for the denominator. This involves thinking about a case-control study as 2 studies. One "study" seeks to estimate the odds of exposure in cases and the other "study" seeks to estimate the odds of exposure in controls. This leads to some additional rules and insights. If the numerator of the odds ratio is too big, the odds ratio will be overestimated. If the denominator is too big, the odds ratio will be underestimated. And there is 1 other possibility: if the odds of exposure are elevated, or diminished, but to the same extent in the cases and controls, then the numerator and denominator are altered to the same extent and the ratio of the odds of exposure in cases and controls (the odds ratio) will not be biased.

In principle, if these 2 odds represent the odds of exposure in the underlying populations of cases and controls, then the expected value of the estimated odds ratio will be the true population value. This is the proof in principle that the case-control design can work. The expectation is:

$$e\left(\text{Odds Ratio}\right) = \frac{e\left(\dfrac{a}{c}\right)}{e\left(\dfrac{b}{d}\right)} = \frac{\dfrac{A}{C}}{\dfrac{B}{D}} = \frac{AD}{BC}$$

Imagine, for example, a hospital-based case-control study investigating association between asthma and smoking. The case group is special in certain respects because its subjects are selected from a hospital. There are many health-related behaviours and characteristics that could increase the chance of hospitalization and hence the probability of selection of cases. For example, people with asthma are more likely to be admitted to hospital if they smoke. The odds of smoking for cases of asthma will be higher if those cases are selected from a hospital. Let's imagine that hospital-based selection doubles the probability of exposure to smoking. If the control group were selected in such a way that its subjects also had similarly elevated odds of exposure (perhaps they are also selected from the same hospital and have other conditions for which smoking doubles their chances of admission), selection bias would not occur. Even though the odds of exposure are twice as high in the cases and controls—indeed, because they are twice as high in both the cases and controls—bias will not occur:

$$e\left(\text{Odds Ratio}\right) = \frac{e\left(\dfrac{a}{c}\right)}{e\left(\dfrac{b}{d}\right)} = \frac{2\times\left(\dfrac{A}{C}\right)}{2\times\left(\dfrac{B}{D}\right)} = \frac{AD}{BC}$$

This is a challenging concept to grasp, but it does lead to a general rule about how a case-control study's estimated odds ratio can avoid selection bias. The rule can be stated as follows: the probability of selection for cases and controls should not depend on exposure in any way that differs between the 2 groups.

This rule can also anticipate the direction of possible bias. For example, if the procedure used to select cases overrepresents exposure, the selection of controls must overrepresent exposure to the same extent. If exposure has an impact on the selection of cases and not on the selection of controls—or not as much—the odds ratio will be biased. In this case, the direction of bias would be positive: the estimated odds ratio would systematically overestimate the population value. As usual, this selection bias comes from a defect in the design of the individual study: increasing the sample size would not fix it. This is systematic error, not random error. The defect is not that the probability of selection depends on exposure, but that it does so in a way that differs between cases and controls. Of course, if the selection of cases and controls did not depend at all on exposure (another way to say this: if the process of selection were independent of exposure), there would be no bias. This is a special instance of the rule stated above: the probability of selection does not depend on exposure in this scenario in a way that differs between cases and controls.

Key point: Selection bias results if selection of cases and controls depends on exposure in some way that is not equivalent between the 2 groups.

Data sources and selection bias in case-control studies

It is easiest to be confident that selection bias has not occurred if the selection of cases and controls does not depend in any way on exposure. If this is the case, it is more obvious that the impact of exposure on selection does not differ between cases and controls.

In Canada, this is sometimes possible due to the existence of population-based data. For example, Canadian cancer registries register all cases of cancer. Registration does not depend on exposure in any way. Case-control studies that use these cancer registries as a source of cases typically use a selection procedure for controls that also does not depend at all on exposure, such as sampling the general population via random digit dialing. For example, Friedenreich et al[110] followed this procedure in their study of alcohol consumption and endometrial cancer risk.

If case-control studies use administrative data to select cases and controls, it is important that coding of disease status (and hence the probability of selection of cases) not depend on exposure status, at least not in a way that differs between cases and controls. A person recorded as having a disease in physician-billing data or hospital-discharge data has seen a physician or been admitted to hospital. Exposure could potentially affect selection among such cases. The selection of the control group would need to include exactly the same impact of exposure.

Several pivotal case-control studies have used administrative data. An example is a case-control study by Rothwell et al,[111] which used Ontario hospitalization records to identify cases of vertebrobasilar dissection or occlusion, and selected controls from the Ontario Registered Persons Database. This database contains a list of everyone covered by the provincial health care insurance plan, which is essentially the entire population. These investigators were interested in whether chiropractic neck manipulation might increase the risk of stroke due to dissection or occlusion of the vertebral arteries. They used administrative data to identify whether cervical visits for chiropractic services had occurred. They reported a fivefold elevation in the odds of this type of stroke when cervical manipulation had occurred in the prior week.

BERKSON'S BIAS

Selection bias that arises from the use of hospitalized cases in a case-control study has a special name: *Berkson's bias*. Berkson published a paper about this form of bias in 1946.[112]

When hospitalized cases are used, it is often difficult to identify an appropriate control group. The controls should be selected such that they would have been cases had they developed the disease. They could, for example, be selected-from the catchment area of the hospital from which the cases were recruited, or from among patients admitted to the same hospital for another reason. This other reason would need to be another disease that is not related to the risk factor in question—a tricky distinction. Some risk factors influence decisions to admit patients with certain diseases to hospital, increasing the odds of exposure among hospitalized cases with those diseases, but not necessarily doing the same thing for controls. If these challenges are not navigated successfully, Berkson's bias will occur.

Misclassification bias in case-control studies

Misclassification bias, like selection bias, is more complicated for odds ratios from case-control studies than for simple parameters such as prevalence.

In simple parameters, insensitive measures of disease status result in frequencies biased downwards: erroneous negative classification of people with a disease moves these people from the numerator to the denominator of the frequency or odds being estimated. Nonspecific measures of disease status result in frequencies biased upwards: false-positive errors result in misclassification from the denominator to the numerator of the frequency or odds, which inflates the estimate compared to the true population parameter.

Where an odds ratio is concerned, the situation is more complex because it involves consideration of 2 elements: the numerator of the odds ratio and the denominator. Again, it is helpful to consider the odds ratio in its raw form as a ratio of 2 odds, rather than in its cross-product form:

$$\text{Odds Ratio} = \frac{\dfrac{a}{c}}{\dfrac{b}{d}}$$

This makes it easier to think of the odds ratio in the same terms as a frequency or odds-based measure—but now with 2 odds of exposure, 1 in the numerator and 1 in the denominator.

If the numerator of the odds ratio is too large relative to the denominator, a positive bias results. This would occur if the specificity of the measure of exposure status were lower in cases than controls: a would be too large (it would be inflated by false-positive exposure assessments that should have been included in c) and, all else being equal, this would bias the odds ratio upwards. By contrast, if the numerator of the odds ratio is too small, a negative bias results. This happens if the sensitivity of the measure of exposure in cases is low: a becomes be too small relative to c, because false-negative classification moves people who should be included in a to c.

Misclassification of exposure can also affect the denominator of an odds ratio estimate. If a measure of exposure is nonspecific among controls, then the number of exposed cases will be inflated by false positives, the denominator will enlarge, and the expected value of the estimated odds ratio will diminish. If measurement of exposure in controls is insensitive, the odds of exposure in the controls will be underestimated, making the denominator of the odds ratio too small, and the odds ratio inflated.

Key point: By considering the effects of misclassification on estimates in the numerator and denominator of an odds ratio separately, the direction of the resulting bias can be anticipated. If the numerator is inflated, the estimate of the odds ratio will be too high. If the denominator is inflated, the estimate of the odds ratio will be too low.

Differential and nondifferential misclassification bias

Our discussion of misclassification bias so far has shown several examples of what is called *differential misclassification bias*, where errors in classification occur at a different rate in the cases and controls. The first example was a lack of specificity for classification of exposure that occurs only among the cases.

This would inflate the estimated odds ratio. The second example was a lack of sensitivity among the cases, which would result in a negative bias.

There are 2 other possible mechanisms of differential misclassification bias. A lack of specificity in the classification of exposure that occurs predominantly among controls would bias the odds ratio downwards (negative bias). A lack of sensitivity for exposure that occurs exclusively among controls would lead to overestimation of the odds ratio (positive bias).

Nondifferential misclassification bias occurs when classification is inaccurate, but equally so for cases and controls. This type of bias cannot be characterized as positive or negative. Instead, it displays a different behaviour: bias towards the null value. Remember that the null value for an odds ratio is 1. Therefore if the exposure is a risk factor, the association will appear smaller than it really is. If the exposure is a protective factor, the odds ratio will be larger than it should be (closer to 1).

RECALL BIAS

Case-control studies are vulnerable to recall bias, a kind of differential misclassification. This is because they assess exposure retrospectively.

Retrospective assessment of exposure does not always depend on the memory of subjects (e.g., the study of ACE inhibitors assessed exposure using administrative record linkage[109]). But when it does depend on the memory of subjects, there is a concern that disease status will affect recall of exposure. The usual concern is that people who are sick are motivated to think harder about reasons for their illness. So, their recall of exposure may be more sensitive than that of controls.

Recall bias creates a tendency for exposed controls to more often be misclassified as false negatives (for exposure), which diminishes the odds of exposure in controls relative to cases and leads to a positive bias (overestimation) of the odds ratio.

Although this type of bias has a name, it doesn't really need a special label. Recall bias can be described as a form of differential misclassification in relation to sensitivity and specificity for exposure classification in cases and controls.

Other aspects of case-control studies

Odds of disease and exposure

In the case-control design, the odds ratio—which contrasts the frequency of exposure in cases and controls—seems to transpose the basic idea of contrasting the frequency of disease in exposed and nonexposed groups. Fortunately, this transposition is not problematic. The reason is a matter of arithmetic related to the properties of this parameter.

Think back to Table 24—the standard 2×2 table from a case-control study. If you base the calculation of the odds ratio on the odds of disease in the

exposed and nonexposed groups—rather than comparing the odds of exposure in cases and controls—the equation would be as follows:

$$\text{Odds Ratio} = \dfrac{\dfrac{a}{b}}{\dfrac{c}{d}}$$

This odds ratio reduces to the following familiar cross-product formula:

$$\text{Odds Ratio} = \dfrac{\dfrac{a}{b}}{\dfrac{c}{d}} = \dfrac{ad}{bc}$$

Fortunately, the odds ratio calculated from case-control data is a valid
means of estimating the association between a risk factor and a disease outcome. The Ontario study about ACE inhibitors, for example, showed lower
odds of exposure to these inhibitors in people with ruptured aneurisms,
which implies that ACE inhibitors lower the risk of ruptured aneurisms.

Incidence and prevalence effects

So far, we have talked about cases and controls with a labelling convention
based on disease-exposure contingencies. However, all cases of disease are
not the same.

A case of disease can be a prevalent case—a person having the disease at a
point in time. Alternatively, a case can be an incident case—a newly developed
case. This distinction is absolutely critical for interpreting the odds ratios that
arise from case-control studies. If a case-control study uses incident cases, the
odds ratio will estimate the ratio of incidence (expressed as an odds rather
than the usual proportion) in the population, and the resulting estimate will
be an estimate of the incidence odds ratio in the population. By contrast, if a
study uses prevalent cases, it will estimate the prevalence odds ratio.

Why is this distinction important? Recall that prevalence reflects the end
result of several underlying dynamics. Partially, it reflects the risk of a person developing a disease (incidence) and partially it reflects the duration of
illness among those developing the disease. Recall also that the purpose of
using ratio-based measures is to create a single parameter that embodies a
comparison between exposed and nonexposed groups. So, a prevalence odds
ratio reflects a comparison of prevalence in exposed and nonexposed people.

Prevalence odds ratios do not directly reflect etiology. Rather, they make a
statement about how common a disease is in people with and without exposure. It is an error to interpret these parameters as if they conveyed information about risk factors. For example, a prevalence odds ratio of 2 does not
mean that the risk factor in question doubles the risk of disease: it only means

that the odds of disease are twice as high in those with the exposure as in those without the exposure. The prevalence odds ratio reflects both the effect of exposure on risk and duration. The implications of this distinction are not trivial. If an exposure is a determinant, this will affect the prevalence odds ratio. If the exposure makes people more likely to die from a disease, it will make the prevalence odds ratio smaller, not larger, because death shortens the duration of disease. If the exposure makes an episode of illness last longer, for example by prolonging survival, it will make the prevalence odds ratio larger even if it has no impact on risk.

If incident cases are used in a case-control study, the resulting incidence odds ratio will reflect an effect of the exposure on the incidence (risk) of the disease.

Key point: The use of incident versus prevalent cases in case-control studies is key to interpreting the resulting odds ratio, even if the formula looks the same in both cases.

TEMPORALITY, INCIDENCE, AND PREVALENCE

Case-control studies can have challenges with temporality similar to cross-sectional studies. As noted in chapter 10 (see page 121), cross-sectional studies are generally precluded from assessing etiology because they cannot clarify the temporal association between disease and exposure. A case-control study that uses incident cases is better able to assess etiology than a cross-sectional study, but this is not true for a case-control study that uses prevalent cases.

In case-control studies that use prevalent cases, questions about temporality can arise and draw into question the cause-effect relationships that the study is attempting to address.

The rare disease assumption

Even though an odds ratio from a case-control study can estimate the odds ratio in a population, debates sometimes arise about whether it can estimate the ratio of 2 frequencies in a population. The key question is: When is an odds ratio a good estimate of the equivalent ratio-based measure that is based on proportions rather than odds? Put into other words, this is the question of whether a prevalence odds ratio can be interpreted as a prevalence ratio, and whether an incidence odds ratio can be interpreted as a risk ratio.

The answer to this question hinges on whether the disease in question is rare. Let's revisit Table 5 (see page 18), the 1×2 table that labels those with a disease as a and those without the disease as b. The odds of disease are very similar to the proportion having the disease when a is small, because the denominator of the odds is b and the denominator of the proportion is $a + b$. These 2 denominators are very similar when a is tiny.

To further illustrate: imagine a sample of $n = 100$ where the proportion with the disease is 1/4 (25%). Here, the odds and the proportion are substantially different: odds = 1/3 (0.333) and proportion = 1/4 (0.25). If the proportion having the disease is 1/100 (1%), however, then the odds are 0.0101, which is almost identical to 1% or 0.01.

This tendency of odds ratios to resemble ratios of 2 proportions only when a disease is rare has a name: the *rare disease assumption*. The term is unfortunate because it seems to suggest that the validity of the odds ratio is dependent on an assumption that a disease is rare. This is not true at all. In epidemiology, valid estimates of a parameter are estimates that do not systematically deviate from the underlying population value. An odds ratio is valid if its distribution does not systematically deviate from the underlying population odds ratio. The rare disease assumption merely points out that an odds-based parameter will only be a close approximation of a related proportion-based parameter if the disease is rare.

Key point: The validity of an odds ratio does not depend on the assumption that a disease is rare.

Induction and latency periods

A case-control study can investigate exposures to risk factors that occur many years before the emergence of the diseases caused by those exposures. This period between exposure to a risk factor and emergence of disease is called the *induction period*. Infectious diseases can have short induction periods: diseases often follow rapidly after exposure to infectious agents. Chronic diseases can have very long induction periods.

A latency period is the time between the onset of a disease and its emergence as a clinically evident entity. Some diseases may exist for years in a latent, or hidden, phase and only become clinically apparent in an advanced stage.

Diseases with long induction or latency periods can pose challenges for epidemiological research. If a study investigating such a disease begins with, say, a random sample, it might need to follow subjects for many years waiting for cases to accrue or become apparent. A case-control study, though, can start with people who are already known to have the disease and enquire retrospectively about their exposures.

In addition, case-control studies allow examination of multiple potential causes of a disease, even a rare disease.

INDUCTION PERIODS AND COMPONENT CAUSES OF DISEASE

Diseases do not usually have a single cause: exposure to a single risk factor is not typically enough in itself to trigger a pathophysiologic disease mechanism. Instead, additional effects from other exposures are usually necessary.

These dynamics have been articulated in a model that posits the existence of multiple component causes for most diseases. This model was developed by Rothman and is therefore often called the *Rothman model*, but is also named (by Rothman) the *causal pie model* of disease etiology.[113] Another name is the *sufficient-component cause model*.

In brief, this model posits that the cause of a disease is a specific combination of component causes. Each component cause is like a piece of a pie: when the pieces fit together into a causal mechanism —a complete "pie"—the disease has its onset. Through the lens of this model, induction periods occur because the completion of a causal mechanism may involve the collection of component causes through time.

Primary, secondary, and tertiary prevention

Primary, secondary, and tertiary prevention are related to induction and latency.

Primary prevention comprises measures to prevent the occurrence of disease. It is a key application of epidemiological research. In the language of the causal pie model, it involves eliminating exposure to component causes (risk factors) for disease, as identified by analytical epidemiological research. By removing a component cause that is a part of 1 or more etiological mechanisms, the onset of disease through those mechanisms is prevented. Primary prevention operates before the onset of disease. For example, reducing the frequency of smoking is primary prevention: it removes a component cause of cardiovascular disease and many types of cancer,[114] and so reduces the incidence of these diseases. Another example of primary prevention is vaccination for human papilloma virus (HPV). HPV is a component cause, and a necessary cause, of certain cancers,[115] meaning that all known causal mechanisms involve the infection. By preventing infection (a component cause) the vaccine prevents the completion of most, or perhaps even all, causal mechanisms leading to those cancers.

Secondary prevention, also known as screening, is based on early detection of established disease. Early detection allows treatment to begin earlier, during the latency phase, before the disease would normally come to clinical attention. In certain instances, this leads to dramatically better outcomes. For example, in congenital hypothyroidism, newborn babies are unable to produce thyroid hormone. Thyroid hormone is essential for development, so this condition leads to serious problems. By the time the condition becomes apparent clinically—through delayed development—irreversible damage has been done. To address this problem, all newborns in Canada are screened for congenital hypothyroidism at birth. Through early intervention, the negative effects can easily be prevented through supplementation treatment.

Tertiary prevention comprises interventions after the overt manifestations of disease have occurred. The goal is to diminish the impact of disease through measures such as treatment or rehabilitation.

Key point: The induction period occurs before disease onset. The latency period occurs after disease onset, but before the disease has become clinically evident.

Strengths and weaknesses of case-control studies

Strengths

Efficiency: Case-control studies are generally viewed as an efficient, and therefore reasonably inexpensive, approach to studying an epidemiological association. Since the orientation of case-control studies is retrospective, the studies can be conducted fairly quickly. Long periods of follow-up are not required, as they are for some other study designs.

Fit with rare diseases: For rare diseases, the efficiency and opportunity (especially the ability to use clinical subjects) provided by the case-control design often make it the most feasible option. However, as with cross-sectional studies, case-controls studies are not necessarily efficient when the exposure is very rare. Even the ability to accrue a large number of cases will not result in precise estimates of association if the number of exposed participants is small.

Fit with long induction and latency periods: In a longitudinal study, induction and latency periods can create long delays and require years of follow-up, which is often impractical. A case-control study, due to its retrospective assessment of exposure, can accommodate long delays.

Ability to examine multiple exposures: With appropriate selection of cases and controls, multiple potential determinants can be examined in a case-control study.

Weaknesses

Vulnerability to selection and misclassification bias: The case-control design is vulnerable to selection bias. To ensure that selection bias does not occur, it is necessary to ensure that any effect of exposure on selection is exactly the same for cases and controls. Yet, cases and controls differ on an important characteristic—whether they have a disease or not. This can affect many aspects of behaviour and function. These, in turn, may relate to both exposure and selection, leading to bias. As a result, it is often difficult to be certain that a case-control study is not biased due to selection.

The case-control design is also vulnerable to misclassification bias—in particular, when these studies rely on the memory of subjects to assess exposure. People with disease (cases) may be more likely to recall exposure than people without disease (controls).

Key point: Case-control studies are vulnerable to recall and selection bias.

Inefficiency for rare exposures: Case-control studies are inefficient for rare exposures.

Limits on estimation: Case-control studies are limited to estimating the odds ratio, which is a measure of association. They cannot estimate actual risks since they cannot estimate incidence proportions or incidence rates.

Can only examine one disease at a time: Since these studies are based on the selection of a case group, a case-control study can only examine risk factors for a single disease at a time.

Thinking deeper

Selection bias and selection odds ratios

One of the most challenging tasks in critical appraisal is the prospect of judging whether an estimate has been systematically distorted by selection bias. The task is easier in descriptive studies, where the parameter being estimated is a frequency or odds. It is always more complex in analytical studies, where the intention is to estimate a complex parameter such as an odds ratio.

So far, we have approached this task by looking at the odds ratio as a true ratio of odds (and setting aside the familiar cross-product equation for calculating this parameter). This breaks the task into 2 parts—since the odds ratio, when considered this way, has a more understandable numerator and denominator—and allows you to connect the assessment of selection bias for this complex parameter to the simpler rules that govern selection bias for odds in general. By considering the effect of selection on the 2 parts individually (the numerator and denominator of the odds ratio), you can begin to approach the problem of whether bias would occur and, if so, in what direction it would tend to go.

Kleinbaum et al[116] many years ago described another approach based on selection probabilities. We introduced the idea of selection probability in chapter 8 (see page 85). There, in a discussion of selection bias in prevalence studies, we identified 2 selection probabilities as important: the selection probability for those with the disease and the selection probability for those without.

In a case-control study, there are 4 relevant selection probabilities, which Kleinbaum et al labelled with the Greek letters α,β,γ and δ. These probabilities can be defined as follows (as usual, uppercase letters signify population data and lowercase letters signify sample-based data):

$$\alpha = \frac{a}{A}$$

$$\beta = \frac{b}{B}$$

$$\gamma = \frac{c}{C}$$

$$\delta = \frac{d}{D}$$

From this set of 4 selection probabilities, you can produce a parameter that Kleinbaum et al called the *selection odds ratio*:

$$\text{Selection Odds Ratio} = \frac{\alpha\delta}{\beta\gamma}$$

This is an imaginary construction in the sense that it would rarely, if ever, actually be calculated. If A, B, C, and D were actually known, there would be little interest in sample-based estimates—the estimates would serve no inferential purpose.

The construction, however, provides an additional framework for evaluating the impact of selection bias in a case-control study. A strong feature of this parameter is that it forces a critical reader to examine a study's design carefully and to think systematically about the probability of selection in each of the 4 relevant contingencies. This, in itself, is a valuable start on thinking through a complex issue such as selection bias.

In addition, the selection odds ratio can help sort out the direction of bias. For example, suppose there is concern that an exposure might favour selection among cases but not controls. This would increase the selection probability for exposed cases relative to other selection probabilities. The equation below clarifies that this methodological flaw would tend to produce a positive bias, because it would inflate the numerator of the selection odds ratio:

$$\text{Selection Odds Ratio} = \frac{(\alpha\uparrow)\delta}{\beta\gamma}$$

If the selection of controls resulted in a similar higher probability of selection due to exposure—in other words, if exposure influenced selection of cases and controls to the same degree—then β would be increased to a similar extent as α, eliminating the bias:

$$\text{Selection Odds Ratio} = \frac{(\alpha\uparrow)\delta}{(\beta\uparrow)\gamma}$$

Some students of epidemiology find this type of schematic useful as a tool for critical appraisal.

Questions

1. List 4 advantages and 4 disadvantages of case-control studies.

2. In infectious disease epidemiology, the period between exposure to an infectious agent and the emergence of signs and symptoms of infectious disease is called the incubation period. Is the incubation period best regarded as an induction or latency period?

3. The table below presents data from the Hackam et al[109] study of ACE inhibitors in preventing rupture of aortic aneurisms. This is the crude 2 × 2 table from the study.

	Cases	Controls
Exposed	665	2761
Nonexposed	2714	9186
Total	3379	11947

a. Calculate an odds ratio from this 2 × 2 table data.
b. Calculate the extent to which the odds of exposure are decreased in the case (ruptured aneurism) group compared to the controls.

4. In plain language, what is your interpretation of the odds ratio calculated in question 3? Do you feel that the odds ratio may be invalidated by the rare disease assumption?

5. Depression is a common health issue in primary care. It is often not detected in clinical practice. Some experts have recommended "screening" to deal with this problem. "Screening" involves the distribution of rating scales to primary-care patients and offering a clinical assessment to people who screen above a threshold score. Would you classify depression screening as primary, secondary, or tertiary prevention?

12

Differential and nondifferential misclassification bias in analytical studies

---

Objectives
- Distinguish differential and nondifferential misclassification bias.
- Explain the effect of differential and nondifferential misclassification bias on the interpretation of epidemiological parameters.
- Describe blinded outcome assessment.

Differential and nondifferential misclassification bias in context

Epidemiology has many study designs, but the 3 major types of study are cross-sectional studies, case-control studies, and prospective cohort studies.

The design of case-control studies and prospective cohort studies give them explicitly analytic goals (which they may or may not achieve). All studies that estimate associations—descriptive and analytic—are vulnerable to differential and nondifferential misclassification bias.

Chapter 11 discussed case-control studies, and introduced the concepts of differential and nondifferential misclassification bias. Chapter 13, on prospective cohort studies, will revisit them.

This chapter discusses these types of bias in more detail because of their key importance in analytical studies.

Bias in review
The types of bias discussed in this chapter have the same characteristics as all types of bias. Here's a review of the key characteristics:

Bias comes from study-design defects. If the classification of study variables is perfect, there can be no misclassification bias. If perfect participation is achieved, there can be no selection bias.

Bias cannot be corrected by increasing the sample size. The occurrence of a study-design defect means that a study is estimating something other than its intended target of estimation. Increasing the sample size will merely result in narrower confidence intervals around an erroneous estimate, providing a false sense of precision.

Bias can be prevented, but not often corrected. Investigators can avoid bias by careful thinking at the stage of study design. Once bias has occurred, it cannot usually be corrected after the fact.

Differential misclassification bias

Let's review how differential misclassification can affect case-control studies.

The retrospective measurement of exposure status in case-control studies often relies on recall. This may result in recall bias. People with a disease (cases) are more likely to recollect exposures. This means that questions and instruments seeking to elicit exposure history are likely more sensitive in cases than in controls, so that misclassification of exposure happens in a way that differs depending on case or control (disease) status. Recall bias typically leads to an overestimation of the odds ratio.

Here's another way of thinking about recall bias, using the classic 2 × 2 contingency table of exposure versus disease. You could say that, in recall bias, misclassification happens across the "exposure" axis of the table and depends on the "disease" axis.

Recall bias is only 1 example of differential misclassification bias. The 2 × 2 contingency table helps us imagine another example, where misclassification happens across the "disease" axis and depends on the "exposure" axis.

In general, misclassification is differential if the misclassification of exposure or disease depends on the other axis.

Magnitude and direction of differential misclassification bias

There are no simple rules for understanding the behaviour of differential misclassification bias. You have to think through the expected impact of the misclassification (see page 130).

In the case of recall bias in a case-control study, since the classification of exposure in the controls lacks sensitivity, the odds of exposure in the controls will tend to be underestimated. This makes the denominator of the odds ratio smaller and consequently the value of the odds ratio larger. This particular mechanism of bias is likely to inflate the observed value of the odds ratio.

> *Key point:* When misclassification is differential, there are no simple rules about the direction or magnitude of bias. Each case needs to be thought through individually.

Nondifferential misclassification bias

Misclassification in general happens because the procedure for classifying exposure or disease has a sensitivity or specificity—or both—of less than 1.

In differential misclassification bias, misclassification occurs and its occurrence depends on the other axis of the contingency table.

In nondifferential misclassification bias, misclassification occurs and its occurrence does not depend on the other axis of the contingency table.

Let's think about this in the context of case-control studies, where most of the concern surrounds the classification of exposure. Nondifferential misclassification bias would mean the frequency with which classification errors occur does not differ depending on case-versus-control status.

This type of misclassification occurs commonly. In a case-control study that measures exposure using a procedure that does not depend on recall, there may be no reason to believe that the errors in classification would depend on outcome (i.e., disease or no disease). In Canada, many case-control studies use record linkage to administrative data to avoid a reliance on recall. However, this is only feasible when the exposure of interest is an event recorded in administrative data.

Magnitude and direction of nondifferential misclassification bias

The direction of bias introduced by nondifferential misclassification errors is always towards the null value of the parameter being estimated.

All of the complex parameters that are intended to embody an association between risk factors and disease have null values. In a case-control study, where the measure of association must be an odds ratio, the null value is 1 because this value implies an absence of effect of the exposure. This means that for a protective association (where the odds ratio is less than 1), the estimated odds ratio will be systematically higher than the true population value. It will appear less protective than it actually is. When a risk factor elevates the risk of disease, the odds ratio is greater than 1, but nondifferential misclassification bias will bring the estimate closer to the null value of 1. (Note that difference-based measures have a null value of 0.)

Nondifferential misclassification bias is unique: other sorts of bias affect estimates by making them too large or too small, and cannot generally be identified as going in any specific direction with respect to a null value. Nondifferential misclassification bias does not inflate or suppress estimates of effects, but rather dilutes the actual effect. The direction is predictable in this sense.

Key point: The effect of nondifferential misclassification is bias towards the null value.

Addressing misclassification bias in critical appraisal

During critical appraisal of a study, it is essential to examine how the study measured disease and exposure variables.

Assessing the quality of measurement strategies

Critical appraisal should include consideration of the quality of a study's measurement strategies. The selection of high-quality measurement strategies is key to avoiding misclassification. Many studies, however, rely on poorly validated scales and measures. They may also fail to employ proper procedures, such as training study staff in the use of measurement instruments.

Blinding: a way to avoid misclassification bias

Critical appraisal also requires careful assessment for differential misclassification bias: Would misclassification of disease occur at a different frequency depending on exposure, or would misclassification of exposure occur at a different frequency depending on disease? In studies that use raters to determine disease or exposure status—for example, through interviews or clinical examinations—the raters can be a source of differential misclassification bias. These studies often use a procedure called *blinding* to avoid differential misclassification. Blinding ensures that raters do not know the disease or exposure status of study subjects. If raters did know, this knowledge could influence their classification. For example, if a rater in a case-control study knew a subject was a case (had a disease), the rater might (perhaps subconsciously) probe more deeply for evidence of exposure.

Interpreting nondifferential misclassification bias

Critical appraisal must finally consider the impact of possible nondifferential misclassification bias. A study that fails to find an exposure-disease association should not be taken seriously if considerable nondifferential misclassification bias may have occurred. This methodological flaw could explain the study's negative result. By contrast, in a study that finds an association, nondifferential misclassification bias would mean that the effect reported is probably stronger than it appears.

Key point: The implications of bias sometimes depend on its direction. A weak (or no-effect) result may not be a credible finding in a study that is biased towards the null, but a strong effect may be even more impressive in the face of such bias.

Thinking deeper

Exploring the mechanisms of differential and nondifferential misclassification bias

Let's do some simple calculations based on hypothetical 2 × 2 tables to more fully understand differential and nondifferential misclassification bias.

Consider a case-control study where a measure of exposure is insensitive. Further imagine that this lack of sensitivity is nondifferential—in other words, the probability of false-negative classification is the same in cases and controls. In this situation, you would expect underestimation in both the numerator (the odds of exposure in the cases) and the denominator (odds of exposure in the controls). You might also expect these underestimations to cancel out—however, they don't. If the odds of exposure are higher in the cases, the extent of misclassification will also be greater in the cases, making them (relatively speaking) more like the controls. In any situation in which there is a positive association (odds ratio > 1), nondifferential misclassification results in bias of the estimated odds ratio towards the null value.

Table 25 presents the first hypothetical contingency table. In Table 25, the odds ratio is 1.

Now, imagine that the method of classification of exposure had a sensitivity of only 0.50, or 50%. You would expect, on average, half of those who really are exposed to be misclassified into the nonexposed group. The expected 2 × 2 table will now look like Table 26—which, however, again has an odds ratio of 1.

Because nondifferential misclassification of this type is always towards the null, it is not surprising that nondifferential misclassification in a situation of no effect does not cause bias.

TABLE 25. 2 × 2 TABLE FOR DATA FROM A CASE-CONTROL STUDY: NO EFFECT OF EXPOSURE, NO MEASUREMENT ERRORS

	Cases	Controls
Exposed	100	100
Nonexposed	100	100
Total	200	200

TABLE 26. 2 × 2 TABLE FOR DATA FROM A CASE-CONTROL STUDY: NO EFFECT OF EXPOSURE, 50% SENSITIVITY FOR EXPOSURE

	Cases	Controls
Exposed	50	50
Nonexposed	150	150
Total	200	200

TABLE 27. 2 × 2 TABLE FOR DATA FROM A CASE-CONTROL STUDY: POSITIVE ASSOCIATION OF EXPOSURE WITH DISEASE

	Cases	Controls
Exposed	150	100
Nonexposed	50	100
Total	200	200

TABLE 28. 2 × 2 TABLE FOR DATA FROM A CASE-CONTROL STUDY: POSITIVE ASSOCIATION OF EXPOSURE WITH DISEASE, 50% SENSITIVITY FOR EXPOSURE

	Cases	Controls
Exposed	75	50
Nonexposed	125	150
Total	200	200

When there is an effect, however, the situation is different. Table 27 shows a case-control study with a positive exposure-disease association and an odds ratio of 3. Table 28 shows the expected 2 × 2 table in the same case-control study with a positive exposure-disease association and a 50% sensitivity for exposure.

In Table 28, the odds ratio is 1.8. The nondifferential misclassification of exposure in this case-control study has resulted in a major dilution of the observed association. Seventy-five of the cases ended up being misclassified compared to only 50 in the control group.

Questions

1. Weintraub et al[108] used various scales to identify impulse-control disorders in their case-control study evaluating the association of these disorders with dopamine-agonist treatment in people with Parkinson disease. One of these was the Minnesota Impulsive Disorders Interview, which was used to assess compulsive buying and sexual behaviour. Such interviews can be embarrassing for respondents to complete, so they may try to withhold their reporting of certain behaviours.
   a. What sort of misclassification errors could embarrassment cause?
   b. What kind of bias would you expect from these errors?
   c. What direction of bias do you anticipate?

2. Case-control studies are considered vulnerable to recall bias.
   a. What subtype of misclassification bias underlies the phenomenon of recall bias?
   b. In what direction does the error associated with recall bias usually go?
   c. Can you think of a disease in which recall bias might make an association appear weaker than it actually is?

3. Hackem et al[109] relied exclusively on administrative data to assess exposure and disease in their study of the association between ACE inhibitors and rupture of

aortic aneurisms. Since they did not need to rely on recall, can their study be considered perfectly safe from misclassification bias?

4. Friedenreich et al[117] conducted a case-control study to evaluate associations between metabolic syndrome (a group of risk factors for diabetes and cardiovascular disease such as large waist size, elevated triglycerides, abnormal lipid profiles, high blood pressure, and elevated blood glucose) and endometrial cancer. The cases were selected from a cancer registry and controls were selected from the general population using random digit dialing to identify people that had not been diagnosed with cancer. Assessment of the metabolic syndrome involved detailed and carefully conducted in-person interviews, anthropometric measurements, and 8-hour-fasting blood draws.

   a. Do you view this study as vulnerable to misclassification bias?

   b. Although the study excluded controls that had been diagnosed with cancer, some controls may have had cancer that was not yet detected. This would result in misclassification of disease status. What are the implications for bias?

5. Villeneuve et al[118] conducted a case-control study to examine the association between lung cancer and long-term exposure to ambient volatile organic compounds and nitrogen dioxide. Cases were recruited from 4 Toronto hospitals. Two sets of controls were selected: a population-based set and a set from a family-medicine clinic. Long-term exposure to ambient pollution is difficult to measure and these investigators needed to rely on models developed during monitoring campaigns to classify exposure. They reported moderate associations (e.g., an odds ratio of 1.59 for increased nitrogen dioxide exposure) in the analyses using population controls. What impact should the possibility of exposure misclassification have on interpretation of the results?

Prospective cohort studies

Objectives
- Define prospective cohort studies.
- Describe measures of association in prospective cohort studies: risk ratios, incident rate ratios, and hazard ratios.
- Explain how to interpret measures of association calculated from prospective cohort data.
- List strengths and weaknesses of prospective cohort studies.

What is a cohort study?
Cohort is an ancient Roman military term, but it has come to mean any group with a shared characteristic. In epidemiology, cohort studies assemble groups of subjects, often based on an exposure, and then compare outcomes in relation to this exposure over time.

There are 2 types of cohort-study designs: prospective and retrospective. These differ in temporal direction: a prospective cohort study looks forward in time (from the present to the future) and a retrospective study looks back in time (from the present to the past).

Temporal direction, logical direction, and study-design classification
Cohort studies can differ in temporal direction, but they always have the same logical direction of inquiry. A study's logical direction of inquiry involves how it explores cause and effect. The logical direction in case-control studies is backward: these studies start with an effect (cases have the disease) and then look for a cause (exposures). By contrast, cohort studies have a forward logical direction: they start with a possible cause (exposure) and then look for effects (disease).

	Logical direction: cause to effect (forward)	Logical direction: effect to cause (backward)
Temporal direction: retrospective	Retrospective cohort study	Case-control study
Temporal direction: prospective	Prospective cohort study	--

FIGURE 6. TEMPORAL AND LOGICAL DIRECTION OF DIFFERENT STUDY DESIGNS

Temporal direction and logical direction are very useful concepts for classifying study designs. Figure 6 presents a classification of study designs according to these key characteristics.

Even though cross-sectional studies do not appear in Figure 6, the concepts of temporal and logical direction are also useful for distinguishing cross-sectional studies from case-control and cohort studies. Since cross-sectional studies begin with a sample intended to represent a population at a point in time, they do not have direction to their logical inquiry. Since they are intended to provide a snapshot at a point in time, they are neither prospective nor retrospective in their temporal direction. This means cross-sectional studies have neither temporal nor logical direction.

The prospective cohort study is a classic analytical epidemiology study, which is why it forms the focus of this chapter. Assessment of causal relationships is the usual reason for choosing this design, so prospective cohort studies almost always have analytic, rather than descriptive, aims.

Don't forget, though, that the analytic-versus-descriptive nature of a study is a soft distinction. Investigators may have a variety of motivations for their research. With prospective cohort studies, they likely have analytical motivations, but they may also have descriptive aims—for example, they may want to generate new hypotheses or describe noncausal associations between some variables. The distinction between analytic and descriptive aims—because soft—is a weak criterion for study-design classification. The characteristics of temporal direction and logical direction—because more tangible—are more useful for study-design classification.

Key point: Temporal direction and logical direction are tangible study-design characteristics that are very useful for study-design classification.

Design of prospective cohort studies

The prospective cohort study design clarifies the temporal relationship between exposure and disease—an important advantage. This type of study can assess risk. Prospective cohort studies can either be based on large multipurpose cohorts, or they may specifically select exposed and nonexposed participants.

To assess risk, it is necessary that the population under study not have the condition under investigation at the start of the observation period. This means that a prospective cohort study needs to eliminate people who already have the disease (or other outcomes) at a baseline time point before commencing follow-up.

Figure 7 presents a schematic of a typical prospective cohort study, as carried out using a data set from a large multipurpose cohort. First, prevalent cases are excluded. Next, the cohort is divided into exposed and nonexposed groups. Then, the "at risk" cohort is followed prospectively to determine the incidence of disease in those that are exposed and nonexposed.

In a study seeking to examine the effects of a single exposure, exposed and nonexposed cohorts may be selected from an underlying source population. In this case, for reasons of efficiency, the selection probabilities for the exposed subjects would generally be much higher than for the nonexposed. However, the key aspects of the study design—its forward temporal direction and logical direction—remain the same (see Figure 8).

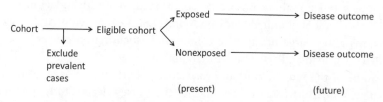

FIGURE 7. SCHEMATIC OF A TYPICAL PROSPECTIVE COHORT STUDY DESIGN: EXISTING MULTIPURPOSE COHORT

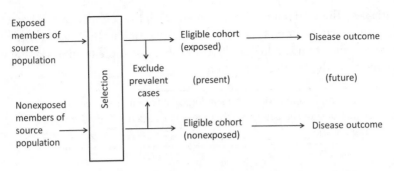

FIGURE 8. SCHEMATIC OF A PROSPECTIVE COHORT STUDY: SELECTION OF EXPOSED AND NONEXPOSED COHORTS

Examples of prospective cohort studies

Prospective cohort studies are expensive to conduct because they usually "follow" cohorts for long periods. So, they need to hire and pay staff for long periods, and they need to maintain contact with study participants for long periods, which is expensive and difficult.

Such large investments of resources need the justification of important goals. As a result, prospective cohort studies typically tackle major analytic questions and often several questions. Multipurpose cohort studies are large-scale projects that address many possible outcomes of many possible exposures.

Prominent examples of multipurpose prospective cohort studies in Canada include the National Population Health Survey (NPHS), and the National Longitudinal Study on Children and Youth (NLSCY). These were large-scale projects that collected baseline data from carefully selected cohorts and then followed the cohorts over time. This allowed for economies of scale and better quality control. Statistics Canada conducted the NPHS and NLSCY. This agency has an established network of interviewers, highly trained personnel, advanced operational systems, and expertise in topics such as sampling and avoidance of attrition. It makes sense that it should play a central role in such national initiatives. Unfortunately, the NPHS and NLSCY were terminated in 2010.

A new and ambitious prospective cohort study of health and aging called the Canadian Longitudinal Study on Aging (CSLA) is currently underway.[119] There is also a large prospective cohort study focusing on cancer etiology called the Canadian Partnership for Tomorrow Project.[120]

Some of the most important prospective cohort studies have been conducted in the United States. These include the Nurse's Health Study, now in its third iteration,[121] and the National Health and Nutrition Examination Survey (NHANES).[122]

Assessing associations in a prospective cohort study using ratio-based measures

Prospective cohort studies exclude cases of disease at a baseline point in time, which makes it possible to assess risk for disease in both the exposed and nonexposed groups.

The parameter that quantifies risk may be a risk ratio (incidence proportion ratio), incidence rate ratio, or a hazard ratio.

RISK RATIOS

Where the incidence proportion is concerned, this leads to the familiar 2 × 2 contingency table of exposure versus disease presented in Table 29. Note, however, that this table only looks familiar: it is very different from a contingency table for a cross-sectional or case-control study. In a prospective cohort study, it includes only study subjects at risk of the disease at baseline. The classification of these subjects as having or not having disease depends on whether they develop the disease during the period of observation of the study. This differs from studies that focus on a point in time (cross-sectional studies) and studies that select participants based on disease status (case-control studies).

As always, there is value in using a single parameter to quantify association between exposure and disease. In cross-sectional studies, the prevalence ratio and prevalence odds ratio function as single quantifying parameters. In case-control studies, the odds ratio does this.

In prospective cohort studies, the odds ratio can work to quantify association—you could derive it from Table 29. Note that this odds ratio is, more specifically, an incidence odds ratio.

TABLE 29. 2 × 2 TABLE FOR A TYPICAL PROSPECTIVE COHORT STUDY

	Incident disease	No incidence disease	Total
Exposed	a	b	$n_{exposed}$
Nonexposed	c	d	$n_{nonexposed}$

Prospective cohort studies can also report estimated association in the form of a risk ratio, which is the ratio of the 2 incidence proportions:

$$\text{Risk Ratio} = \frac{\dfrac{a}{a+b}}{\dfrac{c}{c+d}}$$

The risk ratio could also, and perhaps preferably, be referred to as the *incidence proportion ratio*. This term is not used very often, perhaps because it is awkward to say. The risk ratio is also sometimes also called *relative risk*.

Key point: Superficially similar parameters comprising ratios of proportions have multiple names.

INCIDENT RATE RATIOS

If a prospective cohort study uses a defined risk interval—for example, 16 years (the duration of the NPHS)—not everyone at risk in the cohort at baseline is actually at risk for the whole 16-year period. A study participant who dies after 8 years, for example, is not at risk of disease during the subsequent 8 years.

When there is appreciable movement in or out of the at-risk cohort, the risk ratio is not the ideal parameter to quantify association. It would be better to use a parameter that can account for movement. Rather than calculating the incidence proportion in the exposed and nonexposed groups—as in a risk ratio—it would be preferable to calculate the incidence rate, with its person-time denominator. The person-time denominator of the incidence rate can account for the reality that not every cohort member is followed for exactly the same amount of time.

A ratio of the 2 incidence rates is the incidence rate ratio:

$$\text{Incidence Rate Ratio} = \frac{\text{Incidence Rate}_{exposed}}{\text{Incidence Rate}_{nonexposed}}$$

HAZARD RATIOS

Mortality rate ratio is a more specific term for an incidence rate ratio that compares 2 mortality rates. Relative mortality can also be estimated using hazard ratios.

Hazard ratios are associated with survival analysis, a technique that is commonly used in the analysis of data from prospective cohort studies, even when mortality is not the outcome of interest. A hazard rate is the rate of an outcome at a point in time conditional on the outcome not having occurred to that point in time. A hazard ratio is the ratio of 2 hazard rates: that for the exposed divided by that for the nonexposed.

Survival analysis is a sophisticated way of addressing the issues that arise when at-risk subjects leave the at-risk cohort, either because they develop the outcome or for some other reason. Survival analysis addresses this issue by censoring (removing participants from the at-risk cohort) in the calculation of hazard ratios. This approach can be extended to more elaborate models, such as proportional hazards models, capable of addressing complex methodological problems.

The techniques used in survival analysis are complex, but hazard ratios can be interpreted very much like other relative measures of effect and can be treated as such during critical appraisal.

> *Key point:* Comparisons of incidence in prospective cohort studies can be accomplished using several parameters. Basic techniques use ratios of risks. More advanced techniques use ratios of incidence rates or hazard rates.

Assessing associations in prospective cohort studies using difference-based measures

Ratio-based measures are useful because they produce a single value that embodies a comparison of incidence between exposure groups. These measures include prevalence ratios, odds ratios, incidence proportion ratios, incidence rate ratios, and hazard ratios.

Another way to distill a single value from 2 values is to calculate a difference. In a prospective cohort study, this could involve calculating an incidence proportion difference—usually called a *risk difference*—or an incidence rate difference.

Ratio-based measures have an expected value in the event that the exposure has no impact on risk: the null value of 1. Difference-based measures also have a null value: the null value of 0.

Most prospective cohort studies use ratio-based measures of association, but there is nothing wrong with using difference-based measures.

Selection bias in prospective cohort studies

There are many names for different types of bias.[123] *Selection bias* is an overarching term that simplifies terminology by focusing on a common mechanism through which the bias arises. Selection bias comes from study-design defects that affect who does or does not participate in a study. Factors that affect participation include the formal process of sampling, and procedures for obtaining consent, retaining subjects during follow-up, and collecting information from subjects (for example, if missing data results in exclusion from the calculation of a parameter).

Think back to selection bias in case-control studies (see page 130), which centred on the methods of selecting cases and controls. The key question was whether the selection of cases and controls (based on disease status) depended on exposure in some way that differed between the 2 groups.

The same general considerations apply to the assessment of selection bias in prospective cohort studies, although the story unfolds in a slightly different way.

THE ROLE THAT DISEASE STATUS DOESN'T PLAY

In prospective cohort studies, subjects are selected (or included) in ways that ensure that none of them have the disease at baseline. Also, they are selected (or just divided) into exposed and nonexposed groups. Since the disease is not present at the time of selection, it is not possible for disease status to affect selection (if disease occurs at all, it will occur in the future)—a different situation than in case-control studies. This provides prospective cohort studies with a degree of protection against forms of bias that arise from defective procedures for selecting participants.

ATTRITION

Attrition happens when participants leave a study in ways not planned by the investigators.

People can "drop out" from the sample because they move, are lost to follow-up, withdraw consent, or for many other reasons. Attrition is almost inevitable in real-world research, and may be influenced by disease, or by precursors of disease, or by exposures that affect behaviour. Of particular concern: attrition can depend on factors related to disease in a way that differs depending on exposure. This is the scenario in which selection bias may occur.

Key point: Cohort studies have some protection from selection bias, because disease has not occurred at the time of selection and therefore cannot influence selection. Attrition, however, creates an important vulnerability to selection bias.

MISSING DATA

Missing data is an issue related to attrition.

If there is missing data about the disease outcome, even among respondents who did not withdraw from a study, those respondents are not usually included in the calculation of a study's estimates. This type of bias can be regarded as a defect of participation, because those who do not provide the necessary data cannot be included in the estimate of association and are essentially not participating in its calculation.

Due to this defect involving participation, a study may systematically over- or underestimate the target parameter. If the missing data are unrelated to exposure or disease, and are missing completely at random, bias will not occur. However, if the missing data are related to the disease outcome in a way that differs depending on exposure, selection bias will occur and will follow familiar principles.

Several procedures have been devised for allowing people with key pieces of missing data to participate in the estimation of measures of association. These involve imputation of the missing values—in other words, replacing the missing data with substitute values. Such techniques, however, are beyond the scope of this book and their effectiveness continues to be debated.

Key point: If there are missing data on the study outcome, which can occur in a prospective cohort study even in the absence of attrition, this can introduce systematic error into an estimate of association.

Misclassification bias in prospective cohort studies

Misclassification bias follows similar patterns in prospective cohort studies as in case-control studies. A difference, however, is that it tends to arise from misclassification of disease status rather than exposure status. The mechanism of bias can be differential or nondifferential. In prospective cohort studies, the key distinction is usually whether misclassification of disease status depends on exposure status (differential misclassification of disease status) or not (nondifferential misclassification of disease status). As in case-control studies (see page 133), the behaviour of nondifferential misclassification is predictable. The direction of the bias is towards the null value. For a measure of relative risk, the null value is 1. For a risk difference, the null value is 0. If the misclassification is nondifferential, the bias can go in either direction, depending on the type of inaccuracy in the measures being used.

Key point: The general principles of misclassification bias are the same in prospective cohort studies as in case-control studies. Nondifferential misclassification bias will be in the direction of the null value for a measure of association. The direction of differential misclassification bias depends on the nature of misclassification in a particular study.

In a cohort study, the exposure status of participants can be accurately measured at the time of selection. However, there is likely to be much concern about the subsequent classification of disease status. This is especially true in situations where knowledge of the exposure might affect the accuracy of outcome classification, leading to differential misclassification of outcome.

For example, if there is suspicion among investigators that the exposure in question is a risk factor, this could cause greater attention to detection of the disease in exposed subjects. As a result, the sensitivity of assessment of outcome could be greater in exposed than nonexposed participants. This would make the denominator of the risk ratio too small, increasing the estimate of the risk ratio. The specificity could also be lower in the exposed, making the numerator of the risk ratio too large. Each possibility would result in differential misclassification, because the accuracy of classification of disease is different depending on exposure. The direction of bias in each case would be towards overestimation.

This type of bias—arising from raters having an increased suspicion of disease (and therefore a greater sensitivity and/or lower specificity of assessment of the disease outcome) in exposed subjects—is sometimes called *diagnostic suspicion bias* or *surveillance bias*. Methodologically, blinding is the best safeguard against this type of bias: raters should be unaware of exposure status whenever possible.

Strengths and weaknesses of prospective cohort studies

Strengths

Temporal clarity: The main advantage of prospective cohort studies is their ability to clarify the timing of exposure in relation to disease. This is a major advantage over cross-sectional and case-control studies. Because of the temporal clarity that they can produce, prospective cohort studies are generally more capable identifying causal effects than case-control or cross-sectional studies. A cause must logically precede an effect, so the ability to confirm temporality is an important advantage of prospective cohort studies. Indeed, this strength of the prospective cohort design is related to its temporal direction, which goes forward in time (from present to future) rather than backward (as in a case-control study) or neither (as in a cross-sectional study).

Key point: An advantage of the prospective cohort study is its forward temporal direction and therefore the clarity that it can provide about the temporal relationship between exposure and disease.

Risk measurement: Data from a prospective cohort study can be used to measure the incidence proportion, incidence rate, or hazard rate in addition to making estimates of association. To illustrate this point, imagine a case-control study that produces an odds ratio of 2. If this is an incidence-based case-control study and if the disease is rare, it may be reasonable to accept this incidence odds ratio as a good approximation of the relative risk. However, the odds ratio would not clarify whether the doubling of risk meant that there was a 2% versus 1% risk, or a 0.002% versus 0.001% risk. So, while case-control and prospective cohort studies can both produce information about associations, prospective cohort studies have the distinct advantage of being able to also examine the actual risks.

Key point: An advantage of the prospective cohort design is its ability to measure risk, something that neither cross-sectional nor case-control studies can do.

Some resilience to selection bias: Prospective cohort studies are often considered less vulnerable to selection bias than case-control studies. However, they are vulnerable to selection bias arising from attrition.

Fit with large numbers of outcomes from single or multiple exposures: Prospective cohort studies can be very efficient for studying a large number of outcomes from a single exposure. Multipurpose cohorts, to the extent that they assess multiple exposures, can be useful for studying multiple risk factors and multiple outcomes.

Weaknesses

Expense: Prospective cohort studies are generally expensive. They often take place over long periods, and require investment in strategies that achieve high rates of response, and careful, accurate measurement.

Lengthy time requirement: In addition to being expensive, they are also time-consuming. In situations where the induction and/or latency periods are very long, prospective cohort studies can be especially time-consuming (and expensive).

Lack of fit for rare outcomes: Prospective cohort studies are not very efficient for studying rare outcomes. When the outcome is rare, even a large cohort may produce only a small number of outcome events, which would diminish the statistical power of the study. The case-control design is a more efficient way to study rare diseases. For rare exposures, however—as opposed to rare diseases (outcomes)—the prospective cohort design has advantages: an exposed cohort can be recruited using high probabilities of selection for the exposed cohort.

Attrition: Prospective cohort studies are vulnerable to attrition because of their long time frame. Attrition can result in selection bias, because it can easily depend on exposure and disease. Of course, the exact reasons for attrition are rarely known, since the "drop outs" are no longer in the study. The only sure way to prevent this type of bias is to ensure a very low rate of attrition from the study.

Key point: Like all study designs, the prospective cohort study design has its strengths and weaknesses. There is no generally superior study design. The best study design must be selected for a particular purpose.

Thinking deeper

A closer look at measures of association

Analytical epidemiology studies almost always include measures of association.

Measures of association distill information from 2 risks or rates down to a single number. Something useful is gained from this: a more accessible quantification of the association. Something is also lost, however: the underlying risks or rates. For this reason, epidemiological data analysis generally includes both the generation and reporting of univariate estimates of parameters (e.g., frequencies) and bivariate parameters (e.g., odds ratios, risk ratios, incidence rate ratios, hazard ratios, and risk differences). In fact, it often goes beyond bivariate estimation to report estimates from multivariable models. Multivariable models quantify exposure-disease associations with various adjustments for the possible effects of other variables. Many epidemiological analyses follow a predictable progression from univariate to bivariate to multivariable procedures. Note the term *multivariable*: some people find the word awkward and prefer to say *multivariate*—but *multivariate* refers to models that have multiple dependent and independent variables.

Ratio and difference-based measures of association have null values— another useful characteristic. For a ratio-based measure, the null value is 1. For a difference-based measure, it is 0. Typically, both types of estimates are accompanied by 95% CIs. This makes for a value-added proposition. If the 95% CI does not cross the null value, you can be confident that the association would have been statistically significant had a hypothesis-testing procedure been implemented.

A common mistake among students of epidemiology is to interpret confidence intervals as if they were tests of statistical significance. This is a mistake because it sets aside a more informative approach (confidence intervals) for a less informative approach (statistical tests). The best way to interpret a confidence interval is to consider its width (quantifying the precision of the estimate) together with the location of the upper and lower confidence limits. This provides a lot of information about the estimate, helping to portray the range of possible associations (e.g., from weak to strong, from strong to very strong, etc.).

Here's another mistake associated with interpreting confidence intervals as if they were tests of statistical significance. It is true that the overlap of a confidence interval with a null value is equivalent to a statistical test conducted at that same level of confidence. However, the overlap of 2 confidence intervals has no such implication, despite frequent (erroneous) assertions to the contrary. It is not uncommon for 2 prevalence estimates—for example, 1 for men and 1 for women—to have overlapping confidence intervals and yet be significantly different.

By contrast, nonoverlapping confidence intervals always have statistical significance.

The reason for this inconsistency can be understood by appreciating that the standard error of the difference between 2 proportions is not the sum of the standard errors of the 2 proportions. Recall that the standard error of a prevalence proportion (p) is:

$$\text{Standard Error}(p) = \sqrt{\frac{p \times (1-p)}{n}}$$

But the standard error for the difference between 2 proportions is not just the sum of the 2 standard errors: it is the square root of the sum of the 2 variances (the standard errors squared):

$$\text{Standard Error}(p_1 - p_2) = \sqrt{\text{Standard Error}_1{}^2 + \text{Standard Error}_2{}^2}$$

Key point: The overlap of confidence intervals from estimated frequencies does not indicate that the 2 groups are not significantly different.

Questions

1. List 4 advantages and 4 disadvantages of prospective cohort studies.

2. Provide a critique for the assertion that prospective cohort studies are the "best" study design for making causal inference.

3. In the Canadian Multicentre Osteoporosis Study (CaMos),[124] a randomly sampled cohort that included 9 423 participants was followed for 10 years and assessed twice, at the 5-year and 10-year time points. The CaMos investigators sought to evaluate whether the use of certain antidepressants was associated with an increased risk of fragility fractures. They conducted an analysis of 6 645 subjects who had a baseline bone mineral density measurement. Among these, 4 011 completed all 10 years of follow-up.

   a. The investigators reported that 978 participants experienced at least 1 fragility fracture during follow-up. Calculate the incidence proportion for fragility fractures.

   b. There was an attrition rate of 40%. What characteristics among the study's "drop-outs" would make the parameter you calculated for fragility fractures an overestimation due to selection bias?

   c. The classification of exposure was difficult in the CaMoS study. Antidepressant use was measured at each of the interviews, but a detailed description of exposure over the entire 10 years was not possible. Could this introduce bias? What type of bias do would you suspect?

4. Suppose that you are the principal investigator of a long-term prospective cohort study. You are studying whether an exposure increases the risk of mortality. What would you prefer to employ as a measure of association: an odds ratio, risk ratio, or hazard ratio?

5. Can you think of an advantage of the prospective cohort design for studying recurrent diseases?

14

Confounding and effect modification in analytical studies

Objectives

- Define extraneous variables, confounding, and effect modification.
- Describe key procedures to control confounding: standardization, restriction, randomization, matching, stratification, and regression models.
- Identify strengths and weaknesses of key procedures to control confounding.
- Define effect modification.
- Define external validity (generalizability).

Confounding and effect modification in context

Chapter 9 looked at confounding in the context of descriptive studies. This chapter looks at confounding in the more complex context of analytical studies.

This chapter also covers effect modification. Effect modification and confounding are related because both come from extraneous variables, but beyond this they are completely different. We have not looked at effect modification before, because it is only an issue in analytical studies, not descriptive studies. This is because only analytical studies assess exposure-disease association. Effect modification involves the influence of extraneous variables on exposure-disease association.

What are extraneous variables?

Extraneous variables are variables that occur outside of the exposure-disease relationship.

The effects of extraneous variables can become intermixed with the effects of exposures, leading to confounded estimates of exposure-disease associations.

Confounding is a serious threat to the fundamental assumption of epidemiology: that diseases distribute in relation to their determinants. Analytical studies have to assume that this distribution-by-determinant relationship provides information about the cause of disease—but confounding draws this relationship into question.

Consider, for example, 2 common exposures that are associated: high levels of coffee consumption and smoking. People who drink a lot of coffee are also more likely to smoke. In a study investigating the potential association of coffee consumption and cancer, smoking becomes an extraneous variable that could confound the observed association. Drinking coffee may be associated with a higher risk of cancer, but—etiologically speaking—the association may have nothing to do with coffee consumption itself. It may merely reflect the associated health behaviour (smoking).

Key point: Association does not always mean causation, even if the estimate is free of bias and the temporal relationships are clear.

Confounding in analytical studies

Confounding literally means intermixing. In analytic epidemiology, the issue is whether 2 causal effects have intermixed in a single measure of association. Confounding is not at issue when 2 causes combine to cause a disease—this can certainly happen, but it is not confounding. Confounding is at issue when the intermixing of independent causal effects occurs in a way that makes the interpretation of measures of association difficult.

Key point: Confounding is a methodological flaw that results in the failure of estimated associations to reflect the independent causal effect of exposures.

More technically, confounding is defined as an intermixing of the effect of an exposure with the effect of an independent risk factor for the outcome (disease), leading to an estimated association that no longer reflects the causal impact of the exposure of interest. There are other ways to define confounding, but this definition is a good place to start.

The confounding triangle

A simple schematic can help clarify the problem of confounding: the confounding triangle (see Figure 9). In this triangle, the horizontal arrow from exposure to disease depicts the association of interest (this is the forward type of logical thinking about causation). The question mark indicates that this is a research question. The investigator wants to establish whether an association exists between exposure and disease and, if it does, to quantify

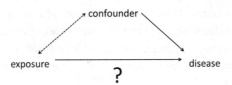

FIGURE 9. THE CONFOUNDING TRIANGLE

the strength of the association. The potential confounder is depicted at the apex of the triangle.

The triangular schematic helps to identify the 3 key characteristics of a confounding variable. First, the potential confounder is a risk factor (hence, the arrow leading to the outcome has no question mark). Second, it is associated with the exposure of interest. Third, it is not a link in a chain of causal events connecting exposure to outcome. In other words, the confounder has effects that are independent of the exposure. Think back to the coffee-cancer example: confounding does not occur because drinking a lot of coffee makes people smoke—it's just that people who drink a lot of coffee are more often smokers. Because the exposure-confounder association is not causal, it is depicted with a dashed line.

Note that the confounding variable is required to have etiological effects that are independent of the exposure. If the effects of the exposure occurred through a chain of events that included the confounding variable (drinking coffee caused people to smoke and smoking caused them to get cancer), this would be an example of mediation rather than confounding. A mediating variable is a link in a causal chain leading from exposure to outcome. This differs from confounding, which is due to an intermixing of independent effects.

Both upper arms of the triangle need to be present for the association to be confounded. If there is an independent risk factor contributing to the etiology of a disease, this will not cause confounding unless it is also associated with exposure. Similarly, many variables may be strongly associated with exposure, but unless these are also independent risk factors for disease, confounding will not occur.

Is confounding a type of bias?

Confounding is not like other forms of bias, even though investigators sometimes use the term *confounding bias*. Bias is a systematic error in estimation of a population parameter such as, for example, an odds ratio. By contrast, confounding has more to do with the interpretation of a parameter than its systematic deviation from a true value. In a study free of defects, with perfect participation and measurement, the odds ratio has an expected value equal to the underlying parameter. It can still be considered unbiased in this sense, even if it represents a mixing (confounding) of independent effects rather than a single causal effect.

In the coffee-cancer example, an elevated risk ratio for coffee consumption may very well centre on the population value for the risk ratio. But the question is: Does that risk ratio reflect an independent effect of coffee consumption or an intermixing of effects of coffee (if any) and smoking?

Key point: Confounding is different than some other types of bias because it does not lead to systematic error in the same way. A confounded estimate can be valid in the sense of not systematically deviating from a targeted population parameter. However, it may nevertheless be misleading if it is intended to represent the causal effect of a single exposure, but actually represents an intermixing of effects of different exposures.

Ways to control confounding

STANDARDIZATION

Chapter 9 covered direct and indirect standardization as procedures to control confounding (see pages 101–106).

To review: chapter 9 discussed a comparison of mortality in 2 geographic areas, Ontario and Nunavut. This was the concern: that the differences observed in mortality between the populations might merely reflect differences in the distribution of age. Age is a nonmodifiable variable, so it doesn't interest epidemiologists very much, at least not where primary prevention is the goal.

Standardization is a way to ensure that such extraneous variables do not become intermixed with variables of interest. Note that standardization is usually used to adjust rates or frequencies, and is most often used with mortality data.

OTHER PROCEDURES TO CONTROL CONFOUNDING

There are 5 procedures beyond standardization to address confounding. These are typically used in studies estimating parameters such as odds ratios, risk ratios, or risk differences.

The procedures fall into categories depending on when, during a study, you implement them: the design stage, the analysis stage, or both.

CONTROL OF CONFOUNDING AT THE STUDY-DESIGN STAGE

RESTRICTION

The classic procedure for preventing confounding at the design stage is restriction. This simply means not allowing people that are exposed to a potential confounder to participate in the study.

Let's take sex as an example of a potential counfounder. Sex is a classic example because it is a nonmodifiable extraneous variable. In addition, sex is an independent risk factor for a large number of diseases, and associated with many exposures of interest. So, investigators are often concerned about its potential to introduce confounding.

If a study used restriction to control confounding by sex, it would restrict participation to either men or women.

Think back to the confounding triangle. The concern is that sex—an independent risk factor for many outcomes—may be associated with the exposure of interest. In this case, an apparent effect of exposure could actually be due to sex. However, if the entire sample consists of either men or women, then the effect of sex cannot be intermixed with the effect of any exposure: there is only 1 sex present. Restriction eliminates any association of exposure and the potential confounder (the left-hand side of the triangle), thereby eliminating any possibility of an intermixing of effects.

The main problem with restriction is that it may affect the applicability of the study results to the real world. After all, the world contains approximately 50% men and 50% women. Study results that derive from men only or women only have questionable applicability to the entire population.

RANDOMIZATION

In randomization, an investigator randomly assigns an exposure to the study participants and then looks for an effect.

Note that randomization is not the same as random selection of a sample—random selection of a sample is a different procedure and has nothing to do with the control of confounding.

Randomization can only be used in studies where investigators assign an exposure, such as a randomized controlled trial. And it is only possible when assigning an exposure is ethically feasible. It is not feasible to randomly assign study participants to harmful exposures, such as smoking. This would violate the ethical principle of nonmaleficence (see page 91). It is likewise unethical to not expose a research participant to a treatment known to be effective—this would amount to another form of maleficence. Generally speaking, the only exposures allowed for random assignment are treatments of uncertain efficacy. This situation—in which there is reason to hope a treatment may be helpful, but not enough evidence to endorse the treatment as helpful—is called *equipoise*. Equipoise is an ethical requirement for randomized controlled trials.

Why is randomization an effective means of controlling confounding? Refer again to the confounding triangle. Due to the law of large numbers, random assignment helps to ensure that the distribution of confounding variables is approximately equal in exposed and nonexposed groups. This eliminates the dotted line on the left-hand side of the triangle, and precludes the occurrence of confounding. Furthermore, the anticonfounding effect can be expected to work both for known and unknown, measured and unmeasured confounders. The law of large numbers distributes all variables with equal effectiveness. Randomization is the only procedure that can control confounders that are unmeasured or even unknown.

MATCHING

Matching ensures that groups being compared are exact matches in terms of the distribution of confounding variables.

Matching is a type of partial restriction: it does not prevent all subjects exposed to a confounder from participating in a study, but it places some restrictions on who can participate.

Like restriction and randomization, matching targets the left-hand side of the confounding triangle. It eliminates any association between the exposure and the matched confounding variables. This can be done at either the individual level (pair matching) or the group level (frequency matching).

In a prospective cohort study, pair matching involves selecting each member of the nonexposed cohort to have the same value of the confounding variable as a matched member of the exposed cohort. If sex is the target confounder in pair matching, here's what this means: for each exposed male a study selects, it also selects a nonexposed male, and for each exposed female, it also selects a nonexposed female.

In a case-control study, pair matching means that each case with exposure to the potential confounder—we'll use sex again—is matched with a control that has the same exposure to that variable. In other words, each male case would have a matched male control and each female case would have a matched female control.

Pair matching at the design stage has implications for the analysis stage (so, matching is regarded as a procedure that controls confounding both at the design and analysis stage). Normally, each observation in a data set is considered independent of the others and conventional statistics can be used in the analysis. When there has been pair matching, each member of a pair is related to the other member in the sense that they have been selected specifically because they share a characteristic. They are not independent, and special analysis techniques must be used to address this.

Key point: Three study design strategies can be used to address the issue of confounding: restriction, randomization, and matching. The last of these creates a requirement for specialized data-analysis procedures.

CONTROL OF CONFOUNDING AT THE DATA-ANALYSIS STAGE

There are 2 procedures to control confounding during data analysis: stratification and modelling. Both counteract the intermixing of effects that cause confounding using the same general approach: unmixing them.

STRATIFICATION

Stratification was introduced in chapter 9 in the context of descriptive studies and basic estimates, such as frequencies or rates (see page 98). Stratification is also commonly used in analytical studies. In analytical studies, it involves stratifying measures of association.

Stratified analysis divides the contingency tables arising from a study into groups (strata). The groups are defined by levels of the confounding variable. In the case of sex, this would mean dividing the data set from a study into sex-specific strata (1 stratum for men and 1 for women) and then examining the effect of exposure separately in each stratum. Since confounding is caused by intermixing, unmixing through stratification will lead to a change in the estimated effect if the unstratified (crude) estimate was distorted by confounding.

Within strata defined by sex, sex can no longer be a confounder (there can be no association on the left-hand arm of the confounding triangle). Therefore, the estimate for each stratum will reflect the effect of exposure and not the effect of exposure mixed with sex.

Stratified analysis leads to a set of adjusted estimates, called *stratum-specific estimates*. Stratum-specific estimates are adjusted for confounding. There is, of course, a drawback to this approach. Since stratum-specific estimates derive from a subset of the sample rather than the whole sample, they are subject to random error to a greater extent. In other words, they tend to be imprecise. Procedures are available to address this problem of imprecision.

REGRESSION MODELLING

Chapter 10 introduced the idea that information about an association could be represented in the form of a linear equation (see page 119). The value of this idea is that regression models based on linear equations have a very important role in the detection of, and adjustment for, confounding.

Regression models produce adjusted estimates. In general, they involve developing a best-fitting linear equation, or a transformed version of such a linear equation. Time-to-event or survival analysis methods are also used for this purpose.

Chapter 10 briefly explored representation of epidemiologic effects in linear models through the derivation of linear equations that basically reproduce the contents of a 2 × 2 table (see page XX). Using statistical software, it is possible to identify an equation of this form that accurately describes more complex data than that of a 2 × 2 table. These more elaborate linear models include not only the exposure of interest, but also potential confounding variables. The estimated effect in such a model (recall that the parameters in these models can be risk differences, log odds ratios, log prevalence ratios, etc.) is adjusted for the effect of the confounders included in the model.

Regression models can separate the independent effects of different variables, and are therefore helpful in identifying and adjusting for confounding effects.

Key point: Procedures to control confounding during data analysis include stratified analysis and regression modelling.

Strengths and weaknesses of procedures to control confounding

Restriction has the advantage of being easily understandable and can, in some instances, be an easy way to allay concerns about confounding. However, it has several disadvantages. The most important disadvantage is the degree of distortion it imposes on population relationships. It makes estimates of association free of the confounding effects of restricted variables, but the frequencies, risks, or rates observed may no longer reflect those of the target population. Restriction can also make it more difficult to find study subjects, since they must be determined to be free of the restricted characteristic. Finally, restriction has a negative effect on the generalizability of estimates (for more on generalizability, see page 174).

Key point: Restriction controls confounding, but at a high cost in terms of generalizability.

Randomization is widely viewed as the best procedure to control confounding due to its unique ability to address both measured and unmeasured confounding variables. Randomization, though, can only be employed in special situations: where equipoise exists. Most randomized controlled trials employ restriction in addition to randomization, and have long lists of inclusion and exclusion criteria to safeguard their internal validity. As in all cases of restriction, this can affect the generalizability of estimates.[125]

Key point: Randomization is the best way to control confounding, but it is often not practical or ethical to use.

Matching has several disadvantages: it distorts population relationships; it can be expensive and inefficient; and in situations where several potential confounders are being matched simultaneously, it can have severe impacts on recruitment into a study.

However, matching can sometimes be easy and inexpensive. And, when the variable at issue is a strong confounder, it can increase efficiency, leading to narrower confidence intervals around a measure of effect than would otherwise occur. Matching can also help control subtle, difficult-to-measure variables—a study can, for example, recruit matched subjects from the same neighbourhood to adjust for effects that can otherwise be difficult to measure (e.g., social standing, living environment). Stratification and modelling, by contrast, can only adjust for quantifiable variables.

Matching, however, should not be viewed as a default procedure for control of confounding: its disadvantages are significant. It is sometimes seen, incorrectly, as a default procedure by investigators who are unfamiliar or uncomfortable with statistical procedures (stratification and modelling).

Key point: Matching can control confounding and sometimes increase efficiency, but these advantages come at the cost of distortion of population estimates. Matching can also lead to operational complexities and extra expense.

Stratification and modelling are closely related procedures. Stratification is a foundational skill for epidemiologists, but in current research it mostly functions as a preliminary procedure for more advanced analysis using statistical models. When these models are encountered in the literature, they can be very complex and difficult to understand. For example, they may include many variables and it may not be clear which, if any, are actual confounders. The procedures for selecting variables to include in the model are often unclear as well. The motivation for presenting complex models is to report estimates that are simultaneously adjusted for many potential confounders, but this approach comes at the cost of diminished transparency. Stratified analysis is much more clear, but it is usually only possible to stratify on 1 or 2 extraneous variables at a time, so it takes a great deal of space to present stratified analyses for a variety of extraneous variables. The needed space often exceeds the limits of journals that publish studies.

Critical appraisal and common models to control confounding

Key models

General familiarity with a small number of modelling approaches is sufficient to critically appraise studies using these tools.

Linear regression models use linear equations to describe data. They predict the mean value of an outcome variable from several predictors included in the model's linear equation. Linear regression models are frequently encountered in the social science literature, where they are usually used to predict the mean value of a continuous variable. A frequency is a type of mean that is calculated from a variable that assumes values of 0 or 1, so it is not surprising that linear regression models are also used in epidemiology. The β coefficients in such models can be interpreted as differences. Depending on the type of frequency data, these may be prevalence differences or risk differences.

Log-transformed models have β coefficients that represent ratios. In logistic regression, the β coefficients are log odds ratios. In models fitting a log frequency rather than a log odds, the coefficients may be log prevalence ratios or log risk ratios, depending on the nature of the underlying data.

Other models produce coefficients that reflect rate ratios and hazard ratios (see page 156). In critical appraisal, the importance of these models is that they contain the exposure of interest as well as other (extraneous) variables.

In each of these approaches to modelling, the method for detecting confounding is the same. The procedure is to examine the parameter quantifying the association without any adjustment, and then to compare this to the estimate after adjustment. If adjustment results in a change of the estimated effect, then confounding has occurred.

An example study

A study by Modgill et al[126] provides an example of models to adjust for confounding. This study used data from the National Population Health Survey to examine the impact of migraine on depression incidence. The investigators used a type of survival analysis called a proportional hazards model and reported an unadjusted (or crude) hazard ratio of 2.1. When sex was included in the proportional hazard model, the hazard ratio (now a sex-adjusted hazard ratio) diminished to 1.9, indicating confounding by sex. Female sex is known to be associated with an elevated incidence of depression and also to be positively associated with migraine. Therefore confounding by sex is expected (see Figure 9). A component of the crude association between migraine and depression reflects that women are more susceptible to migraine and have a higher risk of depression. In the absence of adjustment, therefore, the effect of sex is intermixed with the effect of migraine.

The general approach to confounding is always the same, no matter the details of the mathematical and statistical models a study may employ. A crude estimate is calculated first. Then the estimate is adjusted for the potential confounder (in this case, the adjustment is based on a proportional hazards model and the potential confounder is sex). If the adjustment changes the estimated effect (if the adjusted estimate—a hazard ratio in this case—changes when the potential confounder is included in the model used in making the adjustment), then confounding has been demonstrated. In this study, the effect of migraine, independent of the effect of sex, is represented by the adjusted hazard ratio of 1.9.

Key point: Models detect confounding when they identify a change in the exposure-disease relationship on adjustment for a potential confounding variable.

The limits of models

In critical appraisal, it is important to remember that models can only handle variables that were measured, and only report on variables investigators included in the models. It is therefore important to ask not only whether a variable looks like a confounder in the analysis reported in a study, but also whether all of the most important potentially confounding variables were addressed at all.

Critical appraisal and generalizability

A study is internally valid if it produces unbiased estimates for its target population.

If it is internally valid, it may also be externally valid: its unbiased estimates might apply to other populations. *Generalizability* is another term for external validity.

Consider an epidemiological estimate from a US study. If the study has an adequate sample size (is not vulnerable to random error) and no study-design defects (these would introduce systematic error), the study can be viewed as internally valid. The question of whether the study could be considered valid in another country (e.g., Canada) is question of external validity or generalizability.

Many of the most important national surveys in Canada have used sampling frames that exclude homeless persons, members of the armed forces, residents of aboriginal settlements and remote areas, and residents of institutions. Are estimates arising from these surveys valid for these populations? This is a question of generalizability.

We have explored tools to assess whether bias and confounding have compromised a study's internal validity. Assessing a study's generalizability—its external validity—is different: it is purely a matter of judgement.

Judgements about generalizability that are too restrictive will result in "reinventing the wheel"—unnecessary confirmatory studies in different populations.

Judgements that are too cavalier can lead to actions harmful to public health.

Key point: Internal validity is a necessary but not sufficient condition for external validity.

Effect modification

Confounding is 1 way in which an extraneous variable can enter into epidemiological analyses. The other way is effect modification.

Effect modification, as the name implies, happens when an extraneous variable modifies the effect of the exposure of interest. Unlike confounding, effect modification is not an artifact that can (or should) be adjusted away or controlled. Instead, effect modification is a real aspect of the exposure-disease relationship under investigation.

When effect modification has occurred, there are multiple effects of exposure in different groups, and different measures of effect need to be reported separately.

An example of effect modification

Friedenreich et al[117] reported effect modification in a case-control study of metabolic syndrome and waist circumference as risk factors for endometrial cancer. Odds ratios in this analysis were stratified for menopausal status, creating 2 groups: pre/perimenopausal and postmenopausal. In the postmenopausal group, the odds ratio for metabolic syndrome as a risk factor for endometrial cancer was 1.61 and that for waist circumference ($\geq$ 88 cm) was 2.01. In the pre/perimenopausal group, stronger effects were seen: 1.96 and 2.98 for metabolic syndrome and waist circumference, respectively. Apparently, these exposures produce 2 sets of effects in the population: 1 in pre/perimenopausal women and 1 in postmenopausal women.

Stratification and homogeneous versus heterogeneous estimates

An important skill of epidemiologists is differentiating confounding and effect modification. Stratification is a very useful tool for doing this. After stratification for a confounder, you expect to see 2 stratum-specific (adjusted) estimates that are similar to each another, but different from the unadjusted (unstratified, or crude) measure of effect. If there is effect modification, the 2 stratum-specific estimates will be different from each another, as in the study by Friedenreich et al.

This distinction between similar and dissimilar stratum-specific estimates is key to the analysis of epidemiological data—so key that it has its own terminology. When 2 stratum-specific estimates are similar to each another, they are termed *homogeneous* (or you can say they display homogeneity). When they are different, they are termed *heterogeneous*.

STATISTICAL TESTS FOR HOMOGENEITY

Epidemiological analysis must always consider the role of chance. Saying that 2 estimates are homogeneous does not mean the estimates are exactly the same, but rather that chance can account for their differences.

Statistical tools can help determine whether 2 stratum-specific estimates are homogeneous. In stratified analysis, the Mantel-Haenszel test for homogeneity is commonly employed. In modelling, tests for statistical interaction between exposure and potentially modifying variables are often used. The model-based tests are called *tests of interaction*.

Key point: Effect modification is not a form of bias and cannot be addressed using statistical adjustments. This a real effect and should be reported through presentation of stratum-specific estimates.

Thinking deeper

"Cooking up" some confounding

The ingredients leading to confounding are well known (an independent risk factor associated with an exposure leading to intermixing of effects), but the concept can be difficult to grasp. To clarify how these ingredients produce confounding, let's "cook up" some confounding.

Many cake recipes tell you to mix ingredients in 2 separate bowls and combine them at a later stage. Our recipe for confounding uses the same approach, except the 2 bowls are 2 × 2 tables.

One of these tables depicts the exposure-disease association in the absence of an extraneous variable, and the other depicts the exposure-disease relationship in the presence an extraneous variable. Mixing these tables together is the opposite of stratified analysis, and pursued here for exclusively illustrative purposes. In stratified analysis, the starting point is a crude estimate of effect and stratification unmixes the variables that contribute to the effect.

Imagine an analysis of a sample of 1000 people. To simplify things, we'll ignore the issue of random error. Assume the following:

- The baseline risk of disease in a group not exposed to either the exposure variable—for clarity, let's call this the *target variable*—or the extraneous variable is 5%, or 0.05.
- The frequency of disease in a group that is exposed to the target variable but not to the extraneous variable is 10% or 0.10. (In other words, the target variable is associated with a doubling of risk.) This is the true effect of exposure: the effect that the analysis is seeking to estimate. In the presence of the extraneous variable, the effect of exposure is the same doubling of risk (meaning that we are "cooking up" confounding and are saying that there is no effect modification).
- Twenty percent of the population is exposed to the extraneous variable.

These assumptions allow us to predict what the 2 × 2 tables will look like.

One table will contain 800 people, since 80% of the sample is not exposed to the extraneous variable. The other table will contain the 200 people who are exposed to the extraneous variable.

The table with 800 people (the stratum not exposed to the extraneous variable) can be divided into disease and exposure contingencies based on the assumptions stated above. In this stratum, 10% ($n = 80$) will be exposed to the target variable. This means that there must be 720 in the nonexposed group within this stratum. There will also be 5% of this 720 ($n = 36$) who will have the disease ($720 \times 0.05 = 36$), leaving $n = 684$ who do not have the disease. Since exposure to the target variable is associated with a doubling of risk, there will be 10% of the remaining 80 ($n = 8$) who are expected to have the disease, leaving 72 of those with exposure who do not have the disease. The 2 × 2 table for this stratum—not exposed to the extraneous variable—will look like Table 30.

The other table comprises 200 people (the stratum exposed to the extraneous variable). Since confounding can only occur if the extraneous variable

TABLE 30. FIRST OF 2 STRATIFIED 2 × 2 TABLES: STRATUM NOT EXPOSED TO THE EXTRANEOUS VARIABLE

	Disease	No disease	Totals
Exposed	8	72	80
Nonexposed	36	684	720
Total			800

is an independent risk factor for the disease, and since our goal is to "cook up" confounding, it will be assumed that the extraneous variable is associated with a threefold increase in the risk of disease. The final ingredient for confounding is that the extraneous variable should be associated with exposure to the target variable. To fulfill this requirement, it will be assumed that exposure to the target variable is 3 times as common in the group exposed to the extraneous variable. At this stage, all of the ingredients needed to concoct the second 2 × 2 table have been assembled.

In the stratum exposed to the extraneous variable, we have assumed that exposure to the target variable is 3 times as common, so 30% of these subjects are exposed to the target variable. There will therefore be 60 (200 × 0.30) in the exposed group and 140 in the nonexposed group. In the subjects within this stratum who are not exposed to the target variable, the risk of disease will be 15%, because the risk of disease is 3 times higher due to the independent effects of the extraneous variable. You would then expect that $n = 21$ would develop the disease (140 × 0.15), leaving $n = 119$ in the no-disease group. In the exposed group, the risk is double this (30% instead of 15%) because there is a doubling of risk due to exposure. Since these are independent effects, the joint risk is therefore a sixfold elevation. This leads to an expectation that 18 (60 × 0.30) will have the disease. Consequently, 42 will not have the disease. The 2 × 2 table for this stratum—exposed to the extraneous variable—will look like Table 31.

Note that if an incidence proportion ratio is calculated from each table, the result is the same, an assumption that was built into these calculations:

Incidence Proportion Ratio (Stratum 1) = 0.10/0.05 = 2

Incidence Proportion Ratio (Stratum 2) = 0.30/0.15 = 2

TABLE 31. SECOND OF 2 STRATIFIED 2 × 2 TABLES: STRATUM EXPOSED TO THE EXTRANEOUS VARIABLE

	Disease	No disease	Totals
Exposed	18	42	60
Nonexposed	21	119	140
Total			200

TABLE 32. UNSTRATIFIED 2 × 2 TABLE*

	Disease	No disease	Totals
Exposed	26	114	140
Nonexposed	57	803	860
Total			1000

* formed by adding the values in each of the 4 cells in Table 30 and Table 31

But what if we mix the 2 × 2 tables for stratum 1 and stratum 2 by tossing them into the same 2 × 2 table? The result is presented in Table 32. Each cell of the separate 2 × 2 tables is simply added together to produce this.

If an incidence proportion ratio is calculated from this table, the result is 2.8! Even though the 2 stratified tables had the correct incidence proportion ratio of 2.0, adding them together and calculating the crude incidence proportion ratio results in an incorrect estimate. This is because the 2 × 2 tables were cooked up with all of the ingredients to produce confounding.

In real-world epidemiologic analysis, things would go the other way. Normally, the first calculation would be the crude incidence proportion ratio, which would then be stratified on the extraneous variable. The analyst would notice that the adjusted, stratum-specific, relative risks were similar to each other and that they were different from the crude—thereby identifying the occurrence of confounding.

If you enjoy this kind of methodological unpacking, you could take this exercise further by setting up a spreadsheet to make all these calculations. This would make the calculations less tedious and would allow you to explore numerous scenarios.

Questions

1. List 3 conditions that must be present for a variable to act as a confounding variable.

2. A case-control study by Weintraub et al[108] on the association between impulse-control disorders and dopamine-agonist exposure reported an unadjusted odds ratio of 2.72. To explore confounding effects, a multivariable logistic regression model was produced. This model contained age, marital status, smoking, family history of gambling problems, and levodopa treatment (as well as the exposure variable: dopamine-agonist use). The adjusted odds ratio from this model was 2.72.

   a. What was the β coefficient for dopamine-agonist use in the logistic regression model?

   b. What does this model have to say about the issue of confounding?

3. A case-control study by Hackam et al[109] examined the association between ACE inhibitors and rupture of aortic aneurisms. It reported an odds ratio of 0.82. After adjustment for demographic characteristics, risk factors for rupture,

comorbidities, contraindications to ACE inhibitors, health care use, and aneurism screening (in a logistic regression model), an adjusted estimate of 0.83 was found. What are the implications of this finding for confounding?

4. A case-control study by Rothwell et al[111] examined chiropractic manipulation as a risk factor for stroke. It found a significant association in those younger than 45, but not in older subjects.

   a. Is this an example of confounding?
   b. How should this result be reported?

5. Depression may be a risk factor for mortality. This condition is more common in young people who are, of course, less likely to die than older people. A Canadian study using data from the National Population Health Survey found an unadjusted hazard ratio of 1.0, suggesting no association of depression and mortality. However, with adjustment for age and sex, the hazard ratio doubled.[127]

   a. How can you explain this effect?
   b. When adjusted for other variables that may predict mortality (such as smoking), the association of depression with mortality again disappeared. Can this be explained in terms of confounding?

15

Stratified analysis and regression modelling in analytical studies

Objectives

- Explain the key importance of analysis-stage techniques to control confounding.
- Describe the following aspects of stratified analysis: fit with noncontinuous variables; pooling of estimates for better precision; identification of effect modification; and detection and adjustment for confounding variables.
- List the steps of stratified analysis.
- Describe the advantages of regression modelling over stratified analysis.
- List the steps of regression modelling.

The context for a deeper discussion of stratified analysis and regression modelling

Chapter 14 looked at design-stage and analysis-stage techniques to control confounding, and discussed them in the context of categorical variables, such as sex.

This chapter looks at analysis-stage techniques—stratified analysis and regression modelling—in more detail, and in the context of continuous variables, such as age.

Why provide a deeper discussion of stratified analysis and regression modelling? These techniques play a role in almost every analytical study, even in studies that have also used design-stage techniques to control confounding.

If you want to understand most of the empirical studies published in the clinical and public health literature, you need to understand the goals and strategies of stratified analysis and regression modelling.

Why do studies use design- and analysis-stage techniques to control confounding?

Design-stage techniques to minimize confounding include randomization, restriction, and matching (see pages 167–169). None of them are foolproof (and not all studies use them). So, analysis-stage techniques—stratified analysis and regression modelling—add confidence to conclusions about exposure-disease associations.

Randomization aims to ensure an equal distribution of all confounders, whether measured or unmeasured, between the groups in a study. This strategy even diminishes the effects of unknown confounders. It is the best way to control confounding, when it is feasible. However, it is not always completely effective. An unbalanced distribution of a confounding variable may occur by chance during randomization. This is unlikely, particularly if the sample size is large, but poses problems if it does occur. For these reasons, randomized studies usually strive to measure all potential confounding variables, so that confounding can be detected and appropriate adjustments can be made through stratification and/or modelling, if necessary.

Key point: Randomization is the best way to control for confounding (when feasible), but it is not foolproof.

Detection of, and adjustment for, confounding remain important in the other design-stage strategies, too.

Restriction eliminates extraneous variables by restricting who can participate in a study. A restricted (eliminated) variable cannot be a confounding variable. However, other variables in a restricted study could still confound exposure-disease associations.

Matching eliminates the effect of extraneous variables by balancing their presence in the groups a study compares. Matched variables cannot act as confounders. However, again, other variables can continue to confound results.

Stratified analysis

The principle underlying the use of stratification is straightforward. Confounding is an intermixing of the effects of an exposure with those of an extraneous variable. The goal of stratification is to unmix these effects.

Stratified analysis and categorical variables

Let's review sex as a confounding variable. If sex is a confounder, conducting the analysis separately in men and women will unmix the effect of an exposure from the effect of sex. An independent effect of sex can no longer be mixed up with effects of exposure if the effect of exposure is examined separately in men and women.

Procedures used to control confounding must also be capable of detecting confounding. (After all, there is no need to control confounding that does not exist.) A popular definition of confounding posits that the detection and control of confounding are related. This definition states that confounding occurs when an appropriate adjustment for confounding leads to a change in the estimated effect. Stratification unveils confounding when it leads to stratum-specific estimates that are different from the crude estimate and similar to each another. When an estimate is stratified (into 2 or more estimates), the stratified estimates are a type of adjusted estimate. If they differ from the unadjusted estimate and are similar to each another, then the occurrence of confounding has been demonstrated through stratification.

With sex as a possible confounding variable, stratification would involve: dividing the sample into male and female strata; calculating the stratum-specific estimates; and comparing the stratum-specific estimates first to themselves and then to the crude estimate. This procedure—stratification for sex—figures frequently in analytical studies, because sex is a risk factor for many health problems, potentially associated with many exposures, and usually viewed as an extraneous variable since it is not modifiable. For example, Vinceti et al[128] used a case-control study to examine whether elevated levels of inorganic selenium in drinking water was a risk factor amyotrophic lateral sclerosis in a region of Italy. They reported a crude odds ratio of 4.2, which was found to be 4.3 in males and 4.0 in females. As the stratified estimates resemble each other and also resemble the crude estimate, this stratified analysis shows that sex does not confound the reported association.

Key point: Stratified analysis is used to identify confounding variables and to adjust for their confounding effects.

Stratified analysis and continuous variables

To stratify for a continuous variable, such as age, you begin by creating age categories, and then examine the association within the resulting strata.

There are some practical considerations involved in creating categories for continuous variables. Recall that, to detect confounding, you need to determine that the stratum-specific estimates differ from the crude estimate, yet resemble each other.

If there are too many strata, the number of study participants in each stratum will be small and subject to random variation. As a result, if the study sample is divided into too many strata (e.g., age categories), stratum-specific estimates show wide variation simply due to chance. This can make it very difficult to detect whether effect modification or confounding has occurred.

If strata are too large, another problem arises. In the case of age, larger strata will contain more observations, but there may also be a larger variation of age within each stratum. For example, 5-year age strata may be too narrow to provide decisive evidence of confounding, but 25-year age strata may be too broad because age can vary so much within each stratum. The variation in age within broad strata increases the possibility that confounding effects occur within these strata (broad strata fail to fully control the confounding). A failure to fully adjust for the effect of a confounding variable due to excessively broad strata is called *residual confounding*.

Where continuous variables are potential confounders, stratified analysis must walk a fine line between the problems of residual confounding (when strata are too broad), and random variation of the stratified estimates (when strata are too narrow). This difficult reality means studies prefer modelling over stratified analysis, and almost all published studies now emphasize the use of models. Even so, it is important to be aware of stratified analysis: studies still use it even if they report it less and less frequently.

Stratum-specific estimates and pooling

Stratification breaks down a crude estimate into a series of stratum-specific estimates. These stratum-specific estimates are then adjusted for confounding. But because they are based on subsets of the larger sample, stratum-specific estimates are often imprecise. Precision is important, so techniques have been developed to pool these stratified estimates in a way that preserves control over confounding.

The parameter classically used for this purpose is the Mantel-Haenszel family of estimators. These pooled estimators can be easily calculated across a series of strata. The family includes pooled versions of the risk difference, risk ratio, rate ratio, and odds ratio.

Pooled estimates are only meaningful if the stratum-specific estimates comprise a single underlying effect. Such consistency of effect across strata is called *homogeneity*. A lack of homogeneity—heterogeneity—implies that there are different effects of exposure in different strata—in other words, effect modification (see page 174). Effect modification makes pooling inappropriate.

Key point: While stratification typically results in a major loss of precision of stratum-specific estimates, much of the precision can be regained through pooling procedures. However, pooling should not occur in the presence of heterogeneity. Pooling is a procedure for achieving greater precision while controlling for confounding, whereas heterogeneity suggests effect modification.

The steps of stratified analysis in summary

Stratified analysis follows a classic series of steps.

First, you estimate a crude effect using a risk difference, risk ratio, odds ratio, hazard ratio, or other parameter.

Next, you examine the association within strata formed by levels of the potential confounding variable.

Then, you assess whether the resulting estimates are similar to each another (exhibit homogeneity)—you could do this with a statistical test for homogeneity.

If the estimates are dissimilar (heterogeneous), effect modification has been identified.

If they are similar (homogeneous), you assess whether they differ from the crude estimate. If they do differ, then confounding has been demonstrated. At this stage, you should report an adjusted estimate of effect, such as 1 of the Mantel-Haenszel family of parameters. If the estimates do not differ from the crude estimate, then there was no confounding and it is not necessary to report an adjusted estimate. The crude estimate is good enough.

A STEP-BY-STEP EXAMPLE OF STRATIFIED ANALYSIS

A classic example of confounding from the history of epidemiology is an investigation of Down syndrome published in 1966 by Stark and Mantel.[129]

A component of this work, which was conducted in the state of Michigan, explored the relationship between birth order and Down syndrome.

The study made a detailed tabulation of the data. The data table cross-referenced:

- birth order: first, second, third, fourth, or fifth and above
- maternal age: < 20, 20–24, 25–29, 30–34, 35–39 and 40+
- number of births with Down syndrome and the total births in the population

Dividing the exposure variable (birth order) into 2 categories for reasons of simplicity leads to the 2 × 2 table shown in Table 33.

A crude odds ratio calculated from this table is 1.86 (95% CI 1.71–2.02), suggesting that higher birth order is positively associated with this outcome. However, there is the possibility of confounding by maternal age. Table 34 shows the odds ratios for birth order calculated within each of the 6 strata for maternal age.

TABLE 33. BIRTH ORDER AND DOWN SYNDROME

	Down syndrome	No Down syndrome
Birth order (third or more)	1547	1 328 554
Birth order (first or second)	877	1 400 752

TABLE 34. ODDS RATIOS FOR BIRTH ORDER STRATIFIED BY 6 RANGES FOR MATERNAL AGE

Maternal age category	Odds ratio	95% CI
< 20	0.66	0.21–1.59
20–24	0.85	0.67–1.07
25–29	0.97	0.79–1.20
30–34	0.80	0.65–1.00
35–39	0.89	0.72–1.10
40+	0.90	0.69–1.20

None of the 6 stratum-specific estimates suggest that birth order is associated with increased odds of Down syndrome. The elevated crude odds ratio was evidently due to an intermixing of the effect of maternal age with birth order.

However, the possibility of heterogeneity in these stratum-specific effects has not yet been addressed. With application of the Mantel-Haenszel test for heterogeneity, the result is nonsignificant ($P = 0.82$: a P value of 0.05 is most often used for rejecting the hypothesis of homogeneity). A final step would be to calculate a pooled odds ratio—the Mantel-Haenszel combined odds ratio—to regain precision of the adjusted estimate. The value for this odds ratio is 0.88 and the 95% CI is 0.80–0.97.

This example shows very strong confounding effects. The direction of estimated effect changes with adjustment for maternal age from a crude odds ratio of 1.85 to an adjusted one of 0.88. Such effect reversals due to strong confounding are examples of the so-called Simpson's paradox.[130]

Effect modification in stratified analysis

The pooling strategies employed in classic stratified analysis are predicated on the presence of a single effect of exposure in different strata after stratification for an extraneous variable. If this is not the case—if the stratum-specific estimates are not homogeneous—then something other than confounding is at play.

If the stratum-specific estimates are different to an extent that cannot reasonably be attributed to chance, this means that they are actually providing evidence of differing effects of the exposure in the different strata. Such heterogeneity of effect indicates effect modification. In other words, the effect of exposure is modified by the effect of the extraneous variable.

Key point: Effect modification is distinct from confounding, both conceptually and in the way it appears during data analysis.

The occurrence of effect modification precludes any assessment of confounding. Recall that confounding can be defined according to whether some form of adjustment alters the effect of exposure. If there is effect modification, there is no longer a single effect of exposure on which to make such a determination. The demonstration that effect modification exists confirms that there is more than 1 effect of exposure. For an extraneous variable such as sex, effect modification would imply that the effect of exposure differs between men and women.

AN EXAMPLE OF EFFECT MODIFICATION IN STRATIFIED ANALYSIS

Tjepkema et al[131] used data from the Canadian census mortality and cancer follow-up study (1991 to 2006) to explore the association between socioeconomic indicators and both all-cause and cause-specific mortality.

When they looked at all-cause mortality, the hazard ratio associated with less-than-high-school education was 2.16 (95% CI 1.95–2.39) in their youngest age stratum (25–34), whereas it was only 1.52 (95% CI 1.46–1.59) in the oldest (55–64) age stratum. This suggests effect modification by age: the effect of low education on all-cause mortality is modified by age.

The 2 intermediate age strata had intermediate hazard ratios, suggesting that the effect declined across the studied age range.

It would be a mistake to obscure this kind of relationship by averaging the hazard ratio across these age strata. The authors appropriately presented the stratified estimates.

Unlike confounding, which is an artifact that can be corrected by adjustment, effect modification is something real, not to be hidden or minimized. Effect modification often has implications for public health and clinical practice.

For example, think back to the study that reported stroke as an adverse outcome following chiropractic manipulation (see page 133).[111] This study found a significant effect, but only in those younger than 45. If this study led to clinical recommendations, the recommendations might apply only to the specific age groups where an association occurred.

Another example comes from the study by Friedenreich et al[117] (see page 174) investigating the association of metabolic syndrome and waist circumference with endometrial cancer. This study found a stronger association in pre- or perimenopausal women as compared to postmenopausal women (effect modification by menopausal status). This finding may have implications for priority setting, or in the development of clinical interventions and guidelines.

Key point: Effect modification is a real effect that should be described when it occurs. There is no basis for attempting to control or adjust for effect modification, which is a real effect rather than an artifact.

A NOTE ABOUT TERMINOLOGY: EFFECT MEASURE MODIFICATION

So far, we have used *effect modification* to describe the situation where an extraneous variable changes the strength of an exposure-disease association, manifesting as heterogeneity across strata.

The simplicity of this term is appealing, but it has a weakness.

Consider this hypothetical example. Imagine a stratified analysis with 2 strata. One stratum has a risk of 6% in its exposed group and 2% in its nonexposed group. The other stratum has a risk of 20% in its exposed group and 16% in its nonexposed group. An analysis based on risk differences would conclude that there is no effect modification, since the risk difference in each stratum is 4%. By contrast, a study using risk ratios would find a risk ratio of 3 in the first stratum and 1.25 in the second, strongly suggesting heterogeneity of effect.

So, the determination of whether an effect is modified often depends on the measure of effect used in the analysis—a stratified analysis based on the risk difference might uncover heterogeneity where a ratio-based measure of association would not, and vice versa.

For this reason, many epidemiologists prefer the term *effect measure modification* over the simpler, but less precise, *effect modification*.

Regression models

Chapter 10 introduced regression models in the form of linear equations with or without a log transformation (see pages 119–120). You can use statistical software to identify the equations that best fit an epidemiological data set. These statistical models are very useful for identification of confounding and effect measure modification.

Advantages of regression models

Regression modelling assists with some of the difficulties that arise in stratified analysis.

Regression models deal more effectively with the sparse-data problems that afflict stratified analysis. They are more capable of simultaneously controlling for multiple confounding variables and joint confounding (where several variables act together to produce confounding).

They also deal better with continuous variables, such as age. In stratification, continuous variables must be broken down, often arbitrarily, into categories. Regression modelling can often work with them directly, as continuous variables. This allows a more sophisticated assessment of effect measure modification and confounding while avoiding residual confounding.

Key point: A key advantage of regression modelling over stratified analysis is that continuous variables can be included in the model, and thereby adjusted for, without the necessity of imposing artificial categories onto ranges of continuous variables.

The steps of regression modelling

The steps for stratified analysis also apply to regression modelling.

The purpose of presenting these steps is to outline analytical strategies involved in statistical modelling, so that you can better interpret analyses reported in published studies. The purpose is not to demonstrate how to conduct analyses using statistical models—something that requires advanced training. In addition, the approach to modelling described here may differ from what you have encountered in other fields of study. Epidemiology emphasizes the use of statistical models as tools for handling the issues of effect measure modification and confounding. Other areas of research emphasize the use and development of statistical models to predict outcomes or explain variability in outcomes—a topic not discussed in this chapter, because it plays a smaller role in epidemiological modelling.

In regression modelling, you usually begin by making an estimate of the crude measure of association. This is done using a statistical model that includes only 1 variable: the exposure. Chapter 10 covered this kind of model (see page 120). Here, for example, is a model of the logistic form from chapter 10:

$$\text{Log Odds} = \alpha + \beta X_e$$

where X_e is an indicator variable for exposure with a value of 1 or 0

This model describes a log odds of α for the nonexposed (where $X_e = 0$) and a log odds of $\alpha + \beta$ for the exposed (where $X_e = 1$). In this type of model (since it predicts the log odds, it is a logistic regression model), β is a log odds ratio—so, you can use this kind of model to calculate the crude estimate.

Next, you use a model to assess the possibility of effect measure modification. This kind of model has 3 terms: the exposure variable, the extraneous variable, and a term that represents exposure both to the exposure variable and the extraneous variable—something called an *interaction term*. Here's the example from chapter 10 with these additional terms:

$$\text{Log Odds} = \alpha + \beta_e X_e + \beta_c X_c + \beta_i X_i$$

where X_e is an indicator variable for exposure, X_c is an indicator variable for the extraneous variable (a potential confounder or modifier), and X_i is an indicator variable for joint exposure (interaction) to X_e and X_c

Interaction terms serve the same purpose as the statistical tests for homogeneity routinely employed in stratified analysis. Where the variables are binary—for example with a value of 1 representing exposure to the exposure variable or the extraneous variable, and 0 representing nonexposure—interaction terms are calculated by multiplying the indicator variables together. As a result, interaction terms are often called *cross-product terms*. The significance of such a term (a significant interaction) is the model-based equivalent of heterogeneity. Statistical software produces the β parameters in such models and also evaluates their statistical significance. Note that the same strategy of multiplying the 2 variables is used when the extraneous variable is a continuous variable, such as age.

If effect measure modification is identified, you report stratum-specific estimates.

If there is no effect measure modification, you should assess for confounding.

To assess for confounding, the model is regenerated without the interaction term. The output will be of the form:

$$\text{Log Odds} = \alpha + \beta_e X_e + \beta_c X_c$$

Now that X_c is in the model, β_e is adjusted for its effects—it is adjusted for confounding. If β_e from this type of model is different than β_e from a model that did not include the interaction term, there is confounding. In this specific type of model—a logistic regression model—the inverse logarithm of β_e (from a model containing a term for the confounding variable) provides an odds ratio for the exposure that is adjusted for the effect of the confounding variable. In assessing for confounding, the unadjusted and adjusted odds ratios are easier to compare than the β coefficients from models. If there is no confounding, an adjusted estimate does not need to be reported: the unadjusted estimate is appropriate to report.

TWO STEP-BY-STEP EXAMPLES
Let's return to the study of Down syndrome by Stark and Mantel.[129]

A logistic regression model containing no extraneous variable or interaction terms has an α coefficient of −7.4 and a β coefficient (for being third or higher in the birth order) of 0.62. Recall that in an equation this type, the β coefficient is a log odds ratio (see page 120). Taking the inverse log of this value yields the same odds ratio seen in the tabular analysis: exp(0.62) = 1.86.

Testing for interactions—by adding terms for maternal age and the relevant cross-product terms (the test was performed in this case using a likelihood ratio test)—finds no significant interactions: $P = 0.82$. Note the similarity of this value to that arising from the Mantel-Haenszel test for homogeneity in the stratified analysis.

As there is no evidence of effect measure modification, the next step is to determine an adjusted estimate using a model that includes the birth order variable and the maternal age indicators. Since there is homogeneity, the interaction term can be removed. The β coefficient for the birth-order variable in this model is −0.13, indicating an odds ratio of 0.88, the same as the Mantel-Haenszel combined odds ratio from the stratified analysis.

Key point: Regression modelling, as it is applied in epidemiology, is not fundamentally different from stratified analysis, either in terms of the logic that it follows or the purposes for which it is applied.

Here's another example, from a study covered in chapter 14 (see page 173). Modgill et al[126] investigated whether migraine increased the incidence of major depression using data from the Canadian National Population Health Survey. The investigators used a time-to-event analysis and therefore estimated hazard ratios. A hazard ratio from a model containing no extraneous variables was 2.1. No significant interactions between migraine and age or sex were found. However, when age and sex were included in the model, the effect of migraine diminished to 1.9, a change that provided evidence of confounding. In a model adjusting for sex alone, the adjusted hazard ratio was 1.9, suggesting that sex was the main confounder. This finding was not unexpected, because more women than men have migraine and female sex is a risk factor for depression.

Other examples of studies using regression models

Cheng et al[132] conducted a case-control study of the association between diabetes and colorectal cancer. These investigators identified several genetic variants associated with colorectal cancer risk. When they included these variables in a logistic regression model, they found that the odds ratio for diabetes diminished from 1.2 to 1.15, which (despite being a small change) was interpreted as evidence that the genetic variants confound the relationship between diabetes status and colorectal cancer risk.

Another case-control study evaluated the role of benfluorex (a psychostimulant derivative) as a risk factor for otherwise unexplained valvular heart disease.[133] The study found the crude odds ratio was huge: 40.4. No interactions with extraneous variables were identified during logistic regression analysis. With inclusion of body mass index and diabetes in the logistic regression model, the odds ratio was unchanged, indicating that its elevation was not an artifact due to confounding by these variables.

Critical appraisal and regression models

In critical appraisal, you need to be able to understand analyses that present modelling results to discern whether the data collected in a study advances the state of knowledge about an exposure-disease association.

The most common models encountered in the epidemiological literature are, like logistic regression, based on linear equations.

Models use different transformations so that their parameters reflect different types of epidemiological estimates. Models are available to adjust estimates of incidence rate ratios, risk ratios (including incidence proportion ratios and prevalence ratios), risk differences, hazard ratios, and odds ratios. They produce adjusted estimates when extraneous variables are added.

Thinking deeper

Regression analysis without a log transformation

Let's revisit a scenario from chapter 10.

In this scenario, there is a binary exposure variable (with 1 representing exposure and 0 representing nonexposure) and there is an extraneous variable coded in the same way (1 meaning exposed to it and 0 meaning not exposed to it).

A linear form of an equation including only an exposure and outcome, and without a log transformation—something like the basic unadjusted, or crude, 2 × 2 table of classic analysis—is as follows:

$$\text{Risk of Disease} = \alpha + \beta_e X_e$$

where X_e is an indicator variable for exposure and β_e is a risk difference associated with exposure

The fact that β_e is a risk difference indicates that this is not a log-transformed model. In other words, when a subject is not exposed ($X_e = 0$), the term on the right-hand side of this equation disappears and the risk of disease in the nonexposed is represented by α. When a subject is exposed ($X_e = 1$), the risk of disease is modelled as $\alpha + \beta_e$.

To say "β is a risk difference" alludes to the reality that the modelled risk in the exposed subjects minus the modelled risk in nonexposed subjects is $\alpha + \beta - \alpha = \beta$. Since the equation above takes a linear form, it would also be reasonable to regard β as a slope term: it is the change in risk of disease that occurs with each unit of exposure. In this scenario, there is only 1 unit of exposure since the exposure here is treated as a binary variable.

This revisited scenario is relatively simple. What if we add an extraneous variable?

This new variable produces a slightly expanded linear equation:

$$\text{Risk of Disease} = \alpha + \beta_e X_e + \beta_c X_c$$

where X_e is an indicator variable for exposure, β_e is a risk difference associated with exposure, β_c is a risk difference associated with the potential confounder, and X_c is an indicator variable for exposure to the confounding variable

In this equation, X_c has a value of 0 or 1 depending on exposure to the potential confounding variable.

The logic of stratified analysis points to a problem with this equation. The risk of disease in those not exposed to the confounder and also not exposed to the risk factor is modelled as α, since all of the other terms reduce to 0 in this scenario. When the risk factor is present but not the potential confounder, the risk of disease is modelled as $\alpha + \beta_e$. When there is exposure to the potential confounder but not exposure to the risk factor, the risk of disease is modelled $\alpha + \beta_c$. Finally, among those exposed both to the risk factor and the potential confounder, the risk is modelled $\alpha + \beta_e + \beta_c$.

This yields Table 35—a sort of parallel to the situation in which a 2 × 2 table is stratified according to the presence or absence of a confounding variable.

Each of the 4 risks of disease depicted in the far-right column of Table 35 would be predicted by the linear equations shown in Table 36.

TABLE 35. TWO STRATIFIED TABLES

		Disease	No disease	Risk of disease*
Stratum 1 (not exposed to the potential confounder)	Exposed	a	b	a / (a + b)
	Not exposed	c	d	c / (c + d)
Stratum 2 (exposed to the potential confounder)	Exposed	e	f	e / (e + f)
	Not exposed	g	h	g / (g + h)

*The term *risk* assumes that the study design is capable of determining risk.

TABLE 36. LINEAR EQUATIONS FOR THE RISKS DEPICTED IN TABLE 35

		Risk of disease*	Linear predictions*
Stratum 1 (not exposed to the potential confounder)	Exposed to risk factor	a / (a + b)	$\alpha + \beta_e$
	Not exposed to risk factor	c / (c + d)	α
Stratum 2 (exposed to the potential confounder)	Exposed to risk factor	e / (e + f)	$\alpha + \beta_e + \beta_c$
	Not exposed to risk factor	g / (g + h)	$\alpha + \beta_c$

*where risk of disease = $\alpha + \beta_e X_e + \beta_c X_c$

In a stratified analysis, you would begin by calculating a measure of effect—say, the risk difference for the stratum not exposed to the confounder. However, the modelled values for the 2 risk differences here are the same:

$$\text{Risk Difference (Stratum 1)} = \alpha + \beta_e - \alpha = \beta_e$$

$$\text{Risk Difference (Stratum 2)} = \alpha + \beta_e + \beta_c - \alpha + \beta_c = \beta_e$$

This means that the linear equation as stated above equates to a stratified 2×2 table analysis, but it does so with a constraint. The equation constrains the value of the risk difference to a single value—β_e—in both the stratum with exposure to the confounding variable and the stratum without.

So, the problem lies with the assumption that the 2 risk differences are homogeneous. They should certainly not be constrained to be identical, if they are in fact heterogeneous. The question of heterogeneity is an empirical question that must be answered. This means that there must be a different starting point that is able to accommodate the possibility of effect measure modification.

The solution is a cross-product interaction term. Such a term should be included early in the determination of whether interaction between the exposure and the potential confounding variable exists. This term is denoted i for *interaction*.

Adding this variable—X_i—and its estimated coefficient from the model—β_i—leads to the following expanded linear equation:

$$\text{Risk of Disease} = \alpha + \beta_e X_e + \beta_c X_c + \beta_i X_i$$

where X_e is an indicator variable for exposure, β_e is a risk difference associated with exposure, β_c is a risk difference for a confounding variable, X_c is an indicator variable for exposure to the confounding variable, β_i is the risk difference between the joint exposures and the sum of their effects, and X_i is an indicator of the joint exposure

This equation predicts each of the 4 risks of disease depicted in the far-right column of Table 37.

The 2 risk differences can now be different. The risk difference for stratum 1 has not changed: it is still β_e. However, the risk different for stratum 2 is now $\beta_e + \beta_i$.

This expanded model that includes an interaction term, therefore, can incorporate an assessment of whether the interaction term is important. If the interaction term is important, then $\beta_e + \beta_i$ will be different than β_e.

The test for statistical significance of the interaction term is a way of operationalizing this question, similar to the Mantel-Haenszel test for heterogeneity

TABLE 37. LINEAR EQUATIONS FOR THE RISKS DEPICTED IN TABLE 35: INTERACTION TERM INCLUDED

		Risk of disease	Linear predictions*
Stratum 1 (not exposed to the potential confounder)	Exposed to risk factor	a / (a + b)	$\alpha + \beta_e$
	Not exposed to risk factor	c / (c + d)	α
Stratum 2 (exposed to the potential confounder)	Exposed to risk factor	e / (e + f)	$\alpha + \beta_e + \beta_c + \beta_i$
	Not exposed to risk factor	g / (g + h)	$\alpha + \beta_c$

*where risk of disease $= \alpha + \beta_e X_e + \beta_c X_c + \beta_i X_i$

in stratified analysis. If β_i is determined not to be important, then the more basic model—including a single term for β_e, as summarized in Table 36—is sufficient. Furthermore, the risk difference from this model (β_e) is adjusted for the effect of the potential confounder, because the linear equation includes β_c.

The next step, assuming the interaction term is not significant in the model, would be to determine whether the inclusion of β_c results in a change to β_e. This amounts to an assessment of whether there is confounding.

Questions

1. Ideally, studies should measure all potential confounding variables. This allows confounding to be detected during data analysis. How can this be done? What principles are applicable to the challenge of identifying all potential confounding variables?

2. Jadidi et al[134] were interested in whether there might be an elevated risk of cardiovascular disease after a diagnosis of multiple sclerosis (MS). To address this question, they conducted a retrospective cohort study using linked Swedish databases (an inpatient register, a total-population register, and a cause-of-death register). They identified 8281 people admitted to hospital with MS between 1987 and 2009. They also selected a control cohort of 76 640 patients, matched for sex and date of birth, who did not have MS at the time of MS diagnosis in their matched case. An elevated incidence rate ratio (IRR) was identified for stroke (IRR: 1.7). Subsequently, the IRR was stratified by sex. The stratified estimates for men (IRR: 1.6) and women (IRR: 1.7) remained similar to each another and were also similar to the crude estimate. Keeping in mind that sex is associated with MS (this disease occurs more often in women), state a possible explanation for the lack of confounding.

3. In the Jadidi et al study, the IRR for heart failure, unstratified by sex, was 2.0 (rounded here from the reported value of 1.98). Upon stratification, this was found to be 1.4 in men and 2.3 in women. Does this provide evidence of confounding?

4. List examples of the advantages of modelling over stratified analysis.

5. Do you think that stratified analysis still has a role in epidemiology?

Other study designs

Objectives

- Describe important features of the following study designs: nested case-control studies, case-crossover studies, retrospective cohort studies, randomized controlled trials, case-cohort studies, and ecological studies.
- Discuss advantages and disadvantages of these designs over other designs.

Study designs so far

So far, we have covered the "classic" epidemiologic study designs: cross-sectional studies, case-control studies, and prospective cohort studies.

This chapter looks at other common study designs in epidemiology.

It's important to know these. Identification of study design—through identifying a study's key features—is an early step in the process of critical appraisal: it begins the process of thinking through a study's vulnerability to error.

> *Key point:* Classification of study design is an important step in critical appraisal. While classification does not say anything definitive about the validity of a study, it helps to organize information about the study and to focus critical appraisal on likely vulnerabilities.

Nested case-control studies

Nested case-control studies are not very different from classic case-control studies. They have a special name because of the way they are conducted.

A nested case-control study is a case-control study situated within a prospective cohort study.

To review: case-control studies have a backward logical direction of inquiry (they start with the selection of cases—effects rather than causes) and a backward temporal direction (they assess past exposures). The case-control design is vulnerable to selection bias, and the appropriate selection of cases and controls is often difficult.

Sometimes, a prospective cohort study provides an excellent framework to facilitate valid case-control studies. In these situations, there is a cohort being followed prospectively. This cohort generates cases and potential controls. This provides a well-defined source population from which cases and controls both arise, and a strong context for conducting a case-control study. For example, whenever a case occurs, a control can be selected from among the cohort members who do not have the disease at that point in time (the risk set), providing a firm procedure for control selection.

Key point: A nested case-control study is an ideal kind of case-control study because the source population for the cases and controls is well defined.

A nested case-control study often addresses a research question not posed at the beginning of its "host" prospective cohort study. The exposure variable at issue for the nested study may therefore not have been measured at the time of selection into the prospective cohort study. A nested case-control study can obtain these extra exposure measurements by assessing exposure in the case group and in a sample of the noncase group (controls). By assessing a sample of the noncase group—instead of the entire noncase cohort—the nested case-control approach applies the familiar efficiency of the case-control design in general: samples of controls generally provide comparable precision whether they are smaller (3 or 4 controls for every case) as when they are larger (10 or 20 controls, or more, for every case).

Nested case-control studies have other advantages over classic case-control studies. They can make selection of cases and controls easier, because the cohort is being actively followed and is presumably strongly engaged in research. They can achieve high response rates: in some prospective cohort studies, participants provide consent to be contacted for related studies. They can benefit from work already done by the host study, which may have already measured many relevant confounding or effect-modifying variables. They may find it easier to ensure that cases are incident cases, because of close follow-up in the host study—this leads to greater clarity of the temporal relationship between exposure and disease.

Verhave et al[135] studied the risk of thromboembolism in a cohort of 913 renal transplant patients. They observed an increased risk of thromboembolism relative to the general population (as assessed using Quebec administrative databases). To investigate the determinants of this increased risk, they nested a case-control study within their cohort of renal transplant patients. They used all 68 members of the cohort who had experienced thromboembolism (cases), and a matched group of 260 cohort members free of thromboembolism (controls). The nested study required that the controls were alive at the time of the thromboembolic event in their corresponding matched case. The investigators calculated univariate odds ratios and conducted a multivariable analysis using a form of logistic regression that accounted for the matching (conditional logistic regression). The study found that increased risk of thromboembolism was associated with low hemoglobin levels, use of sirolimus (a drug used to prevent rejection), and hospitalization. It found lower risk was associated with use of drugs inhibiting the renin-angiotensin system.

Case-crossover studies

Case-crossover studies are another variant of case-control studies.

Like case-control studies, they have a backward logical direction of inquiry. The investigation begins with the identification of a series of cases and then (this is the logically backward part) assesses exposure.

Unlike case-control studies, case-crossover studies use the same people for cases and controls.

The focus of a case-crossover study is the timing of exposure. Instead of comparing a group with disease to a group without the disease, a case-crossover study assesses the frequency of exposure in the cases immediately before the onset of disease, and compares this to another time when the same people did not develop the disease. In this sense, these studies also have a retrospective temporal direction. The underlying logic is this: if an exposure precipitates disease, that exposure should occur more frequently during the interval before disease onset than during some other interval when disease did not occur.

The case-crossover design is used to study outcomes that rapidly, and typically temporarily, follow exposure—for example, the transient risks that follow alcohol consumption.[136]

Key point: Case-crossover studies are a case-control variant that emphasize the timing of exposures within people, rather than the differences in the frequency of exposure between groups of people.

In a classic case-control study, the cases and controls are different people and the observations made by the investigators of the frequencies of exposure in cases and controls are independent observations. In situations where they are not independent, such as when pair-matching has been implemented, different methods of analysis are required to account for this (e.g., conditional logistic regression). In some ways, the case-crossover design is the ultimate form of matching. Because the comparisons occur within individuals, all of the individual characteristics that don't change over time and might contribute to the outcome are "matched" and, therefore, cannot act as confounders of the exposure-disease relationship. Matching eliminates confounding that arises from fixed characteristics such as genetic factors, stable psychological characteristics (personality), education, and stable aspects of health status. Much like pair-matched data in case-control studies, the nonindependence of these observations requires an approach that accounts for nonindependence, so case-crossover studies use analysis statistics that are designed for matched data.

Key point: Analysis of data from a case-crossover study closely resembles that of a pair-matched case-control study.

Redelmeier et al[137] used the case-crossover design to investigate whether driving convictions were effective in preventing traffic fatalities. They identified licensed drivers in Ontario who had been involved in fatal crashes, and examined whether these drivers had received traffic convictions in the month before their fatal crashes, as compared to the same month a year prior. They also examined additional referent periods. They used analysis procedures for matched data and determined that a conviction within the previous month resulted in fewer fatal accidents.

Retrospective cohort studies

Prospective cohort studies have a forward logical direction and a prospective (forward) temporal direction. They start with exposure, measuring this in the present, and then follow participants into the future and determine their disease outcomes.

Retrospective cohort studies have a forward logical direction—starting with exposure and asking whether an increased risk of disease follows exposure—and a retrospective (backward) temporal direction.

Key point: Retrospective cohort studies have the same logical direction as prospective cohort studies, but differ in temporal direction. Retrospective cohort studies look back in time.

Retrospective cohort studies require exposure data from the past. Many use data from occupational settings. Some occupational exposures can be defined by participation in a particular industry (e.g., uranium mining). Sometimes, exposure data may have been measured routinely for safety purposes (e.g., radiation exposure badges). In other instances, a group may have been exposed to a disaster or accident (e.g., a nuclear meltdown), which qualifies the group as an exposed cohort.

After finding a data source, a retrospective cohort study must then find a way to measure the relevant health outcomes from the time of exposure to the present day. This can often be accomplished through record linkage.

Because retrospective cohort studies are often conducted in occupational settings, the selection of referents (the nonexposed group) is challenging—doubly so, because working people (in occupational studies, the exposed group comprises only working people) may differ in many ways from non-working people (possible members of the nonexposed group). The most obvious concern is that jobs require good health, since workers must be able to function at their jobs. Workers, therefore, tend to be healthier than people who are not working—a problem called the *healthy worker effect* (we also discussed this effect on page 104).

In addition, workers are likely to differ from the general population—the most common referent in retrospective cohort studies—in many ways other than the healthy worker effect. For example, some occupational groups tend to be dominated by young people. Some may have an imbalanced sex ratio. This produces an obvious vulnerability to confounding by the nonmodifiable variables of age and sex. Typically, retrospective cohort studies use indirect standardization to address this vulnerability: they most commonly report measures of effect as standardized mortality ratios (SMRs), standardized morbidity ratios (also SMRs), and standardized incidence ratios (SIRs).

Key point: Retrospective cohort studies are very useful for studying occupational cohorts. These studies often use indirect standardization to support comparison to general population referents.

Retrospective cohort studies do not always rely on general population referents. Some use referent cohorts consisting of other workers—for example, people who have worked in a similar setting or who have been employed by the same company. In the best-case scenario, the study uses the same exposure measures to assess the exposed and referent cohorts, and can track both cohorts effectively over (past) time. These studies employ the same measures of association typical of prospective cohort studies: incidence proportion ratios (risk ratios), incidence rate ratios, and hazard ratios.

Examples of retrospective cohort studies

An early retrospective cohort study examined cancer risk and mortality in Air Canada pilots[138] using SMRs and (for cancer incidence) standardized incidence ratios. For all cancers, the SMR was 0.63, likely indicating a healthy worker effect. The study identified an elevated standardized incidence ratio for acute myeloid leukemia and an elevated SMR of 26 for aircraft accidents.

Dimich-Ward et al[139] examined cancer mortality and incidence among nurses in British Columbia. They found low SMRs and standardized incidence ratios for most cancers. Malignant melanoma, however, had a standardized incidence ratio of 1.3.

Villeneuve and Morrison[140] studied a cohort of fluorspar miners in Newfoundland to examine a possible association between radon exposure (which had been measured in the cohort) and subsequent coronary heart disease mortality. To account for the healthy worker effect, these investigators based their analysis on relative risks associated with different levels of radon exposure within the same cohort. The results suggested a possible association: the relative risk for the highest level of radon exposure was 1.5, but the 95% CI included the null value (the reported CI was 0.77–2.75)—so the result was not statistically significant. The investigators extended the follow-up for another 10 years and eventually concluded that there was no evidence of association.[141]

Randomized controlled trials

Randomized controlled trials have a forward logical direction: they start with an exposure and then determine outcome. They also have a forward temporal direction: they follow their participants from the present into the future. So, they are similar to prospective cohort studies in these ways, but they are fundamentally different in a key way.

Randomized controlled trials, unlike prospective cohort studies, are not observational studies: they are interventional studies. The investigators assign subjects to the exposure, and they do this by a random process.

All randomized controlled trials are interventional studies, but not all interventional studies are randomized controlled trials. Interventional studies that use nonrandom procedures to assign exposure are called *quasi-experiments*. In classifying studies, you need to be careful about the concepts of random and nonrandom: some authors describe randomization as a key feature of experimental studies. This is not a good use of terminology. The term *experiment* typically connotes a study conducted in a highly controlled setting, such as a laboratory. In an experiment, the effect of an independent variable on a dependent variable is examined with everything else held constant. Such studies are really the antithesis of epidemiological research, which seeks to investigate real-world problems in real-world settings. It is better to classify studies as interventional if the investigator assigns the exposure, and also to specify whether this assignment occurred randomly (randomized controlled trial) or nonrandomly (quasi-experiment).

Key point: Randomized controlled trials are a form of interventional prospective cohort study in which the exposure is randomly assigned by the investigators.

What is so special about randomization? Recall that confounding occurs when an independent risk factor is unequally distributed between exposure groups. Randomization helps to ensure that there is no inequality in the distribution of extraneous disease determinants. The law of large numbers helps to ensure that all extraneous variables will be equally distributed among the exposure groups. Restriction is another strategy to control confounding. By simply eliminating participants exposed to a potential disease determinant, the possibility of confounding by those determinants is eliminated. Randomized controlled trials tend to liberally employ restriction, before randomization. Other methods to detect and control confounding variables—stratification and modelling—may also be used in such studies during data analysis. However, they can only be used for variables that are known to be potential confounders and that were consequently measured. The unique power of randomization is its ability to control for the confounding effects of variables that are not measured, including those that are not even known.

Key point: The unique power of randomization is its ability to control for the confounding effects of variables that are unmeasured and perhaps not even known.

Selection bias in randomized controlled trials

It is sometimes said that randomization controls for selection bias. There is some truth in this assertion.

For selection bias to occur, a process affecting participation in a study must unfold in a way that depends both on exposure and disease.

Normally, a prospective cohort study is protected from such bias because the outcome has not occurred at the time of selection.

Randomized controlled trials are usually conducted to evaluate treatments, putting a different twist on this situation. The treatment is administered in such trials by clinicians working in clinical settings. A methodological concern is that this allocation of exposure may occur in a way that depends on the expected treatment outcomes. For example, in a randomized controlled trial, clinicians might try to get patients whom they think will respond well to a treatment into the treatment arm of a placebo-controlled trial. They could do this, for example, by gaming or distorting the allocation procedure. If the allocation is randomized, this is—in theory—impossible to do. Since randomization ensures that the allocation of exposure cannot depend on outcome, it should prevent such selection bias from occurring. However, in practice it is important not only that a study be randomized, but also that the procedure used for randomization be of sufficient quality that it cannot be subverted. Usually the random allocation is done using a computer generated sequence of random numbers. This sequence should be concealed from the clinicians and participants involved in the trial. Also, the allocation should occur after the participants have provided consent, so that there cannot be selective non-consent depending on assignment.

If the outcome of randomization is not adequately concealed, it can be subverted. For example, if outcomes are provided to investigative sites in envelopes, clinicians might simply open several of the envelopes and select the allocation they want for their patient. For these reasons, it is best if randomization is applied at a remote site, and communicated to investigators by some means (such as interactive voice response or a secure website) that they cannot subvert. If such design procedures are used, they must also be reported so as to be accessible to critical appraisal.

Key point: Randomization can prevent selection bias and confounding if it is implemented properly.

Critical appraisal and randomized controlled trials

Well-established standards of methodology and reporting are available for randomized controlled trials.[142] These can be helpful as guides to critical appraisal.

In addition, randomized controlled trials have methodological resemblances to prospective cohort studies, so critical appraisal follows familiar principles.

Even though randomization provides protection against selection bias, attrition can still lead to the occurrence of such bias. Attrition must therefore be minimized in randomized controlled trials. An interesting way to deal with attrition in randomized trials is to conduct an intention-to-treat analysis. This means that everyone randomized is included in the analysis, even if they do not actually comply with the treatment or if they leave the study. This requires the use of an imputation procedure to complete the data set, such as carrying forward the last available observation. This strategy is believed to help prevent the occurrence of selection bias resulting from attrition.

Measurement bias can also compromise the validity of randomized trials: trials must use blinding to prevent raters who are classifying outcome status from knowing treatment status. Trials should be double blind, which means that both participants and the trial staff are blinded. This will prevent the type of differential misclassification bias that could otherwise occur if outcome raters tended to rate randomized groups differently.

Examples of randomized controlled trials

Randomized controlled trials are among the most frequently published studies. A typical example is the Can-SAD trial by Lam et al[143] at the University of British Columbia. These investigators compared bright light therapy for winter depression to a standard antidepressant medication in 4 Canadian centres. They used the following procedures: a computer-generated code for random allocation, centralized allocation to treatment, double-blinded outcome assessment, and an intention-to-treat analysis. They found few differences in the effectiveness of the 2 treatments.

The Women's Health Initiative Randomized Controlled Trial was an important randomized controlled trial from the point of view of public health.[144] This study sought to clarify uncertainties in a literature of observational studies that had evaluated combined estrogen and progestin (hormone replacement therapy) in postmenopausal women for prevention of heart disease and certain cancers. The trial included 16 608 women between the ages of 50 and 79, randomized either to hormone treatment or placebo. The results indicated that health risks (an elevated risk of cardiovascular disease) exceeded the benefits of treatment. Because equipoise was lost, the trial was stopped after 5 years when these risks became evident to a monitoring committee.

Case-cohort studies

A drawback of the prospective cohort study design is its inefficiency. It needs a large investment of resources to track cohorts over time—and, typically, only a small proportion of a cohort will ever develop the outcomes under investigation. The case-cohort study design seeks to improve efficiency by making a subcohort its focus, rather than the entire cohort.

A case-cohort study compares a series of cases to a subcohort. The subcohort is drawn from the larger cohort that gives rise to the cases. As the name suggests, the study design is a kind of hybrid between case-control and cohort methodologies.

To make the design clear, let's compare it to the nested case-control study design. In a nested case-control study, the controls are selected from cohort members who do not have the disease at the time when each case develops the disease (the risk set). In a case-cohort study, the subcohort represents the entire cohort from which the cases arose. This is done by selecting the subcohort from the population at risk at the start of the cohort's follow-up interval. Typically, such studies are analytic in their orientation and therefore select incident cases for their case groups. The subcohort is representative of the larger cohort comprising people at risk of developing the disease. The subcohort does not include prevalent cases, but because the subcohort is selected at the beginning of follow-up, some of its members may develop the disease during follow-up.

Van Lonkhuijzen et al[145] used a case-cohort design to investigate meat consumption and endometrial cancer risk. They identified 26 024 residents of Ontario who had participated in a prospective cohort study called the Canadian Study of Diet, Lifestyle, and Health. They linked their study data, which included a dietary questionnaire assessing meat consumption, to the Ontario Cancer Registry and the national mortality database to determine outcome.

The study included 116 cases diagnosed with endometrial cancer during, on average, 11 years of follow-up. The subcohort consisted of a random sample of the entire at-risk cohort and included 1830 respondents. Notably, 19 members of the subcohort were also cases because they developed endometrial cancer during follow-up. Van Lonkhuijzen et al used modified proportional hazards models to estimate hazard ratios for the exposure. The hazard ratio for a comparison of the highest-to-lowest quartile of red meat consumption was 1.6, but the result was not statistically significant. The 95% CI was 0.86–3.08.

Ecological studies

Ecological studies are a distinct type of study design, differing from all of those discussed so far. They use a unit of analysis not based on individual people. The unit of analysis in ecological studies consists of groups of people, such as the population of neighbourhoods, cities, or countries.

Ecological studies assess correlation between exposure and disease, both measured at an aggregate level. Because correlation is so often the method of analysis in such studies, they are sometimes called *correlational studies*. Examples of aggregate measures of exposure include mean sodium consumption per person in different countries, and average number of grams of fish consumed in different provinces. Typical aggregate outcomes might be age-standardized mortality rates in different countries or cancer incidence in different provinces.

Examples of ecological studies

Ecological research mainly focuses on hypothesis generation. It is also a way to engage aggregate statistics. Many suitable aggregate statistics are routinely available. For example, the World Health Organization reports mortality statistics for almost every country in the world.[146]

Cheng et al[147] used mortality data for 193 countries in an ecological study showing that country-level measures of water sanitation were negatively correlated with infant and maternal mortality.

Durbin et al[148] correlated hospital admission rates for psychosis and mood disorders with the percentage of immigrants in the population of 507 census-derived geographic areas in Ontario. They found a positive correlation (Pearson correlation coefficient: 0.22) for the percentage of first-generation immigrants in these areas and rates of first admission for psychotic disorders. However, the association was attenuated when adjustments were made for population density and average income—2 potential confounders—in the geographic areas.

Strengths and weaknesses of ecological studies

Most ecological studies have descriptive aims. If suitable aggregate data are available, ecological studies provide an inexpensive study design for generating hypotheses. However, these studies are not entirely limited to descriptive aims. Some investigators are interested in evaluating etiological hypotheses through ecological studies. In other words, they are not merely concerned with aggregate statistics as an easily accessible proxy for individual exposures, but with characteristics that are best conceptualized at an aggregate level, such as income inequality. For example, Auger et al[149] examined the extent of income inequality in 143 Quebec communities, using a variety of indicators, and examined the relationship of this variable to mortality rates in those communities. Although the correlations differed depending on the definition of income inequality, alcohol-related mortality was found to be significantly associated with income inequality.

When it comes to causal reasoning, ecological studies have notable deficiencies. A particularly important concern is the ecological fallacy. This concept emphasizes the danger of making inferences about individual people based on correlations between aggregate units of individuals. For example, the observation that higher rates of admission for psychotic disorders tend to occur in areas with a higher percentage of immigrants does not necessarily mean that immigrants have higher rates of admission. Individual-level data would be required to confirm this.

Ecological studies also have a very limited ability to address the issue of confounding, owing to their lack of individual-level data.

A large drawback to ecological studies is that their target of estimation, usually a correlation, is not easily interpreted in terms of risk and probability. A correlation between aggregate exposures and outcomes does not have the same intuitive meaning as many of the other parameters encountered in the epidemiological literature. A correlation coefficient simply describes the tendency of 1 variable to vary with another.

Key point: The most prominent methodological concern with ecological studies is their vulnerability to the ecological fallacy. However, some exposures are ecological characteristics (e.g., income inequality) and here, the concern does not apply.

Thinking deeper

Statistical analysis in case-crossover studies

Most standard approaches to statistical analysis assume that the observations in a sample are independent of each other.

In case-control studies, observations often consist of matched pairs, which are nonindependent. Specialized statistical procedures have been designed for this situation.

Case-crossover studies also have nonindependent observations, since they compare exposures during different time periods within the same person. For example, di Bartolomeo et al[136] compared the following in the same people at different times of day:

- the frequency of alcohol consumption in the 6 hours before an episode of driving ending in a crash
- the frequency of alcohol consumption in the 6 hours before an episode of driving without a crash

The data consisted of pairs of observations and the approach to analysis needed to reflect this. Table 38 presents a 2 × 2 table for a paired analysis. Note that the table differs from usual 2 × 2 tables: the counts within its cells are pairs of observations rather than individual people. The table shows the results for 752 observations made in 326 people recorded by di Bartolomeo et al.

Note that Table 38 resembles the table used for pair-matched case-control studies. In pair-matched case-control studies, however, each cell contains a count of pairs of people rather than pairs of observations within a single person.

Table 38 contains paired observations of 2 types: concordant and discordant.

The concordant pairs include the 3 respondents who reported consuming alcohol before both of the driving episodes and the 281 respondents who did not drink before either driving episode. These pairs provide no information about the association under investigation.

The discordant pairs, however, do provide information. Drinking before the occurrence of a crash, and not drinking before an episode of incident-free driving, suggests an etiologic role for alcohol. By contrast, drinking before an episode of incident-free driving, and not drinking before an episode with a crash, gives the opposite impression. If drinking contributes to the risk of a crash, then the former type of pairing should be more common than the latter. As it turns out, the ratio of these 2 discordant pairs is the odds ratio for this association. In this case, the odds ratio is 24/18 or 1.33, as reported in the original study.[136]

TABLE 38. 2 × 2 TABLE FROM A CASE-CROSSOVER STUDY BY DI BARTOLOMEO ET AL[136]

		Alcohol consumption in 6 hours before driving episode without a crash	
		Yes	No
Alcohol consumption in 6 hours before driving episode with a crash	Yes	3	24
	No	18	281

Questions

1. What is the main difference between a nested case-control study and a case-cohort study? Identify key advantages of case-cohort studies over:

    a. nested case-control studies

    b. prospective cohort studies

2. Reich et al[150] sought to determine whether the introduction of better options for medical management of ulcerative colitis (e.g., ciclosporin and tumour-necrosis-factor alpha inhibitors) had reduced the frequency of colectomy surgery (a type of treatment reserved for patients whose disease cannot be managed medically). They used administrative data in Alberta to address this question. They determined the rate of surgery per year, before and after the new treatments were introduced. An increasing rate of surgery was seen up to the introduction of the new medications, followed by a decline. The investigators concluded that the rate of surgery was declining as a result of improved medical therapies.

    a. What kind of study design is this?

    b. Do you believe that showing a decline that starts at the introduction of a new treatment confirms a causal impact of that treatment?

3. What are the key differences between a retrospective cohort study and a case-cohort study?

4. Describe the main advantage of the case-crossover design compared to other study designs.

5. What, in your opinion, is the biggest advantage of randomized controlled trials over nonrandomized interventional studies and observational studies?

17

Other measures of association in epidemiology

Objectives
- Define the following measures of association: attributable risk among the exposed, attributable risk percent, population attributable risk, and population attributable risk percent.
- Describe how to interpret these measures of association.

Measures of association so far

So far, we have discussed the measures of association most often used in classic epidemiological studies. These include:

- prevalence differences, prevalence ratios, and prevalence odds ratios in cross-sectional studies
- odds ratios in case-control studies
- risk differences, risk ratios, incidence odds ratios, incident rate ratios, and hazard ratios in prospective cohort studies

This chapter covers other measures of association that convey important and useful epidemiological information. Most of these measures are estimates based on risk differences, but they seek to quantify more than just an association. They seek to quantify the causal impact of a risk factor on a population. They comprise types of attributable risk.

Attributable risk among the exposed

You can quantify an association by subtracting a frequency from another frequency. The proper interpretation of the resulting difference depends on the nature of the frequencies.

If the frequencies are incidence proportions, which quantify risk, the difference would be a risk difference. If a risk difference is believed to represent a causal effect, you could call it an *attributable risk among the exposed*—a member of the family of attributable risk parameters.

$$\text{Attributable Risk}_{exposed} = \text{Incidence Proportion}_{exposed} - \text{Incidence Proportion}_{nonexposed}$$

Labelling this risk difference an *attributable risk* clearly gives it a causal interpretation. There are situations where this is not justified. For example, if the difference between the 2 incidence proportions could arise from a confounding variable, the risk may not be attributable to the exposure.

If the exposure truly is causal, however, the attributable risk among the exposed reflects the extent of risk in exposed subjects due to the exposure. The formula makes the basis of this interpretation evident: if the difference in risk is attributable to the exposure, removing the effect of that exposure would render the 2 incidence proportions equal to each another. The risk difference, therefore, quantifies the extent to which risk in exposed subjects could be diminished if the effects of the exposure were eliminated.

Attributable-risk measures have value in public health because they help quantify the impact of a risk factor. Attributable risk among the exposed and several related parameters (discussed below) are therefore measures of impact as well as measures of association.

Attributable risk percent

Some epidemiologists prefer to present estimates of attributable risk among the exposed as percentages rather than simple risk differences. It would be accurate to call this parameter *attributable risk among the exposed percent*— but the shorter name (*attributable risk percent*) is easier.

Instead of quantifying how much risk of disease could be diminished by eliminating (or ameliorating) the effect of exposure in the exposed subjects (attributable risk among the exposed), the attributable risk percent quantifies the percentage of risk among the exposed that could be eliminated by doing so.

The first step is to change the risk difference into a proportion of the incidence among the exposed, and then to multiply the proportion by 100 to create a percentage.

$$\text{Attributable Risk \%} = \left(\frac{\text{Incidence Proportion}_{exposed} - \text{Incidence Proportion}_{nonexposed}}{\text{Incidence Proportion}_{exposed}} \right) \times 100$$

Note that attributable-risk measurement has importance for primary prevention. Primary prevention involves eliminating an exposure or ameliorating its effects (e.g., through reducing rates of smoking, correcting lipid imbalances, implementing appropriate occupational safety measures, etc.) to diminish incidence of disease. In other words, it targets risk factors with the goal of reducing incidence. Attributable-risk measurement helps quantify the potential impact of primary preventive interventions.

A small amount of algebra provides another formula for the attributable risk percent among the exposed:

$$\text{Attributable Risk } \% = \left(\frac{\text{Risk Ratio} - 1}{\text{Risk Ratio}} \right) \times 100$$

This is a handy formula because it allows attributable risk percent to be calculated from an approximation of the risk ratio, such as an incidence odds ratio from a case-control study (see "Thinking Deeper" in this chapter).

There is a lot of variability in the terminology for attributable risk. Some epidemiologists refer to the attributable risk percent as the *attributable fraction*, and do not necessarily express it as a percentage. Or they may use a similar term: *attributable proportion*. Others use *attributable fraction for the exposed* to clarify that it reflects impact on those who are exposed and not the entire population. When you read a study that reports these parameters, it is important to look carefully at the how the study uses the term *attributable risk*.

Key point: Attributable risk parameters combine risk differences with a judgement that those differences reflect a causal effect. They help to predict the potential impact of primary prevention on the health status of an exposed population.

Preventive fraction

Some exposures decrease risk, rather than increase risk. For example, a diet high in fruits and vegetables has many health benefits, leading to a lower incidence proportion for several outcomes (e.g., heart disease and cancer) among those exposed. In this scenario, the formula we have presented for attributable risk percent would result in a negative number—which could complicate its interpretation. The preventive fraction is a way of calculating an attributable fraction for a protective association:

$$\text{Preventive Fraction} = \frac{\text{Incidence Proportion}_{\text{nonexposed}} - \text{Incidence Proportion}_{\text{exposed}}}{\text{Incidence Proportion}_{\text{nonexposed}}}$$

The formula for the preventive fraction differs in 2 ways from the formula for the attributable fraction. First, in the numerator, the incidence in the proportions is reversed. This means that the preventive fraction will be positive for a protective association. Second, the demominator has changed and now contains the incidence in the nonexposed, rather than the exposed.

Epidemiology has different goals for risk factors versus protective factors. For protective factors, the goal is to increase exposure among those not exposed. We want to quantify the reduction in incidence that would occur through exposure to the protective factor. Attributable risk answers the question: How much disease could be prevented among the exposed by removing a harmful factor (risk factor)? Preventive fraction answers the question: How much disease among the nonexposed could be prevented by adding an exposure?

This fraction may also be expressed as a percentage, according to preference. Here's another way to state this formula (see "Thinking Deeper" in this chapter):

$$\text{Preventive Fraction} = 1 - \text{Risk Ratio}$$

Population attributable risk

It is sometimes valuable to understand the effect of primary-prevention interventions on an entire population. This requires a parameter beyond attributable risk among the exposed, which can only quantify the effects of primary prevention among the exposed.

Elimination of a risk factor, even a factor strongly associated with disease, will not prevent very many cases of disease if only a small subset of the population is exposed to the risk factor. For example, due to strict regulation, the frequency of exposure to asbestos is low in developed countries. As a result, even though asbestos is a strong risk factor for lung cancer among those exposed to it, asbestos does not have a large impact at the population level.

Population attributable risk is a composite parameter that incorporates the prevalence of exposure and its strength of association. The most intuitive formula is:

$$\text{Population Attributable Risk} = \text{Incidence Proportion}_{\text{total}} - \text{Incidence Proportion}_{\text{nonexposed}}$$

Here, the effect of exposure in the population is represented as the difference between incidence in the total population (which in turn reflects the effect of the exposure in question and all other factors) and incidence in the nonexposed (which reflects the risk of all other factors in the absence of the exposure). If the exposure could be eliminated, or all of its effects ameliorated, the incidence in the total population would be that of the nonexposed. Population attributable risk represents the extent of change in incidence that would occur in a population if the effects of the exposure were eliminated.

Population attributable risk percent

Population attributable risk can also be expressed as a fraction or a percentage:

$$\text{Population Attributable Risk \%} = \left(\frac{\text{Incidence Proportion}_{\text{total}} - \text{Incidence Proportion}_{\text{nonexposed}}}{\text{Incidence Proportion}_{\text{total}}} \right) \times 100$$

A cautionary note: some epidemiologists use *attributable fraction* to refer to population attributable risk percent. It is always important to understand what investigators actually did in an analysis: don't assume that all investigators use terms the same way.

Key point: Population attributable risks are a family of parameters that combine risk differences with judgements about causation to predict the potential impact of primary prevention on the health status of the total population.

Thinking deeper

Estimating attributable risk without incidence data

The formulas presented in this chapter are standard for dealing with incidence data and best convey the meaning of the parameters.

However, it may be useful to estimate such parameters even in situations where incidence data are not available. For example, a case-control study may produce a valid approximation of a risk ratio that reflects a causal association. Nevertheless, it is not obvious how to calculate the attributable risk percent from the case-control data.

In considering this problem, the basic formula for attributable risk percent is a good place to start:

$$\text{Attributable Risk \%} = \left(\frac{\text{Incidence Proportion}_{\text{exposed}} - \text{Incidence Proportion}_{\text{nonexposed}}}{\text{Incidence Proportion}_{\text{exposed}}} \right) \times 100$$

Next, recall the basic formulation of the risk ratio as the ratio of 2 incidence proportions:

$$\text{Risk Ratio} = \frac{\text{Incidence Proportion}_{\text{exposed}}}{\text{Incidence Proportion}_{\text{nonexposed}}}$$

This means that the incidence proportion for the exposed can be written a different way:

$$\text{Incidence Proportion}_{\text{exposed}} = \text{Risk Ratio} \times \text{Incidence Proportion}_{\text{nonexposed}}$$

Then, substitute this expression for *incidence proportion*_{*exposed*} in the equation for attributable risk percent:

$$\text{Attributable Risk \%} = \left(\frac{[\text{Risk Ratio} \times \text{Incidence Proportion}_{\text{nonexposed}}] - \text{Incidence Proportion}_{\text{nonexposed}}}{\text{Risk Ratio} \times \text{Incidence Proportion}_{\text{nonexposed}}} \right) \times 100$$

Incidence proportion$_{nonexposed}$ can now be factored out of the numerator of the equation:

$$\text{Attributable Risk \%} = \left(\frac{\text{Incidence Proportion}_{nonexposed} \times (\text{Risk Ratio} - 1)}{\text{Risk Ratio} \times \text{Incidence Proportion}_{nonexposed}} \right) \times 100$$

Finally, *incidence proportion*$_{nonexposed}$ cancels out, leading to a formula for calculating the attributable risk percent from the risk ratio:

$$\text{Attributable Risk \%} = \frac{\text{Risk Ratio} - 1}{\text{Risk Ratio}} \times 100$$

As an intuitive confirmation of the formula, note that the equation indicates that when the risk ratio is 2—indicating that the exposure doubles the risk—the attributable risk percent will be 50%. Attributable risk percent can be estimated from a case-control study in situations where the odds ratio is considered a good estimate of the risk ratio.

In the case of the preventive fraction, it is possible to follow the same reasoning. Consider this formula for the preventive faction:

$$\text{Preventive Fraction} = \frac{\text{Incidence Proportion}_{nonexposed} - \text{Incidence Proportion}_{exposed}}{\text{Incidence Proportion}_{nonexposed}}$$

You can write this formula as 2 fractions:

$$\text{Preventive Fraction} = \frac{\text{Incidence Proportion}_{nonexposed}}{\text{Incidence Proportion}_{nonexposed}} - \frac{\text{Incidence Proportion}_{exposed}}{\text{Incidence Proportion}_{nonexposed}}$$

This leads to the alternative formula:

$$\text{Preventive Fraction} = 1 - \text{Risk Ratio}$$

Questions

1. Shiue et al[151] estimated that the population attributable risk percent was 9% for the effect of low indoor room temperature (< 18 degrees) on high blood pressure. They based their calculation on an odds ratio derived from the 2010 Scottish Health Survey, a cross-sectional study.
   a. Taken at face value, what does this estimate mean?
   b. Do you have any reservations about the estimate?

2. Kuendig et al[152] used hospitalized cases and controls to estimate odds ratios quantifying the association of alcohol exposure and injury. They estimated what they called the alcohol attributable fraction (AAF) using the formula:

$$\text{AAF} = \frac{\text{Odds Ratio} - 1}{\text{Odds Ratio}}$$

What type of parameter is the AAF?

3. Based on case-control data, Yusuf et al[153] estimated a population attributable risk of 35.7% for currently smoking versus never having smoked as a risk factor for myocardial infarction. Explain the meaning of this parameter in plain language.

4. Here is a table from a study describing incident depression in medical inpatients in relation to a set of drugs believed to contribute to depressive symptoms.[154]

	Depressed	Total Cohort
Exposed to a potentially depression-causing drug	17	86
Not exposed to such a drug	5	92

   a. Using the formula provided in this chapter, calculate attributable risk among the exposed.
   b. Calculate attributable fraction among the exposed (express the parameter as a percentage).
   c. Calculate the population attributable risk.
   d. Calculate the population attributable risk percent.
   e. The data presented in the table are unadjusted, yet associations between drugs and depression are likely to be confounded by the severity of the illness being treated. In pharmacoepidemiology, this phenomenon is called *confounding by indication*. How does this affect your interpretation of the parameters calculated from the table?

5. Arseneault et al[155] followed a birth cohort to determine whether cannabis use increased the risk of psychosis. They assessed a particular psychotic disorder, schizophreniform disorder, which is often a precursor to schizophrenia. They categorized 730 children who reported no use or minimal use as nonexposed. Of these, 22 developed a psychotic disorder by age 26. Among 29 exposed subjects, 3 developed psychosis. What is the population attributable risk?

PART V

Evaluating epidemiological studies

18

Causal judgement in epidemiology

Objectives
- Describe the role of judgement in causal reasoning in epidemiology.
- Describe causal reasoning in the context of primary, secondary, and tertiary prevention.
- List classic criteria for weighing judgements about causality.
- Describe how greater-than-additive-risk helps identify causal mechanisms.

Critical appraisal and causal judgement

This chapter presents criteria for evaluating findings of causality in epidemiological studies—a key and complicated task in critical appraisal.

Findings of causality first require valid epidemiological estimates—estimates, in other words, that arise from properly conducted, well-designed studies. This book has described the characteristics of properly conducted, well-designed studies.

Findings of causality also require judgement. Causal significance is never self-evident—so, in critical appraisal, judgements about causation must always be carefully weighed.

In weighing judgements about causation, thousands of specific considerations could come into play. You risk paying too much attention to certain issues, and not enough attention to others.

The criteria in this chapter help clarify issues of concern. They do not provide a method or formula for determining causality, and they should not be regarded as a source of evidence for causation. Rather, they provide a framework to guide the task of weighing.

This chapter takes direction from the most widely used criteria, which appear in 2 classic sources: a 1965 paper by British epidemiologist

Bradford Hill,[156] and a 1964 report on smoking and health from the US surgeon general.[157]

> *Key point:* Causality in epidemiology is an issue of judgement. These judgements are complex and can be facilitated by a framework.

Causation and validity

In critical appraisal, you start by assessing the validity of a study's estimates of epidemiological effect before you consider any claims it makes about causality. This is a hierarchical relationship: valid estimates of exposure-disease association precede conclusions about exposure-disease causality (disease etiology).

It's important not to be too dogmatic about this, though. Many studies are vulnerable to nondifferential misclassification bias. The direction of the resulting bias is predictable and towards the null value (see page 135). A study vulnerable to this type of bias, and reporting a strong association, needs careful consideration. The estimate may not be valid in the strictest sense, but it may be clear that it underestimates an effect that exists—so, in this case, the association is stronger than the estimate suggests.

As a task of critical appraisal, assessing a study's conclusions about causality differs from assessing its vulnerability to random error and bias. Random error and bias are relatively objective concepts: confidence intervals quantify vulnerability to random error, and concrete mechanisms link methodological features (e.g., classification error rates and selection probabilities) to systematic error.

Causality, however, is more subjective. Critical appraisers often find themselves taking issue with investigators' judgements about the causal implications of their findings—even findings based on valid estimates. For example, investigators sometimes overlook the limitations of their work, and critical appraisers sometimes conclude such investigators are "biased." This is a different use of *bias* than in the technical context of systematic error and internal validity.

> *Key point:* Validity and etiology are hierarchical considerations. Consideration of causality cannot move forward until the existence of an association has been confirmed through a valid estimate.

The concept of causation in epidemiology

The concept of causation, as it applies in epidemiology, differs from concepts of causation encountered in other types of scientific research. Rather than searching directly for the underlying pathophysiological events that lead to disease, epidemiologists seek modifiable links in specific causal chains of events that ultimately lead to diseases and other adverse health outcomes.

The ultimate test for an epidemiological finding is its ability to make a difference in clinical practice or public health—so, in terms of primary, secondary, and tertiary prevention.

Primary prevention seeks to interrupt a destructive chain of causal events. For example, if people are becoming sick from drinking contaminated water, it may seek to provide clean drinking water, because the quality of drinking water is a modifiable link in a causal chain. Chains of causality leading up to this modifiable link may explain why a population has become exposed to unclean water: these may involve war, or a lack of effective civil institutions, or a faulty monitoring system. Additional links in the causal chain may also explain why the unclean water makes people sick: these links may involve reproduction of microbes in the gastrointestinal tract and the molecular actions of toxins produced by those microbes. But primary prevention focuses on links in chains of causality it can modify.

Secondary prevention, which involves screening for diseases, also brings a narrow focus to chains of causality. The links between screening activities and improved health depend on many factors—for example, whether people participate in screening, whether screening tests are accurate, and whether follow-up treatments are effective. So, secondary prevention identifies and fosters chains of causality that may make screening activities effective in improving the health of populations: administration of accurate screening tests, leading to earlier detection, leading to earlier treatment, leading to better outcomes.

Tertiary prevention—reducing negative impacts of established disease—targets specific links in chains of causality that lead to better outcomes for clinically established diseases (e.g., the administration of drugs or delivery of other treatment or rehabilitative practices). The effectiveness of a treatment—a drug, for example—depends on chains of causal events including regulatory and economic issues (both strongly related to availability of a drug), prescription of the drug by a physician, purchasing the drug from a pharmacy, adherence to the treatment regime, absorption of the drug, interaction of the drug with biological processes, and subsequent actions that diminish the impact of the disease or cure it. Tertiary prevention targets modifiable factors within this chain of causality such as whether a treatment is administered or not.

Chains of causality link together into causal webs. Within this universe of causality, epidemiological studies tend to be opportunistic. They look for best opportunities to intervene in processes of causation.

Criteria for weighing causality

Temporality

Temporality refers to the question of whether exposure to a risk factor precedes the disease outcome. Temporality is the most important criterion for weighing causality, because a cause must precede an effect. Studies that fail to clarify the temporal relationship between exposure and disease therefore fail to quantify a necessary feature of a causal relationship.

Some study designs are inherently better at clarifying the issue of temporality than others. Cross-sectional studies and ecological studies tend to be particularly weak in this regard. Case-control studies can be just as weak on temporality if they fail to use truly incident cases.

Key point: Temporality is the most important and useful causal criterion, since a cause must logically precede an effect.

Strength of association

Strength of association is a causal criterion identified by Hill. It says that strong associations are more likely to indicate causality than weak associations.

This criterion draws attention to some of the practical realities of epidemiological research. Epidemiological studies are almost always subject to some source of error, such as random error, bias, or confounding. The possibility always exists that data indicating a weak association could arise by chance, or from some minor defect in study design or analysis. However, it is less likely that data indicating a strong association would arise from such circumstances. So, although a weak association does not preclude causality, a strong association is more strongly suggestive of causality.

Note that strength of association does not reflect a single metric. Associations can be measured using either difference or ratio-based measures, and a strong association on 1 scale may be weak on another.

Key point: The value of strength of association as a determinant of causality reflects practical realties of epidemiological research. Strong associations are less likely to arise from minor defects in study design.

Also note that precision affects this criterion. You need to check the confidence intervals of a study reporting a strong association. If the point estimate is large, but the lower limit of the confidence interval is near the null value (a value of 1 for a relative measure and a value of 0 for a difference-based measure), it is not possible to be confident that an association really is strong.

Consistency

The criterion of consistency refers to consistent findings among many studies investigating a possible association (i.e., within a literature of studies), not to the findings of any particular study.

Again, this criterion reflects some of the practical realities of epidemiological research. No single epidemiological study is perfect. All studies are vulnerable—in varying ways and degrees—to random and systematic error. However, different studies are likely to have somewhat different vulnerabilities to error. For example, case-control studies tend to have different vulnerabilities than prospective cohort studies. Also, different populations may embody different distributions of potentially unknown or unmeasured confounding variables. They may also differ in factors that affect the probability of recruitment, consent, and participation. Measurement instruments may perform differently in different populations because of language and culture. For all of these reasons, a result consistent across different types of studies conducted in different times and places is more likely to be a causal effect.

Key point: The casual criterion of consistency does not refer to the results of a particular study, but rather to the level of consistency seen in a literature of studies.

Like assessing strength of association, assessing consistency requires nuanced consideration. For example, inconsistency within a literature of studies may result from inconsistent quality among the studies (e.g., some studies are better resourced than others, some use more accurate measures of disease and exposure). In this situation, it would be a good idea to look for consistency in the highest-quality studies, rather than the entire literature. Another concern is that a literature of studies may appear more consistent than it really is. For example, if a drug company conducts multiple studies, some of which are positive and some of which are negative, it may choose to publish only the studies with the most favourable results. This would make the literature look falsely consistent.

Specificity
This criterion is rarely used. However, it was included in Hill's paper and also in the surgeon general's report.

The specificity of an association refers to whether a risk factor is associated specifically with a disease outcome, or nonspecifically with several or many outcomes. This criterion relates to important ideas early in the history of epidemiology about linking infectious agents to disease (see Koch's criteria, page 6).

When an infectious agent causes a disease, it may be possible to find that agent in all cases of the disease, and not in people without the disease, as Koch postulated. This idea no longer has power for causal reasoning. Some examples illustrate why:

- Infectious agents that cause serious disease in vulnerable individuals (e.g., the immunocompromised) may exist as normal flora in healthy individuals.
- The most important risk-factor associations for chronic diseases tend not to be in any way specific. For example, obesity is a risk factor for type 2 diabetes, but lots of obese people do not have diabetes and lots of people with diabetes are not obese.

- Carcinogens, such as those contained in cigarette smoke, increase the risk for multiple cancers (including cancers of the mouth, pharynx, larynx, and esophagus) and also chronic conditions such as coronary artery disease, emphysema, chronic bronchitis, and asthmatic bronchitis.

Even so, in a widely cited study discussing the evidence for causality in the association between human papilloma virus and cervical cancer, Bosch et al[158] identified lack of evidence for the virus's involvement in other cancers as evidence of specificity.

Key point: Hill's specificity criterion in not very important for causal judgement.

Biological gradient

Sometimes, biological evidence suggests that a higher level or intensity of exposure leads to greater incidence of disease. This effect is sometimes referred to as a *dose-response relationship*. In such cases, a biological gradient may provide supportive evidence for causation.

However, biological gradients pose many problems for identifying causal relationships. Most of these relate to situations where a biological gradient might not be seen even if there was a causal effect.

This would happen in a saturation effect. In this case, some level of exposure has a causal impact on risk, but higher levels of exposure do not create higher levels of risk. Presumably this happens because the underlying biological effect is occurring through a saturated mechanism.

It could also happen where a range of exposures occurs below a threshold demarcating a harmful level of exposure. There may not be a biological gradient below this threshold.

The US surgeon general's report did not include biological gradients among its criteria for weighing causality, and a biological gradient is not a strong indicator of causality. Epidemiological publications, however, frequently mention biological gradients as evidence supporting causal interpretation.

Key point: While a biological gradient may be viewed as supporting the idea of causation, particularly if biological theory suggests that such a gradient should exist, the absence of such a relationship does not usually provide evidence against causation.

Biological plausibility

This criterion links the interpretation of epidemiological information to biological data from basic science. If an epidemiological estimate suggests an effect that is not very plausible according to other elements of current biological knowledge, it is likely that the finding represents an artifact rather than truth.

The biggest problem with this criterion is philosophical. Epidemiology is an empirical science that depends on the law of large numbers to produce informative estimates from samples representing populations. This is based on the fundamental assumption that the distribution of diseases in populations reflects the determinants of those diseases. It seems illogical, given this perspective, to discount estimates based on the supposition that they do not align with known biological mechanisms. Thinking back to the story of John Snow (see page 5), it would have been a mistake to dismiss the link between sewage-contaminated water and cholera just because the biological agent (the cholera bacillus) was unknown.

Like all causal criteria, this criterion requires careful consideration. A plausible association is less likely to be an artifact than an implausible association—but a biologically implausible finding, if replicated, requires biological investigation.

Coherence

This criterion is similar to biological plausibility, but engages a wider field of inquiry, beyond biology. Coherence refers to the fit of an epidemiological estimate with results from any type of scientific research or theory. As with the issue of biological plausibility, such considerations are important, but should not be viewed as necessary features of a causal association.

Experimental evidence

Hill's paper referred to experimental or "semiexperimental" evidence as a criterion for weighing causality.

In current epidemiology, researchers sometimes use the phrase *experimental evidence* to indicate that a study has employed randomization. Randomization is a uniquely powerful strategy for addressing the issue of confounding in epidemiological research. For this reason, judgements about causality from interventional studies—which use randomization—carry a lot of weight.

Ethics disallows the assignment of potentially harmful risk factors to study subjects, so interventional studies do not have routine use in epidemiological research. In the only area where they can be used (the evaluation of treatments), randomized controlled trials have become the most important type of epidemiological study.

All strategies to control confounding—not just randomization—are central to causal reasoning in epidemiology. These strategies seek to confirm that an observed effect arises from particular exposure-disease associations, and not other, independent risk factors.

Analogy

Analogy refers to causal inference drawn from comparison or correspondence to other causal associations. Hill listed this criterion, but its usefulness is questionable and it is rarely used.

Key point: Coherence, experimental evidence, and analogy are not very useful criteria for supporting causal judgements in epidemiology.

Thinking deeper

Greater-than-additive risk and causality

Kenneth Rothman's causal pie model (see page 139) has some interesting implications for causal reasoning. Other names for the causal pie model are the *Rothman model* and the *sufficient-component cause model.*[159]

The core concept of the causal pie model is this: diseases arise from component causes that, in various combinations, form a causal mechanism that leads to disease onset.

Component causes are exposures or risk factors. Rothman calls them *component causes* because, as a graphic, his model presents exposures or risk factors as "pieces of pie" in a causal mechanism presented as a "whole pie." There may be several combinations of component causes that can lead to a disease. If 1 of these component causes is present in all possible causal mechanisms, it can be regarded as a necessary cause. If there is a necessary component cause, it will be seen as an exposure in every person with the disease.

The causal pie model views the induction period of a disease as the time between exposure to a component cause and the completion of the causal mechanism through addition of other component causes. The model simplifies the ideas of "triggering or precipitating events," and "vulnerability or predisposing factors." In the causal pie model, a triggering or precipitating event is a final component cause that completes a causal mechanism. Vulnerability and predisposing factors are component causes that have not yet (and may never) participate in completed mechanisms.

In epidemiological studies, the causal pie model—though very interesting in theory—has much less currency than causal criteria in discussions of causality. Despite this, it has some interesting real-world implications.

Consider a study investigating the effects of 2 component causes (labelled *A* and *B*) on disease incidence. In this study:

- Some cases of disease may occur among people who are not exposed to either component cause. This would confirm that there are causal mechanisms that do not involve either A or B.

- Some cases may occur among subjects with exposure to A but not B. The incidence in this group reflects the existence of causal mechanisms that involve A and other, presumably unknown, component causes.

The risk difference for A is the difference between these first 2 groups. A similar situation would apply to those who have exposure to B but not A, and this also leads to a risk difference.

The interesting group is the group with exposure to both A and B. If there are no specific causal mechanisms that require A and B, the risk difference for this double-exposure group will equal the sum of risk differences for the single-exposure groups (A-not-B and B-not-A groups), because the cases of disease in this group will arise by 1 of these 2 types of mechanism. By contrast, if there are specific mechanisms that require both A and B, the risk difference for this double-exposure group will be greater than the sum of risk differences for the single-exposure groups.

Greater-than-additive effects would manifest as interactions in models based on risk differences, suggesting that such models, and interaction terms nested within them, may be particularly useful for exploring causal effects. Statistical tests based on this theory have even been developed.[159]

The important link between absolute changes in risk and causality highlights the importance of being able to translate relative measures into absolute measures. This can easily be done if the resulting absolute difference is reported as a percentage or fraction. Here is the formula:

$$\% \text{ Change in Risk} = (\text{Relative Risk} - 1) \times 100$$

In other words, a relative risk of 2.0 indicates a 100% increase in risk, and a relative risk of 1.5 represents a 50% increase in risk.

Au et al[160] examined whether there was a greater-than-additive effect of elevated C-reactive protein and depression on diabetes incidence. They found no significant interaction. Their study reported that the hazard ratio (a relative measure of effect) for elevated C-reactive protein only was 1.43, that for depression only was 1.63, and that for both exposures was 2.03. Converting these relative measures to absolute change, the absolute change associated with C-reactive protein was 43%, that for depression was 63%, and that for both was 103%. Notice that the additive effects of the individual exposures (43% + 63% = 106%) are almost identical to the absolute effect of the double exposure. This suggests that both factors elevate the incidence of diabetes, but does not suggest that there are specific causal mechanisms for diabetes that require both factors to be present.

Questions

1. A review of the association between cannabis exposure and psychosis referenced a dose-response relationship as evidence in support of a causal connection.[155] How strong do you think this argument is?

2. Mente et al[161] sought to evaluate evidence for a causal association between dietary factors and coronary heart disease by conducting a systematic review of the literature. In general, do you feel that it is appropriate to address questions of causation with literature reviews?

3. In their review of dietary factors and coronary heart disease, Mente et al adopted a criterion-based strategy for their assessment of causation, but decided to emphasize only 4 of Hill's criteria: strength, consistency, temporality, and coherence. Do you agree with their choices? Can you guess their reasons for not addressing biological plausibility, analogy, and dose-response relationships?

4. Since Hill's classic paper,[156] biological plausibility has been viewed as a causal criterion. However, in that same paper, Hill seems to dismiss it: "It will be helpful if the causation we suspect is biologically plausible. But this is a feature I am convinced we cannot demand. What is biologically plausible depends upon the biological knowledge of the day."

   a. In your own words, state a reason not to include consideration of biological plausibility.

   b. Hill seems to argue that strength of association is the most important criterion for causation: "First upon my list I would put the strength of the association." Can you produce a counter argument?

5. Hill alludes to how causation is conceptualized in epidemiology with the following statement: "How such a change exerts that influence may call for a great deal of research. However, before deducing 'causation' and taking action we shall not invariably have to sit around awaiting the results of that research. The whole chain may have to be unravelled or a few links may suffice. It will depend upon circumstances." What does he mean by "links in a chain"?

19

Steps in critical appraisal

Objectives
- Describe the goals of critical appraisal.
- List steps for critical appraisal, and describe their hierarchy.
- Explain critical appraisal as a skill honed with practice, feedback, and knowledge.

The goals of critical appraisal

Critical appraisal forms part of the necessary work of researchers, clinicians, and public health professionals.

Researchers need to understand the existing state of knowledge before they can strive to add to that knowledge. They must be able to tell when a reported finding is completely wrong, when it needs further substantiation, or when it can reasonably be accepted as a fact.

Clinicians need to keep up with scientific developments in their fields of practice. They need to know when a new approach to treatment or a new method of assessment can be implemented or, perhaps even more importantly, when evidence in support of its implementation is lacking. They need to be able to see through exaggerated claims and distorted conclusions.

Public heath professionals need to identify solid, up-to-date information to shape decisions about public policy, regulation, health surveillance, primary prevention, and health promotion.

None of these challenges can be addressed by accepting what researchers claim to be true. They can only be accomplished by critical examination of the scientific literature. Making the right decisions depends on being able to determine which assertions are supported by evidence and which are not.

If it is accepted (as it should be, see page 14) that the law of large numbers is the main driving force for scientific progress in the health sciences, then critical appraisal safeguards its integrity. Real evidence comes from the processes described in this book: sampling, measurement, detection of effect measure modification, control of confounding, and appropriate interpretation of the resulting estimates (if they are valid) in terms of their causal significance and generalizability.

Research is a conduit for information and knowledge. Critical appraisal gauges the success of research in achieving this goal. Critical appraisal is, therefore, an important part of channelling the mathematical reality of the law of large numbers through observation and analysis, which delivers real scientific progress.

The process of critical appraisal unfolds at all levels of scientific inquiry, millions of times every day, all around the world.

Consider the typical process for undertaking a study, which often begins with a grant proposal. Researchers typically ask colleagues to read and criticize their grant proposals before submission. By providing criticism of research methods, this type of internal peer review helps to identify and correct study-design defects—for example, vulnerability to random error from inadequate sample size—that could otherwise lead to erroneous results. When proposals are submitted to funding agencies, peer reviewers again critically appraise proposed research methods, seeking defects that could render the results vulnerable to error. This critical peer review helps to ensure that studies likely to produce erroneous results (either as a result of random error or systematic error) are not funded. If funded and implemented, studies are written up and submitted to journals. Peer reviewers, again, critically appraise studies to assess whether to publish them. This ensures that the limitations of studies are openly acknowledged. If published, studies undergo assessment by those who read them—such as researchers, clinicians, and public health professionals. Study methods, analysis, results, and interpretations must again pass the test of critical appraisal.

The default position in critical appraisal is, of course, a critical stance. Results are not accepted as true because investigators assert that they are true. It is better to assume that results are false, and to only grudgingly accept them if vulnerabilities to random error, systematic error, and confounding cannot be uncovered. If the methods of a study allow the possibility of serious error, a critical appraiser should reject the results unless convinced that potential errors—whatever they might be—would not substantially distort the study results. If a study does not provide enough information to support critical appraisal—in other words, if the quality of its reporting is low—critical appraisers should question the veracity of the reported results.

Critical appraisal step by step

The parts of a published study

Published studies usually include a statement of purpose for the research they report. This is almost always supported by a discussion of relevant background literature, which aims to demonstrate that the study engages important questions that prior studies have not addressed, or have insufficiently addressed because of faulty methodology.

Next, there is typically a summary of the methods employed, perhaps with some words of justification for decisions about study design and procedures. This summary usually includes information about the selection of subjects, measurement of study variables, and procedures to assess vulnerability to random error and to control confounding.

This is followed by presentation of the study results and discussion of the implications of the findings for causality and generalizability, and for clinical practice and public health.

Finally, there is usually an acknowledgement of the limitations of the study.

The value of an organized approach to critical appraisal

Critical appraisal usually needs to address all aspects of published studies (although studies may assert they have already addressed all relevant issues). The exception is when a study flaw makes further appraisal irrelevant. For example, invalid estimates make questions of causality and generalizability unimportant.

Critical appraisal is a complex task: it is easy to get off track and miss important points. It helps to structure the task.

The steps presented here provide a coherent framework for the principles and strategies covered in this book.

Step 1: Identifying the study's research question or hypothesis

A study's topic of inquiry should be clearly stated in a form that aligns with an estimate or comparison.

It should be stated either as a hypothesis (e.g., that an exposure is significantly associated with a disease, that a treatment leads to better outcomes than placebo) or a question (e.g., Does this exposure increase the risk of this disease? Does this treatment lead to a better outcome than treatment with placebo?). An example of a research question is: "What is the distribution of deaths due to cerebrovascular disease in Ontario?"[162] An example of a typical hypothesis is: "We hypothesized that COX-2 inhibitor use would be associated with increased bone mineral density (BMD) in postmenopausal women not using estrogen therapy."[163]

Some published studies are poorly conceptualized. Investigators (authors) may not express goals in a way that fits the needs of critical appraisal. For example, they may state that their goal was to "explore" or "look at" an issue. They may then present various estimates or models, and attempt to form conclusions based on interpreting these estimates and models. In this situation, it is it best to set aside the authors' narrative, and focus on a particular estimate or result reported in the study. Sometimes, you may need to state a coherent hypothesis or research question that the authors themselves did not state. At least then, the study can be critically appraised in a coherent fashion. In essence, this converts the authors' vagueness into real methodological issues: vulnerability to type I error or other problems that emerge with the selective reporting of exploratory or descriptive results.

Let's consider an example. A study by Agrawal and Ebrahim includes the following statement in the background section of its abstract: "It is postulated that a diet high in legumes may be beneficial in preventing diabetes. However, little empirical evidence on this association exists in developing countries. We aimed to examine the association."[164] If critical appraisal took this vague statement as its focus, it would do no more than evaluate an opinion. As it turns out, though, this was a cross-sectional study that used the odds ratio as its measure of association—so, a coherent approach to critical appraisal would assess the validity of the prevalence odds ratio, and then critique the authors' conclusions about causality in view of the cross-sectional design. This orients critical appraisal towards the tractable goals of appraising the validity of a prevalence odds ratio and perhaps assessing the extent to which it can support a causal interpretation.

Some studies state objectives in a way that serves as an excellent starting point for critical appraisal. Consider the statement of objectives in the abstract of a study by Cedergren and Källén: "This study determined whether obese women have an increased risk of cardiovascular defects in their offspring compared with average weight women".[165] Although the statement does not have a question mark, it clearly represents a research question: Do obese women have an increased risk of cardiovascular defects in their offspring? Critical appraisal can then evaluate how well the study answers that research question.

A study by Petitti et al states this objective: "To assess the risk of environmental heat-associated death by occupation."[166] Yet, the study was a case-control study, a design that cannot assess risk. Rather, the study reported age-adjusted odds ratios, which provide estimates of relative risk. In this case, critical appraisal should begin by noting the true focus of the study (estimating relative risk), and proceed by assessing the validity of the reported odds ratios and the causal interpretations associated with them.

> *Key point:* The results of a study generally relate to a research objective. Identification of a study's objective is a good early step in critical appraisal.

Step 2: Identifying the exposure and disease variables

You can easily get off track in critical appraisal without a clear sense of the exposure and disease of interest.

For example, the stated objective of an analysis arising from the Women's Health Initiative was: "To assess the major health benefits and risks of the most commonly used combined hormone preparation in the United States."[144] This study examined many health outcomes—so, many possible exposure-disease associations. Critical appraisal, however, requires a more precise focus. A precise focus on specific exposure-disease associations allows evaluation of issues such as measurement accuracy, or attrition related to disease and exposure status. In the case of this study, it would be best to gain a clearer picture of the specific outcomes of interest before proceeding further with critical appraisal.

> *Key point:* Identify the exposure and disease variables early in the process of critical appraisal.

Step 3: Identifying the study design

Once you have identified the exposure and disease variables, it is usually quite easy to identify the study design.

If the study is observational and the measures are aggregate, the study is ecological. If the measures are individual, examining the temporal direction and logical direction of the study's inquiry should help clarify the study design.

Often, of course, the authors have already classified the study design and made a statement about what sort of study they have conducted. However, a little skepticism makes sense here, because authors may use terminology incorrectly or choose terminology that they think will put a positive spin on their results.

While different study designs have different strengths and weaknesses, there are no absolute rules about what designs are better or worse overall. For a particular question, for example, a case-control design may lead to a more valid answer than a prospective cohort design, even though prospective cohort studies are often viewed as more robust in their methods. Even a randomized study, often regarded as the gold standard in study design, can be inferior to other types of studies if it is poorly conducted.

So, classifying the design of a study should not lead directly to conclusions about the quality of the study. The point of classification is to add structure

TABLE 39. "RED FLAGS" CLASSICALLY ASSOCIATED WITH PARTICULAR STUDY DESIGNS

Study design	Red flags
Case-control studies	Recall bias (differential misclassification of exposure) Selection bias
Cross-sectional studies	Lack of temporal clarity
Ecological studies	Ecological fallacy Difficulty detecting and controlling confounding
Prospective cohort studies	Bias due to attrition (selection bias) Differential misclassification of outcome
Randomized controlled trials	Diminished generalizability

to the task of critical appraisal. As soon as you determine, for example, that a study is cross-sectional, you can immediately flag difficulties that the study may have in determining temporality—an issue with implications for causal reasoning. Other designs raise other red flags (see Table 39).

> *Key point:* Classifying study design does not in itself identify methodological problems, but it can help to organize critical appraisal and often points to potential methodological problems.

Step 4: Assessment of selection bias

Why selection bias first?

There are 2 main sources of error in epidemiological research—random error, and systematic error leading to bias. Which should you consider first in critical appraisal?

Systematic error comes first. The logic behind this assertion is that systematic error and random error have a hierarchical relationship. Random error is quantified using techniques such as statistical tests and confidence intervals—but if an estimate is invalid in the first place, these quantifications of the role of chance are pointless. No one cares whether an invalid (biased) estimate is statistically significant. Indeed, P values and confidence intervals have little meaning in the face of systematic error. Therefore, systematic error (bias) is the best place to start.

Of the 2 main categories of bias—misclassification bias and selection bias—selection bias is probably the best to consider first, since the subjects for a study must be selected before measurement can occur.

> *Key point:* Selection bias is a good place to begin addressing the issue of bias, because—methodologically—selection occurs before classification of disease and exposure status.

To assess selection bias, you need to conceptualize the selection probabilities and apply the rules that determine when selection bias will occur. With selection probabilities, it is important to think broadly. Selection probabilities are influenced by more than just sampling. They are also influenced by factors such as provision of consent, provision of information, and attrition. Anything that affects participation must be considered.

Selection probabilities, however, are almost never known—not to critical appraisers, and generally not to researchers either. Therefore, the assessment of selection bias involves a qualitative assessment of the likely values of selection probabilities.

In a study that is estimating a frequency such as prevalence, the rules governing the assessment of selection bias are simple. If the selection probability depends on the attribute whose frequency is being assessed, bias will occur.

The rules are more complex in analytical studies, in which the targets of estimation are population parameters such as odds ratios and risk differences. Here, the selection probabilities will often depend explicitly on disease (e.g., in a case-control study) or on exposure (e.g., in many prospective cohort studies). This in itself does not cause selection bias. However, selection bias will occur if the probability of selection of cases and controls—in a case-control study, for example—depends on exposure in some way that differs between the cases and controls. Similarly, in a prospective cohort study, attrition may introduce bias if it depends on disease in a way that differs between those with and without exposure.

Selection bias in schematics

Figures 10, 11, 12, and 13 express these principles in schematics. They use arrows to represent movement from the population (where disease-exposure contingencies are represented by uppercase letters) to the sample (where they

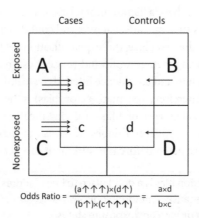

Odds Ratio $= \dfrac{(a\uparrow\uparrow\uparrow)\times(d\uparrow)}{(b\uparrow)\times(c\uparrow\uparrow\uparrow)} = \dfrac{a\times d}{b\times c}$

FIGURE 10. SCHEMATIC OF AN UNBIASED CASE-CONTROL STUDY

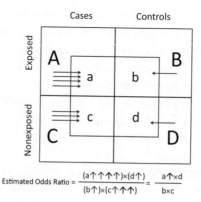

$$\text{Estimated Odds Ratio} = \frac{(a\uparrow\uparrow\uparrow\uparrow)\times(d\uparrow)}{(b\uparrow)\times(c\uparrow\uparrow\uparrow)} = \frac{a\uparrow\times d}{b\times c}$$

FIGURE 11. SCHEMATIC OF A BIASED CASE-CONTROL STUDY

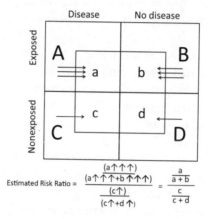

$$\text{Estimated Risk Ratio} = \frac{\dfrac{(a\uparrow\uparrow\uparrow)}{(a\uparrow\uparrow\uparrow+b\uparrow\uparrow\uparrow)}}{\dfrac{(c\uparrow)}{(c\uparrow+d\uparrow)}} = \frac{\dfrac{a}{a+b}}{\dfrac{c}{c+d}}$$

FIGURE 12. SCHEMATIC OF AN UNBIASED COHORT STUDY

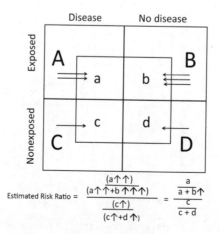

$$\text{Estimated Risk Ratio} = \frac{\dfrac{(a\uparrow\uparrow)}{(a\uparrow\uparrow+b\uparrow\uparrow\uparrow)}}{\dfrac{(c\uparrow)}{(c\uparrow+d\uparrow)}} = \frac{\dfrac{a}{a+b\uparrow}}{\dfrac{c}{c+d}}$$

FIGURE 13. SCHEMATIC OF A BIASED COHORT STUDY

are represented with lowercase letters). A formula for the odds ratio—at the bottom of each figure—shows another way to describe these principles.

Figure 10 and Figure 11 describe selection effects in a case-control study. In a case-control study, the selection probabilities for cases are much greater than controls (shown by more arrows for cases than controls). In Figure 10, these probabilities vary in exactly the same way for cases and controls. In an odds ratio calculated from this study, the arrows occur to the same extent in the numerator and denominator, cancelling out, and demonstrating that selection bias does not occur in this scenario.

In Figure 11, the selection probabilities for cases vary by exposure. This can happen if a case-control study has flawed methods that result in a greater probability of selection for exposed cases than nonexposed cases, and do not result in the same influence of exposure in selection of controls. The odds ratio ends up having too large a numerator, leading to bias. Figure 11 describes the process by which sets of selection probabilities translate into bias in an estimated odds ratio.

Figures 12 and 13 describe selection effects in cohort studies. Note that in Figure 12—an unbiased cohort study—overrepresentation of exposed subjects does not result in bias. One of the advantages of cohort studies is that they can oversample from groups with a rare exposure. Figure 12 shows that this in itself does not cause bias.

Figure 13 shows a biased cohort study, where attrition results in an underestimation of the effect of exposure: attrition has occurred to a lesser extent among exposed subjects with disease than among exposed subjects without disease, whereas the same effect does not occur in the nonexposed cohort.

Figure 14 depicts selection bias in a risk difference. This mirrors the bias in Figure 13, except the measure of effect is now a risk difference rather than a

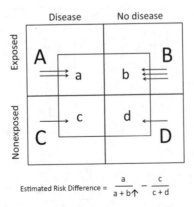

$$\text{Estimated Risk Difference} = \frac{a}{a+b\uparrow} - \frac{c}{c+d}$$

FIGURE 14. SCHEMATIC OF A BIASED COHORT STUDY: RISK RATIO AS MEASURE OF EFFECT

risk ratio. In the risk difference in Figure 14, the first risk in the risk difference is too small, resulting in an underestimation of this effect.

The 2 parts to bias assessment

Critical appraisal of selection bias—and all bias—has 2 parts. First, you determine if a source of vulnerability to bias exists. If a source exists, you then determine the expected direction and magnitude of bias.

Note that the schematics presented in this section can clarify the direction of bias. They can also indicate magnitude. For example, Figure 14 could have indicated bias of a greater magnitude by depicting the underrepresentation of exposed cases with 2 arrows rather than 1 arrow.

Decisions about the direction and magnitude of bias represent judgements made by critical appraisers. The representation of these judgements using visual aids such as the schematics presented here adds structure to the critical-appraisal process.

Key point: By considering probability of selection in relation to disease-exposure contingencies and study designs, the direction and magnitude of selection bias can be anticipated.

Step 5: Assessment of misclassification bias

If a study is vulnerable to selection bias—and the vulnerability arises from a defect that would lead to serious over- or underestimation of the target parameter—then the task of critical appraisal might stop there. There's no point looking for more flaws if the flaw you've found is fatal. However, if the impact of selection bias is posited to be negligible or at least modest, then there is value in continuing.

For studies estimating a frequency, the rules governing misclassification bias are again fairly straightforward. Insensitivity of the measure used to classify the attribute will lead to false negatives, deflating the numerator and leading to underestimation of the frequency. A lack of specificity in such a measure will predictably lead to false-positive results. These can be expected to inflate the numerator of the frequency with a resulting tendency towards overestimation.

Again, the situation is more complex when the goal of a study is to estimate a complex parameter such as a ratio or a difference between frequencies. Misclassification can then be differential or nondifferential. If nondifferential, the direction of bias is predictably towards the null value. If differential, you need to determine its direction and magnitude.

Differential misclassification bias in schematics

Figure 15 describes an unbiased study. It contrasts with Figure 16 and Figure 17, which describe the effects of misclassification bias.

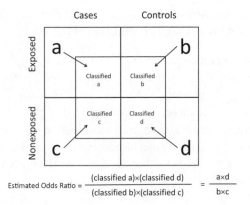

FIGURE 15. SCHEMATIC OF AN UNBIASED CASE-CONTROL STUDY: ODDS RATIO AS MEASURE OF EFFECT

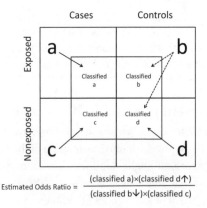

FIGURE 16. SCHEMATIC OF A BIASED CASE-CONTROL STUDY: RECALL BIAS, ODDS RATIO AS MEASURE OF EFFECT

Note that these schematics do not use uppercase and lowercase letters to distinguish populations and samples—after all, selection plays no role in the mechanisms leading to misclassification bias. Misclassification bias results from classifying members of the study sample into the wrong categories in the classic 2 × 2 contingency table.

Figure 15 represents the process of classification of exposure in a case-control study where there are no classification errors. The outer box of the schematic represents the actual status of the sample (depicted with lowercase letters since these are sample values). Here, all of the exposed subjects are true positives for exposure and all of the nonexposed subjects are true negatives for exposure. The contingencies according to the classification are the same as the real contingencies in the sample and there is no bias introduced into the estimate.

Figure 16 describes a case-control study where misclassification from recall bias has taken place. In recall bias, people with a disease tend to think harder about possible causes of their condition. They are more likely to recall exposures than members of the control group. Here, the misclassification is due to a lower sensitivity for classification of exposure among the control group. So, some of the exposed persons in the control group are misclassified as nonexposed, moving people from the upper-right contingency cell to the lower-right cell (depicted as a dashed line in Figure 16). When the odds ratio is calculated, there will be too few in the upper-right cell and too many in the lower-right cell, leading to an overestimation of the odds ratio.

Key point: Critical appraisal must distinguish differential and nondifferential misclassification bias in analytical studies, because these different forms of bias have important implications for the direction of bias.

Figure 17 presents another classic form of differential misclassification bias: diagnostic suspicion bias (surveillance bias) in cohort studies. The idea is that the measure of disease status may be less sensitive in the nonexposed than in the exposed. Because there is a higher index of suspicion among the exposed, they are followed more closely. Some of those in the nonexposed group are sometimes misclassified as nondiseased because they are not followed closely enough for all cases to be detected.

The risk ratio will be overestimated in the scenario in Figure 17 because the denominator of the risk ratio will be too small:

$$\text{Estimated Risk Ratio} = \left[\frac{\left(\dfrac{\text{Classified } a}{\text{Classified } a + \text{Classified } b}\right)}{\left(\dfrac{\text{Classified } c \downarrow}{\text{Classified } c \downarrow + \text{Classified } d \uparrow}\right)}\right]$$

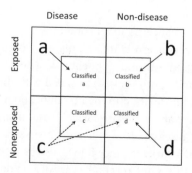

FIGURE 17. SCHEMATIC OF A BIASED COHORT STUDY: DIAGNOSTIC SUSPICION BIAS

As with selection bias, the assessment of misclassification bias should also include an assessment of the magnitude of bias. The assessment is again a matter of judgement, but the schematics can help structure it. For example, Figure 17 depicts the misclassification of nonexposed cases due to low sensitivity of diagnostic procedures in the nonexposed cohort. You can look up what is known about the accuracy of the diagnostic procedures used in a study. For example, if a diagnostic procedure is expected to achieve only 50% sensitivity in the nonexposed cohort, the arrow (dotted line) leading to the "classified d" cell will move half of those who should be in the "classified c" cell to the "classified d" cell. Assuming that other aspects of classification are accurate, this would make the value of c in the denominator of a risk ratio about half as large as it should be, thereby doubling the value of the risk ratio.

Step 6: Assessment of confounding and effect measure modification

Effect measure modification first

The issues of effect measure modification and confounding always go together. Confounding cannot be considered unless effect measure modification has been assessed.

An obvious question for critical appraisal concerns whether a study has addressed these issues properly. If you are concerned that an extraneous variable may have modified the effect of the exposure variable in a study, then you will want to see that the study has assessed this possibility. A study would normally do this with a test for heterogeneity or with an interaction term in a model. If effect measure modification has not been assessed, then the study's estimates may be meaningless averages of the effect in people with or without the modifying variable.

Confounding next

If a study has addressed effect measure modification—or if effect measure modification is not a concern—then your next focus is how the study controls confounding.

There are usually 2 concerns about confounding.

The first common concern is that a potential confounder exists that the study has not addressed. Any independent risk factor for the study's outcome may act as a confounder, if it is also associated with the disease in question. It is unusual to find information in the literature about associations between potential confounders and exposure variables, but many studies have identified risk factors for diseases. Any independent risk factor for a disease is a potential confounding variable, since it may also be associated with exposure (note, however, that this is unlikely in the case of a randomized study). Ideally, you would want to see every independent risk factor addressed in some way as a potential confounding variable, either at the design stage or in the analysis. If you can identify a potentially confounding variable that has not been addressed, you have identified a methodological weakness of the study.

The second common concern arises if confounding has been poorly dealt with in an analysis. For example, an analysis that is based on broad stratification across arbitrary categories for a continuous variable may leave residual confounding within its strata. When there is residual confounding, pooling procedures, such as the Mantel-Haenszel family of pooled estimators, will not fully adjust for those confounding effects. Another example: a study has measured a confounding variable, so that the variable can be controlled in the analysis, but the study has measured the variable inaccurately. This will result in inadequate control of the effects of the confounding variable.

A final concern about confounding is whether variables controlled in an analysis were not confounders but mediating variables. Recall that a confounding variable must be an independent risk factor for the outcome under study. If both exposure and confounder exist on the same causal chain of events, adjustment for confounding may attenuate the effects of the exposure, creating the false impression that the exposure is not causally related to the disease. Discerning whether a variable is an independent risk factor or a mediator of the effects of the exposure must often come from the literature. An interesting example has unfolded in a debate about whether very strenuous physical activity may have negative health implications. O'Keefe et al[167] described a U-shaped relationship between running distance per week and all-cause mortality. Runners had lower mortality than nonrunners, but runners covering distances greater than 20 miles per week had increased mortality, similar to nonrunners. These estimates were adjusted for body mass index, blood pressure, diagnosis of hypertension, lipids, glucose, and psychological factors.[168] Pointing out that many of these variables are beneficial effects of running, Weber[169] later argued that the U-shaped curve may have been exaggerated because these adjustments may have removed (or adjusted away) many of the beneficial effects of running. Consistent with this, the authors subsequently repeated their analysis with adjustment only for age and sex. While a U-shaped pattern was still evident, it was "blunted" compared to what had been previously reported.[168]

Key point: Assessment of the control of confounding in a study should assess whether potential confounding variables were treated correctly (e.g., during stratification or modelling), and also whether all important potentially confounding variables were included.

Step 7: Assessing the role of chance

In epidemiology, the role of chance is assessed using either statistical tests or confidence intervals. Confidence intervals are the preferred procedure. Unlike *P* values, confidence intervals do not confound the effect of sample size with that of effect size. Instead, they provide a plausible range of values for an estimated epidemiologic parameter. However, *P* values continue to be commonly reported. This produces a temptation to interpret confidence intervals as if they were tests of significance. Keeping in mind, for example, that an odds ratio has a null value of 1, it may be tempting to interpret a 95% CI primarily by whether it crosses the null value, as this would indicate statistical significance. However, this would be a mistake because confidence intervals have much to say beyond statistical significance. To interpret a confidence interval, it is a good idea to look at 2 different things: the location of the interval and also its width. The location of the upper and lower confidence limits provides information about the smallest and largest population values that are consistent with the observed data. Anything between these 2 limits is a plausible value for the population parameter. The width of the interval quantifies the precision of the estimate.

When *P* values are reported in a study as indicators of statistical significance, critical appraisal needs to focus on the vulnerability of the study to type I or type II error, depending on the results the study reports.

If a study reports a significant result, the concern is with type I error. If a study has a small number of tests (ideally, 1 test to evaluate a single well-defined primary hypothesis), the *P* value quantifies the risk of type I error. However, if the analysis is poorly structured and there are multiple hypotheses, or ill-defined hypotheses, then the risk of type I error is decidedly higher. Remember that, when using tests based on a 5% level of confidence, there is a 5% chance of type I error. If a study uses multiple tests, there is a much higher probability of type I error: the risk for each specific test is 5%. There is no way to know which of the significant tests are type I errors, so a shadow is cast over all the results.

If a study reports a statistical test that is not significant, the possibility of type II error must be considered. The probability of type II error is related to the power of the study. It is therefore very helpful if studies report a justification for their chosen sample size, such as a power calculation.

Of course, if the estimate is biased then confidence intervals are of little interest—nor are *P* values. In this situation, confidence intervals do not quantify the role of chance properly, nor does their width reflect the precision of the estimate in a meaningful way. When an estimate is biased and the sample size for the study is very large, the confidence intervals are likely to be extremely narrow and are unlikely to include the actual population at all.

Given this state of affairs, the naive interpretation of a 95% CI (or, of course, a *P* value) in the presence of bias is internally contradictory.

Key point: Interpretation of a confidence interval involves consideration of the location of the confidence limits and the width of the interval.

Step 8: Addressing causality

The concept of causality is hierarchically related to the concept of validity. If an estimate is invalid, there is often no point in considering its causal significance. Note, however, that this is not always the case. For example, consider an estimate that suggests a strong effect, but that may be affected by nondifferential misclassification bias—it is safe to say that the actual estimate is stronger than reported. Here, it may make sense to consider questions related to causation.

Key point: If an estimate is unbiased, causation may be considered. A common approach is to consider causal criteria, as described—for example—by Bradford Hill.

Step 9: Assessing generalizability

If an estimate is judged to be invalid, then there is no point assessing its generalizability. Internal validity is a necessary precondition for any consideration of external validity.

Keep in mind the distinction between internal and external validity. Internal validity can be defined in a technical sense as the absence of bias—it is something you can assess objectively in critical appraisal. External validity is a study's applicability to populations beyond its target population—its assessment is entirely a matter of judgement.

If you are reading a study from the United States, for example, you can reasonably ask whether the study applies to Canada (as long as its estimates are judged valid). This assessment—as in all considerations of external validity—would be a matter of considered opinion, not fact.

In general, epidemiological findings that involve biological aspects of disease etiology (such as the increased risk of cardiovascular disease associated with smoking) are likely to be readily generalizable, whereas associations that involve culturally sensitive or health system–related estimates are less likely to be generalizable.

Key point: Consideration of *P* values and confidence intervals, as well as issues of causation and generalizability, are important when an estimate is internally valid. When an estimate is invalid, these considerations are not usually important at all.

Step 10: Reporting a critical appraisal

A critical appraisal can usually be written up in a few pages, or provided verbally in 5 to10 minutes. It should normally follow the steps presented in this chapter. This means that it would often start with a brief summary of the work: the objectives of the study, the exposure and disease variables, and the study design. This would be followed by an examination of the key issues of bias, effect measure modification, and confounding, as outlined above. If the results of the study are considered invalid, the appraisal may end there. If the estimates are determined to be valid, a discussion of their causal significance and generalizability are often pursued.

Critical appraisal as a skill

This chapter has presented a series of steps to guide critical appraisal, but critical appraisal is too complex to be simply a technical procedure.

Critical appraisal is a skill and, like all skills, requires practice and feedback.

It also requires knowledge. For example, consideration of biological plausibility often depends on knowledge of physiology, and judgements about external validity require knowledge of different populations.

The best way to develop the skill of critical appraisal—to build your fluency with study designs and types of error, to identify critical gaps in your knowledge—is to apply it in settings where feedback is available, such as peer-review groups and journal clubs.

Questions

1. Identifying a study's design can help to focus critical appraisal on the potential vulnerabilities of a study because specific methodological vulnerabilities tend to be associated with specific study designs. Identify the single most notorious vulnerability of each the following study designs:
   a. ecological studies
   b. cross-sectional studies
   c. randomized controlled trials
   d. prospective cohort studies
   e. case-control studies

2. Do you think there are any situations in which an invalid estimate can be generalized to another population?

3. Can a study conducted in Newfoundland be generalized to British Columbia?

4. Many contemporary studies present complex models that simultaneously adjust for multiple potential confounding variables.
   a. These studies often fail to report whether they evaluated interactions between these variables and the exposure of interest. In your opinion, is this a problem?

    b. Sometimes, the authors defend the inclusion of variables in these models based on whether they are statistically significant. Does this seem to you like the best way to decide what variables should be included in a regression model?

5. All major medical journals have web pages where they post online versions of studies. It is usually possible for authors to publish supplementary materials relevant to their studies. What kinds of materials provide assistance to critical appraisers?

ANSWERS TO QUESTIONS

Chapter 1

QUESTION 1

a. There are different types of administrative data. In Canada, provincial public health insurance plans are widely available sources of data. These data include diagnostic codes that fee-for-service physicians submit to provincial plans to get paid, and summaries that are completed by hospitals when discharging patients. These data may not be accurate for some conditions—for example, for conditions where people do not seek assistance from physicians or hospitals. They may also lack accuracy where several diagnoses might be relevant. For example, physicians often only need to report a single diagnosis to receive payment, yet many people have more than a single disease. Also, some provinces require only "rough" diagnostic codes (e.g., the first 3 codes of the International Classification of Disease, or ICD, which sometimes represent a group of diseases rather than a single disease).

b. The study seeks to quantify the amount of disease in the population, so it has primarily descriptive aims.

c. For a condition that may have a different prevalence in different provinces, pooling estimates from different provinces to produce a national prevalence estimate would be a major concern. Extending results that are based on 5 provinces to all 10 provinces would amount to assuming that the prevalence is the same in all provinces.

d. This kind of information is important for 2 main reasons. First, those planning health services need to know how much disease is in a population, so they can anticipate the quantity of resources needed. However, if differences were observed among provinces, this might generate hypotheses about risk factors for the disease. In turn, this might lead to additional studies (analytical studies) seeking to determine why the prevalence is higher in some regions of the country than in others.

QUESTION 2

a. The study does not target a population that is entirely geographically based, but it still targets a well-defined population. This is a population-based study.

b. This study is concerned with the distribution and determinants of health issues (pain, undertreatment of pain) in a defined population, so it is an epidemiological study. Some might call this *health services research* to emphasize that it is focused on a health-system performance issue—the proper management of pain—but it is not necessary to make this distinction.

c. Epidemiological studies need large samples so that they can see patterns of disease and exposure in populations. The "noise" of random variation often obscures these patterns when samples are small.

d. They have identified a problem. Further understanding the basis of this problem, or doing something about it, will improve the health of members of this population.

e. Like all descriptive studies, this study has value in identifying a problem, which makes it possible for health services to address the problem. The study has also quantified the extent of the problem—another valuable piece of information for administering health services. The study may also lead to analytical studies that investigate why the problem is happening.

QUESTION 3

a. This study is concerned with whether a particular risk factor (fewer years of education) increases the risk of Alzheimer disease. The study is evaluating a hypothesis about disease etiology, so it is an analytical study.

b. In this case, it is not easy to discern how this information would be useful for prevention through public health action. However, identification of this association could prove valuable for understanding the disease, and a better understanding of the disease could ultimately play a role in prevention.

QUESTION 4

These studies share the following focus with the work of John Snow: examining patterns of distribution of diseases in populations. They seek to identify the burden of disease, generate hypotheses about disease etiology, or test hypotheses about disease etiology.

QUESTION 5

a. If this association can lead to actions that will diminish mortality due to cholera, then those actions are valuable. This kind of information can lead to fruitful public health actions, saving lives and preventing suffering. Such actions do not always (indeed they rarely) depend on a full understanding of each step in the pathophysiology of a disease.

b. Diseases occur as a result of an intermixing of many component causes. *Vibrio cholerae* is obviously a key component cause, but it is only 1 step on a causal chain of events. Intervening at other places along that chain (e.g., the safe disposal of fecal waste and protection of drinking water supplies) can effectively control cholera.

Chapter 2

QUESTION 1

The prevalence is 2 363 010/35 158 300, or 0.067, or 6.7%.

QUESTION 2

a. The prevalence is 9/401, or 0.022, or 2.2%.

b. The standard error is 0.007.

QUESTION 3

Point prevalence estimates the proportion in a population with a disease. This parameter is of clear value for descriptive epidemiology because it quantifies the burden of disease. If point prevalence is particularly high or low in a particular population, it may also generate hypotheses about etiology, another important descriptive goal. However, point prevalence is less useful for analytical epidemiology because it does not quantify the risk of developing a disease—it is merely the proportion having a disease.

QUESTION 4

Basic epidemiological parameters are intended to quantify probabilities and risks. When a risk does not apply to a segment of the population, such as women in this case, that segment would not usually be included in the calculation.

QUESTION 5

In principle, there is no reason to quantify the precision of an estimate that actually is the population estimate. In practice, when a parameter such as prevalence is measured at several different times, some degree of random variation will likely affect the estimates. This is especially true for rare diseases. As a result, procedures such as confidence intervals are commonly used to assess the "stability" of proportions and rates in entire populations.

Chapter 3

QUESTION 1

a. Of the 10 people, there are 4 who become ill during the observation period. Therefore, the annual period prevalence is 4/10.

b. In August, there are 3 people with the disease. The population at this point in time consists of 9 people, since 1 has died. The point prevalence is therefore 3/9.

c. This is the proportion of people at risk of the disease who develop the disease during the defined interval of follow-up. There are 2 people that have the illness at the baseline time point and who are therefore not at risk. Two of those who are at risk develop the disease, which makes the cumulative incidence proportion 2/8.

d. Since this is a mortality rate, all 10 subjects contribute person-time observations to the calculation, regardless of whether they have the disease at baseline. Everyone alive is at risk of death. However, person-time after death is not counted because it does not exist. The total person-years of observation is 105 (the grid potentially holds $10 \times 12 = 120$ person-months of observation, but there are 15 white squares) and there are 3 deaths, so the rate is 3 per 105 person-months, or 0.029 per person-month, or 0.029 month^{-1}. To convert this value to person-years, multiply it by 12 (months per year): 0.343 year^{-1}.

e. Since the disease is a recurrent disease, people reenter the population at risk after they recover. Therefore, even person number 4 provides person-time at risk starting in April. The only person contributing no person-time is person number 9, because that person is ill throughout the entire interval. However, people who are ill do not contribute to person-time at risk. The total person-time at risk is 82 person-months. Since the disease is recurrent, there can be more than 1 episode of illness in a given person. Therefore, person number 7 contributes 2 episodes to the numerator of the incidence rate. So, there are 3 incidents per 82 person-months, or 0.037 month^{-1}, or 0.439 year^{-1}.

QUESTION 2

a. Of the 10 people, there are 3 who become ill during the observation period. Therefore, the annual period prevalence is 3/10.

b. In August, no one has the disease. The point prevalence is therefore 0.

c. Of 9 persons at risk at the baseline time point, 2 develop the disease during follow-up. The incidence proportion is therefore 2/9.

d. There are 85 person-months of observation and 4 deaths, so the mortality rate is 4/85 person-months, or 0.047 months^{-1}. This corresponds to 0.565 years^{-1}.

e. There are 82 person-months at risk of the disease, contributed by the 9 people free of disease at the baseline time point. Two incident cases arise from this person-time at risk. The incidence rate is therefore 2/82 person-months, or 0.024 months^{-1}, which is 0.293 years^{-1}.

QUESTION 3

a. There are 2 people affected during the 1 year of observation. Therefore, the period prevalence is 2/10.

b. The point prevalence is the same in each month: 1/10.

c. Eight of the 10 people contribute 12 person-months of observation. The other 2 contribute 6 person-months each. The incidence rate is therefore 12/108 person-months, or 0.111 months^{-1}, or 1.33 year^{-1}. Note that it is possible for an incidence rate to have a value greater than 1: this is a rate, which can be associated with different units, not a proportion.

d. The prevalence odds equal the incidence rate multiplied by mean duration. Each episode has a 1-month duration. So, the prevalence odds are the same as the incidence rate, except that the units disappear during the process of multiplying 1 month by 0.111 month^{-1}. Of course, you could also calculate the prevalence odds by dividing the number of people with an episode by the number of people without an episode: 1/9 = 0.111. In addition, you could calculate the prevalence odds from the prevalence proportion using the formula for this purpose (odds = proportion / 1 – proportion), which is 1/10 / (1 – 1/10) = 0.111.

QUESTION 4

a. 0.0009

b. 0.0091

c. 0.0989

d. 9

QUESTION 5

Prevalence (which quantifies how common a disease is) is approximately equal to incidence (expressed as a rate with time^{-1} units) multiplied by the duration of illness (in time units). Since insulin is a life-saving treatment for people with insulin-dependent diabetes, its discovery lengthened the duration of illness and has increased its prevalence.

Chapter 4

QUESTION 1

Approximately a quarter of a million people die in Canada from all causes each year. This is the numerator of a crude prevalence calculation. Statistics Canada produces annual population estimates—the 2014 population estimate was approximately 35 million. Crude mortality in Canada is therefore approximately 250 000 divided by 35 000 000 or approximately 700 per 100 000. Consistent with this, Statistics Canada reported a 7 per 1000 population crude mortality rate for 2014. This can properly be called a rate, because the midyear population (July 1) was used in the calculation. The midyear population is a good approximation of person-years of life within the population during that year.

QUESTION 2

The cause-specific mortality rates for tuberculosis and malignant neoplasms can be estimated using the same procedure described for question 1. You also need to decide how to report the estimate. Dividing 70 by 35 million leads to a cause specific mortality of 0.000002 or 0.002 per 1000 (here, the units are omitted: it would perhaps be misleading to represent this "quick and dirty" calculation as a rate because the midyear population was not used in the calculation). However, this is a difficult number to digest. It would perhaps be better to report this as (roughly) 2 per million since this immediately suggests the number of expected deaths in a country of approximately 35 million.

QUESTION 3

a. In Canada, age 75 is most often used as the index age against which to determine potential years of life lost (PYLL). In this collision, 2 people died, losing 55 and 48 potential years of life, respectively. The total lost is therefore 108 PYLL. The vulnerability of young people to traumatic deaths, particularly motor vehicle–related deaths, accounts for the major contribution of trauma to PYLL in Canada.

b. Since this person was more than 75 years old, his or her death is not considered to have caused any premature mortality. The contribution to PYLL is 0.

QUESTION 4

a. The conditions that kill the most people in Canada are cancer, heart disease, and stroke.

b. The 3 leading causes of premature mortality are the same as the leading causes of overall mortality. Other conditions such as road injury, congenital malformations, and self-harm are, however, highly ranked in terms of premature mortality because they afflict young people. The Global Burden of Disease (GBD) study has produced a country-specific report for Canada that includes "years of life lost" as a measure of premature mortality.[170] This is similar to PYLL, although the GBD uses slightly different definitions than those adopted by Statistics Canada in CANSIM.

c. According to the GBD, the top contributors to years lived with disability in Canada (as of 2010) were low back pain, major depressive disorder, and musculoskeletal disorders other than low back pain.

QUESTION 5

This rate describes the proportion of people with a specific disease that die from it and is therefore a case-fatality rate. For infectious diseases, the case-fatality rate is often a simple proportion. For other illnesses, it may be reported as the proportion dying during a specific time interval, as in this study.

Chapter 5

QUESTION 1

The key feature of critical appraisal is that it adopts a critical stance towards research results. A critical appraiser does not read a study under the assumption that it was done correctly and that the results are valid. Instead, a critical appraiser looks for problems that may have introduced errors into the reported results (and also interpretations, conclusions, etc.). The popular media often do not approach health studies from a critical stance (although good reporters will seek opinions from several experts as they develop their stories). This sometimes leads to uncritical reporting of a "finding" (often an interpretation by an investigator) from a major study.

QUESTION 2

Random error is error that results from sampling variability. According to the law of large numbers, and assuming that there are no defects in a study's design, the extent of random error will predictably diminish with increasing sample sizes. The extent of random error can be quantified during the process of estimation by confidence intervals. The width of confidence intervals is the precision of the estimate.

QUESTION 3

The standard error of 0.42% (or 0.0042) indicates that an approximate 95% CI should be the point estimate (3%, or 0.03) plus or minus 2 times this quantity (roughly 0.8%). Therefore, an approximate 95% CI would be 2.2%–3.8%.

QUESTION 4

If the method of data collection (self-report over the phone) fails to detect some cases, the prevalence estimate will be too low. Increasing the sample size will not correct this problem, so this is not a form of random error. Rather, this is a form of systematic error (more specifically, a measurement bias). Consistent with the possibility of underreporting, a study conducted by Maclaren and Best[171] at the University of New Brunswick and Thompson Rivers University reported a higher prevalence. However, there are many other possible explanations for the divergent results.

QUESTION 5

Technically, it would be correct to say that, were this study conducted many times, the confidence intervals calculated from these repetitions would include the population value 95% of the time. However, this definition seems excessively technical, because studies are never conducted many times. A usual interpretive statement would be (assuming that the study methods are considered valid) that the study shows with 95% confidence that the population value is between 0.11 and 4.15 per 100 000.

Chapter 6

QUESTION 1

There are 21 subjects that have DVT according to the gold standard test. Of these, 8 are positive on the colour Doppler ultrasound test, which means the sensitivity is 8/21, or 38.1%. There are 298 that are negative for DVT, of whom 275 test negative, which means the specificity is 275/298, or 92.2%.

QUESTION 2

The odds of DVT are 21/298 or 0.07. These are the pretest odds: they represent the odds in the absence of any information about the test results. The pretest probability (or prevalence) of DVT can be calculated from these odds using the formula: proportion = odds ÷ (1 + odds). For this study, the result is 0.07 ÷ 1.07 = 0.066. Because the outcome is fairly uncommon, the prevalence proportion is quite similar to the prevalence odds.

QUESTION 3

The likelihood ratio positive can be calculated as: sensitivity ÷ (1 − specificity). In this study, the result is 0.38 ÷ (1 − 0.92) = 4.9.

QUESTION 4

The posttest odds are the pretest odds multiplied by the likelihood ratio positive, or 0.07 × 4.9, which is 0.35. Without knowing the test result, the best guess about the probability of DVT was the pretest odds of approximately 7%. The likelihood ratio positive indicates that a positive test increases this fivefold.

QUESTION 5

If the pretest odds are 1.0, then the likelihood ratio positive indicates that the posttest odds would be 4.94. Converting this to a proportion—so, proportion = odds ÷ (1 + odds)—results in a positive predictive value of 83%. Bayes' theorem, as always, produces the same result: (0.38 × 0.50) ÷ [(0.38 × 0.50) + (1 − 0.92) × (1 − 0.5)] = 0.83, or 83%.

Chapter 7

QUESTION 1

a. The performance of the algorithm in this sample is good. However, the sample is small ($n = 20$ with parkinsonism and 20 controls). The actual sensitivity and specificity of the algorithm may differ from the 100% estimates due to random error. As a result, the future use of the algorithm could nevertheless contribute to misclassification bias in assessment of the prevalence of parkinsonism.

b. All cases of diabetes will be detected since the sensitivity is 100% (note, however, that the 100% sensitivity is itself an estimate). Seventy percent specificity means that false positives are expected to occur with this particular algorithm. This will inflate the estimated prevalence because the false positives will occur in the numerator of the formula for prevalence.

QUESTION 2

a. Imperfect measurement creates vulnerability to bias. Because the sensitivity for this particular condition was quite low, it is likely that the majority of cases would be missed, which would likely lead to bias. It should be noted that the interRAI rating system had excellent performance for several other conditions. Traumatic brain injury stood out in the Foebel et al study as a specific condition where the performance of interRAI was not very good.

b. Since interRAI was highly specific, few false positives are expected. Because its sensitivity for traumatic brain injury was low, those with traumatic brain injury will be underrepresented in the numerator of the prevalence formula, leading to a negative bias. The expected value of the estimate is too low.

QUESTION 3

a. This type of bias (where people hide an attribute due to an awareness that it is negatively perceived by others) is called *social desirability bias*. If the level of stigma reported by people is lower than the level of stigmatizing beliefs that they actually hold, this will introduce bias.

b. This would be a negative bias: the mean level of stigma that is estimated will be lower than the actual level in the real population. Notably, during the development of the scale, Kassam et al measured the effect of social desirability on the scores and argued that the scale was not highly vulnerable to this type of bias.

QUESTION 4

a. It is doubtful that even those mothers searching their memories for a cause for the malformation would produce false-positive recollections. The tendency to focus on such issues would, therefore, likely improve the sensitivity of their reporting of such exposures. If their sensitivity of recollection was 100% and if no false-positive reports occur (specificity = 100%), bias would not occur.

b. The best way to control misclassification bias is when the study is designed. By ensuring accurate measurement (e.g., built-in double-checks of the self-report, or cognitive interviewing techniques that provide cues to ensure highly accurate reporting) the possibility of misclassification bias is minimized.

QUESTION 5

This is a matter of opinion. In the past, there has been much criticism of the quality of information on medical charts. However, electronic medical records are evolving and may (or may not) contain better information than the old paper charts of the past. Marrie et al also reported kappa statistics, which quantified the level of agreement between the 2 data sources without assuming that the chart review was a gold standard. This assumption is built in to the definitions of sensitivity and specificity.

Chapter 8

QUESTION 1

a. An unwillingness to disclose excessive use of substances could lower the sensitivity of the interview to detect these conditions. This could introduce bias, but it would not be selection bias. This would be a form of misclassification bias.

b. The fear of stigma may have caused people with mental illnesses to be less likely to participate in the survey than people without such difficulties. This would result in the numerator of the prevalence equation being diminished and in estimates that are negatively biased.

c. If there is no selection, then selection bias cannot occur. However, bias could still arise from problems affecting participation—for example, from problems with missing data. Investigators don't generally label bias due to missing data *selection bias*, although both types of bias occur through similar mechanisms if investigators handle missing data by excluding those participants from the calculations. *Bias due to missing data* is a better, descriptive label.

QUESTION 2

The question appears to state that the selection probabilities would be lower in people with dementia. Therefore, participation in the survey is related to the attribute whose frequency is being estimated. This is a typical situation in which selection bias could occur. However, if the target population is the household population, then the target of estimation is the prevalence of dementia in the household population (not the entire population, which would include household residents and others, such as residents of institutions and homeless people). For this reason, bias would not occur, at least not through the mechanism specified.

QUESTION 3

Such studies typically use the entire population in their denominator. This is the correct denominator, because universal health care in Canada essentially ensures that the entire population is registered with a provincial, or territorial, health care insurance plan. There are a few exceptions, such as members of the armed forces. The fact that some people with this condition may not have seen a physician during the study period (nor been admitted to hospital) would not be a cause of selection bias. This would be a form of misclassification bias: some of those people would have been misclassified as not having the illness, but they would still be included in the prevalence calculation (they would appear in the denominator).

QUESTION 4

a. Yes: if symptoms of the illness cause people with schizophrenia to be less likely to provide consent than others, selection bias would result.

b. The numerator of the prevalence equation would be too small, so that the prevalence of schizophrenia would be underestimated. The direction of bias is negative.

QUESTION 5

Yes: attrition affects participation in prospective studies. If an illness-related characteristic increases the risk of attrition, bias could occur in the estimated parameter—in this study, an incidence proportion. Bias due to attrition—because it is related to participation in a study and behaves similarly to other forms of selection bias—is often classified as a form of selection bias in epidemiology.

Chapter 9

QUESTION 1

a. This is indirect standardization. Note that values for the number of observed and expected cases have been reported.

b. The standardized mortality ratio (SMR) is $42/46.28 = 0.91$

c. This SMR does not suggest that increased mortality from this particular cause is associated with this exposure. An SMR less than 1 may reflect a healthy worker effect.

QUESTION 2

a. This a hugely elevated SMR. It indicates that these women are dying at a rate nearly 50 times that of the general population, after adjustment for age.

b. Intravenous drug use itself is dangerous. Many of these women would have also been homeless, and therefore vulnerable to violence, victimization, and many other risk factors for mortality (exposure, malnutrition, etc.). Socioeconomic deprivation is a major risk factor for mortality. HIV and sex-trade involvement were strongly associated with mortality in this analysis.

QUESTION 3

Indirect standardization can control for the effects of basic demographic variables such as age and sex (and also race, see question 4) because mortality rates for the general population are usually known for such variables. This allows an expected number of outcomes to be calculated for the exposed group. However, other confounders (e.g., smoking status) could account for an elevated SMR and are not addressed during the standardization procedure.

QUESTION 4

According to the authors: "Given that illicit drug users are often unaware of or misperceive the impacts of drug use on safe driving, it may be important for health-service or public-health interventions to address such biases and improve road safety." Long-term record linkage studies of this type may not provide the detailed information needed to formulate such interventions, but they do produce evidence relevant to the generation of such hypotheses.

QUESTION 5

Direct standardization is often used with mortality data, which is merely a specific type of incidence data. Direct and indirect standardization can both be used with other types of incident events. In this case, the value of the procedure is that the 3 ethnic groups can be compared without worrying that differences merely reflect the demographic characteristics adjusted for in the standardization (sex, and age based on 10-year age increments).

Chapter 10

QUESTION 1

Advantages:

- Provides a snapshot of disease burden at a point in time, which is valuable information for those planning and administering health services. As cross-sectional studies often take the form of surveys they can adopt sampling procedures that are well suited to making population inference about prevalence.
- These studies can be completed on a shorter timeline and often with less expense than longitudinal studies of a comparable size and complexity.
- As examples such as the Canadian Community Health Survey attest, it is often possible to incorporate multiple exposures and multiple disease outcomes in a single cross-sectional survey.
- Since the data are collected at a single point in time there is not an issue with loss to follow-up in cross-sectional studies, as there may be in longitudinal studies.

Disadvantages:

- Only prevalence can be estimated from a cross-sectional survey, not incidence. Therefore, such studies cannot usually provide information about risk.
- The results of a cross-sectional study can be misleading if there are changes over time (e.g., seasonal changes) in prevalence.

- The design is not strong for determining causation because the temporal relationship between exposure and disease can generally not be elucidated by cross-sectional studies.
- These studies are inefficient for rare diseases and rare exposures since even large samples may include too few cases to allow precise estimation.

QUESTION 2

This statement is sometimes made, usually based on the (generally true) assertion that the temporal sequence of exposure and disease cannot be clarified from cross-sectional data. However, cross-sectional data provide clear temporality in some situations—for example, studies of the adult outcomes of birth or childhood-related exposures, genetic inheritance, and congenital malformations.

QUESTION 3

a. The prevalence calculation includes all those with the disease in the numerator, regardless of their exposure status[108]: 420/3090, or 0.136.

b. An approximate 95% CI can be calculated using the normal approximation of the binomial distribution. The standard error of the estimated proportion is:

$$\text{Standard Error} = \sqrt{\frac{p \times (1 - p)}{n}}$$

For this study, the standard error is 0.006. The approximate confidence limits are then 0.136 +/− 1.96 × 0.006, leading to a 95% CI of 0.124–0.148. Of course, an exact confidence interval is always preferable and in this case the result (from statistical software) is 0.124–0.149. In this case, the approximate formula performed quite well.

QUESTION 4

The prevalence difference is the prevalence in the exposed (0.171) minus the prevalence in the nonexposed (0.069), which is 0.102, or 10.2%.

QUESTION 5

a. The odds in the exposed is 348/1692 = 0.21 and ln(0.21) = −1.58. Among the nonexposed, the odds are 72/978 = 0.074 and ln(0.074) = −2.61.

b. The first step is to calculate a. The indicator variable representing exposure has a value of 0 in the nonexposed group, which means −2.61 is a. The log odds in the exposed are −1.58. Since $a + \beta$ must be −1.58 and a is −2.61 (see above), β must be 1.03. The linear equation is therefore: log odds of impulse control disorder = −2.61 + 1.03X_e.

c. The inverse log of β (which has a value of 1.03 in the equation above) is 2.79. This is the odds ratio. In this kind of equation, β is a log odds ratio.

Chapter 11

QUESTION 1

Advantages:

- Very efficient for rare diseases.
- Can easily examine multiple exposures for a single disease.

- Compared to longitudinal studies they are inexpensive and can be relatively quick to complete.
- Able to cope with long induction and latency periods.

Disadvantages:

- Vulnerable to bias due to selection and misclassification.
- Cannot study multiple diseases.
- Inefficient for rare exposures.
- Cannot assess risk—only exposure-disease associations.

QUESTION 2

The incubation period is a period during which the infection has become established but has not yet progressed to where it is clinically evident. Therefore, this is best regarded as a latency period. In infectious diseases, the offending microbe is a necessary component cause, by definition, but is rarely sufficient. Since some exposed persons do not contract infectious diseases, there must be other component causes that these resilient individuals do not have.

QUESTION 3

a. The odds ratio is 0.82, as reported in the study.[109]

b. To calculate the percent reduction from a relative measure such as an odds ratio or risk ratio, subtract 1 from the odds ratio or risk ratio and multiply by 100. An odds ratio of 1.5 implies a percent increase of $(1.5 - 1.0.) \times 100 = 50\%$ in the odds of disease. An odds ratio of 0.82 implies a $(0.82 - 1.0) \times 100 = -18\%$ reduction in the odds of rupture among those treated with angiotensin-converting enzyme (ACE) inhibitors.

QUESTION 4

The odds of rupture in those being treated with ACE inhibitors is only 0.82 that of those who are untreated. The results are interpreted in terms of odds, so there is no concern about the rare disease assumption. This assumption only reflects the extent to which odds and odds ratios can serve as an approximation of proportions and relative proportions.

QUESTION 5

This is not screening in the sense used in epidemiology and public health, where screening means secondary prevention or early intervention (during a detectable preclinical or latent phase of the disease). A better term for the effort described in the question is *case finding*. Underdetection is not a de facto reason for screening, although it is occasionally regarded as such. A critique of "screening" for depression has been published by Thombs et al.[172]

Chapter 12

QUESTION 1

a. Social desirability bias occurs when people attempt to present as normal by providing inaccurate answers. This would result in false-negative classification, or low sensitivity.

b. It seems unlikely that the sensitivity of these instruments would be affected by exposure, so the most likely type of bias would be nondifferential misclassification bias. However, since the investigators are concerned that impulsive behaviour may be caused by these drugs, it is conceivable that the exposure could change the measurement properties of the diagnostic instruments. For example, people might impulsively provide certain answers when taking these medications.

c. Nondifferential misclassification bias is predictably in the direction of the null value of the parameter being estimated. In the case of the odds ratio, the estimates would be biased towards the null value of 1.

QUESTION 2

a. Recall bias refers to increased recollection of past exposures among people with a disease. The term can mean other things, so more specific terminology is preferable—e.g., differential misclassification of exposure with greater sensitivity in the cases.

b. This type of bias in case-control studies tends to inflate the value of the odds ratio.

c. In a disease that causes cognitive problems (such as dementia), those with the disease may be less likely to recall past exposures than controls. Their defective recall could lead to bias in the other direction. This possibility illustrates the hazards of using nonspecific terminology such as *recall bias*.

QUESTION 3

Any type of misclassification can introduce bias. Administrative data are not collected for research purposes and may therefore be inaccurate. Such inaccuracy introduces bias into the estimation of epidemiologic parameters. The fact that inaccuracy of exposure classification would not depend on disease status in most situations does not mean that bias will not occur, only that the misclassification bias will be nondifferential.

QUESTION 4

a. The study used careful measurement strategies, so it is not vulnerable to misclassification bias. Theoretically, any degree of imperfection in measurement can introduce bias, but minor inaccuracy will normally be a minor threat to the validity of the study. No epidemiologic study is perfect.

b. Similarly, this form of bias is possible in theory, but only a tiny proportion of the population are likely to fall into this category. The impact of such bias will be negligible.

QUESTION 5

This is a situation where the type of misclassification bias is of critical importance. Because the bias is almost certainly nondifferential, the expected direction of bias is towards the null value and it is likely that the actual associations are stronger than reported.

Chapter 13

QUESTION 1

Advantages:

- They can clarify the temporal relationship between exposure and disease.

- They allow an assessment of risk as well as association.
- They can look at multiple outcomes of an exposure.
- Prospective cohort studies are protected from selection bias since, in order for selection bias to occur, participation must be affected both by exposure and disease. This is unlikely to occur in a prospective cohort study since the disease (or other outcome) has not occurred at the time of selection.

Disadvantages:

- They tend to be expensive, since subjects must be tracked prospectively over time.
- They can take a long time to produce results, especially in situations where induction periods are very long.
- They are usually not an effective way to study very rare outcomes.
- They are vulnerable to bias resulting from attrition.

QUESTION 2

It is too simple to say that one study design is better than another. The best study design must be chosen for a particular research question. A prospective cohort design may be impossible to apply for certain diseases (such as those with a very long induction period). A poorly conducted prospective cohort study may yield lower quality estimates than a higher quality case-control study.

QUESTION 3

a. $978/6\,645 = 14.7\%$, which is the 10-year incidence proportion reported in the study.[124 (p1476)]

b. To cause selection bias, attrition must be related to both exposure and disease. It seems plausible that people in poorer health, perhaps those having more fractures, would be more likely to drop out of the study. This would result in an underestimation of the incidence proportion, but would not necessarily cause bias in a measure of association. If multiple fractures tended to lead to drop out in the nonexposed subjects, but did not do this to the same extent in the exposed subjects, then the estimate could be biased in a positive direction: the incidence of fractures in the nonexposed group would be underestimated to a greater extent than in the exposed, diminishing the denominator of the risk ratio relatively more than the numerator. This would increase (inflate) the value of the estimated risk ratio. While this could occur in theory, it does not seem likely to occur. It seems perhaps more likely that depressed people (including many more of the exposed group) might be less able to cope with the pain of the fractures and more likely to drop out, which would create a negative bias in the risk ratio.

c. There is no reason to expect that the measurement of antidepressant use would be more or less accurate depending on subsequent fractures. Inaccurate classification of exposure could lead to bias, which would be nondifferential and in the direction of the null value. Bias of this type cannot explain the association observed, but leads to suspicion that it might be stronger than reported.

QUESTION 4

Any of these measures could be chosen. Since most people understand proportions better than odds, the odds ratio may not be the best choice. The risk ratio would be a good choice, but a long-term study may experience attrition from its sample, which is difficult to deal with using a risk ratio. A hazard ratio derives from survival analysis methods and can accommodate attrition by censoring observations at the time subjects leave the sample.

QUESTION 5

A recurrent disease is very difficult to study cross-sectionally or retrospectively. It can be difficult for people to remember the onsets and remissions of their illness. The prospective cohort design allows this information to be collected prospectively, allowing much more accurate measurement.

Chapter 14

QUESTION 1

A confounding variable:

- must be a risk factor for the outcome under investigation
- must be associated with the exposure
- must not occur on the causal pathway under investigation

QUESTION 2

a. The β coefficient in the logistic regression model is a log odds ratio. Since the odds ratio is 2.72, the β coefficient is 1.001 (the log of 2.72).

b. The lack of change in the crude odds ratio with adjustment for these covariates indicates that these variables did not confound the association under investigation.

QUESTION 3

Since the adjusted odds ratio is essentially the same as the crude (unadjusted) odds ratio, the model shows that these variables did not act as confounding variables in the analysis.

QUESTION 4

a. This is not confounding. In confounding, the stratified estimates differ from the crude estimate, but resemble each another. Here, the stratum-specific estimates differ from each another, which indicates effect measure modification by age.

b. When there is effect measure modification, the stratum-specific estimates should be reported, as was done by these investigators.

QUESTION 5

a. Age is a strong determinant of mortality. If depression is more common in young people, age could be a strong confounder of the depression-mortality association. Since depression is most common among young people, and younger people are much less likely to die, the possible effect of depression may be masked by the effect of age.

b. If variables such as smoking, which are independent determinants of mortality, are associated with depression, they may act as confounding variables. What appears to be an effect of depression in age- and sex-adjusted estimates may actually be due to the effect of variables such as smoking.

Chapter 15

QUESTION 1

The best strategy is to measure all suspected or known risk factors for the outcome under study. Potential confounders must be associated with exposure as well as outcome, but there is rarely sufficient information to make a firm determination about whether a potential confounder is or is not associated with exposure.

QUESTION 2

A confounding variable must be associated with exposure and must be an independent determinant of disease. Female sex is associated with multiple sclerosis. However, in this study the exposed and nonexposed groups were matched on sex, so there will be no association between exposure and this potential confounding variable in the sample. Sex can therefore not act as a confounding variable.

QUESTION 3

This pattern is suggestive of effect measure modification and not confounding. After stratification for a confounding variable, the stratum-specific estimates should be different than the crude estimate and similar to each another. In this case, they appear to differ from each other.

QUESTION 4

Models can sometimes avoid the need for arbitrary stratification—for example, when a continuous variable such as age is a potential confounder. In doing so, they avoid the sparse-data problems that plague stratified analysis. They are better for examining multiple strata of a single potential confounding variable or for simultaneously examining the effects of multiple confounding variables.

QUESTION 5

Most epidemiologists believe that stratified analysis continues to play an important role. Stratified analysis involves making tables, so it may offer a better connection to the data than the more abstract output of regression modelling. In practice, many analysts carry out stratified analysis, but often include only model-based output in published studies.

Chapter 16

QUESTION 1

The key difference between a nested case-control study and a case-cohort study is that the case-control study selects a referent, or control, group that includes only respondents who do not have the disease. In contrast, a case-cohort study selects a subcohort representative of the entire cohort from which the cases later arose.

   a. Case-cohort studies have an important advantage over nested case-control studies. In the nested case-control design, a new set of controls needs to be selected for each outcome examined. If a single control is to be selected for each case, controls should be selected from among those without the disease at the time when an incident case emerges. With the case-cohort design, multiple outcomes can be examined using the same subcohort as a referent group. This counteracts a limitation of the case-control design—its usual ability to examine only a single outcome.

b. The main advantage of case-cohort studies over prospective cohort studies is efficiency. Case-cohort studies take measurements only in the cases and the subcohort, not the entire cohort.

QUESTION 2

a. This kind of study design is sometimes called an *interrupted time series*, since it looks for a change in the pattern of an outcome before and after some key event (in this case the introduction of sophisticated medical treatments). However, the study design is ecological. Ecological studies use aggregate units of analysis, which can be geographic areas, political units, or units of time. They are comparing a set of years before and after the introduction of the new treatments and are examining whether a difference in exposure within these years is associated with the rate of surgery (an aggregate measure).

b. Always be careful about making causal inference from ecological data, because of the possibility of ecological fallacy. Here, even though the rate of surgery declined in association with the introduction of the new medical therapies, the study does not actually confirm that the people who are avoiding surgery are getting the medical treatments instead.

QUESTION 3

In a retrospective cohort design, selection is usually based on an assessment of exposure. Typically, a comparison is made to the general population using an SMR, although some retrospective cohort studies have both exposed and nonexposed cohorts, which allow them to calculate parameters such as risk ratios or hazard ratios. These studies have a forward logical direction, from exposure to disease. In contrast, the case-cohort design has a backward logical direction, comparing a series of cases to a referent cohort in terms of their exposure frequency.

QUESTION 4

The main advantage of the case-crossover design is that—because this design makes comparisons within the same people, often over a short period—it can account (essentially through matching) for a large number of time-invariant personal characteristics that might otherwise act as confounding variables.

QUESTION 5

The key advantage of randomized controlled trials is the unique ability of randomization to address both measured and unmeasured confounding variables, by helping to ensure that any such variables will be approximately equally distributed between the comparison groups.

Chapter 17

QUESTION 1

a. The implication is that 9% of high blood pressure could be avoided if people kept their indoor living temperature above 18 degrees.

b. This interpretation depends on a series of assumptions, including that the cross-sectional estimate of association reflects a relative risk. Generally, prevalence ratios or prevalence odds ratios should not be accepted as a measure of relative risk. Risk cannot be estimated from cross-sectional data. Also, it must be assumed that the effect is causal, which is dubious in this case and cannot generally be determined from cross-sectional data at any rate.

QUESTION 2

Based on the formula used, the alcohol attributable fraction (AAF) is the attributable fraction (among the exposed). The formula presented is predicated on the idea that the odds ratio provides a good estimate of the relative risk.

QUESTION 3

It is not easy to explain. If all current smokers could be changed to never smokers, the incidence of myocardial infarction in the population could be reduced by 35.7%. In this case, the population attributable risk is a theoretical parameter, since current smokers can become former smokers, but they cannot become "never smokers."

QUESTION 4

a. Attributable risk among the exposed: 0.14

b. Attributable fraction among the exposed: 0.725

c. Population attributable risk: 0.07

d. Population attributable risk percent: 56.0%

e. Confounding by indication may mean that the observed effect is not causal. The effects (if any) of the drugs are probably mixed with the effects of the illnesses that they treating. If this is the case, the effects should not be attributed to the drugs and the above parameters should not have been calculated.

QUESTION 5

The population attributable risk (PAR), expressed as a percentage, is the total population incidence (25/759) minus the incidence in the nonexposed (22/730), all divided by the total population incidence and multiplied by 100.

$$PAR\% = \frac{\left(\dfrac{25}{759} - \dfrac{22}{730}\right)}{\dfrac{25}{759}} \times 100 = 8.5\%$$

Chapter 18

QUESTION 1

Causal judgements are always somewhat subjective, so the weight placed on specific criteria varies by context. In general, a dose-response relationship is viewed as providing supportive evidence for causation, but due to the existence of threshold and saturation effects, the lack of a biological gradient does not usually provide evidence against causality.

QUESTION 2

Questions of causation cannot usually be settled by a single study and usually require accessing the broader literature. A case in point is the criterion of consistency, which requires examining the results of different studies.

QUESTION 3

They argued that all of the associations between diet and coronary heart disease investigated in this literature were biologically plausible, and therefore that this criterion was satisfied by default. They argued that analogy was too subjective to be useful. They also noted that most risk factors for coronary heart disease were inevitably nonspecific, so this criterion was not very meaningful to them.

QUESTION 4

a. Hill argues that important risk factors may not seem plausible when first reported in epidemiological studies. Epidemiological studies sometimes drive biological research and should therefore not be subordinated to it.

b. The counter argument is that temporality is the most important criterion, because it alone is a logical requirement for causation. In his discussion, Hill describes several situations in which extremely strong associations led to decisive conclusions—for example, the observation that mortality from cancer of the scrotum occurred 200 times more often in chimney sweeps. Such observations are indeed compelling, but they are not encountered very often in modern epidemiology.

QUESTION 5

This is a profound statement about the way in which causality is conceptualized in epidemiology. The word *links* refers to the concept of a causal chain. The opportunistic and pragmatic perspective adopted by epidemiologists is highlighted by optimism that disrupting key associations along causal chains are often sufficient to make a positive impact on population health.

Chapter 19

QUESTION 1

a. Ecological studies: the ecological fallacy.

b. Cross-sectional studies: their (usual) inability to clarify temporal effects.

c. Randomized controlled trials: external validity. These studies typically apply multiple inclusion and exclusion criteria, and often unfold in an idealized environment, which can draw their external validity into question.

d. Prospective cohort studies: selection bias, which can be introduced through attrition from the study cohort.

e. Case-control studies: misclassification and selection bias.

QUESTION 2

It is difficult to argue that there can be external validity of an estimate that is invalid. If an estimate is wrong, it has no value in the population in which it was estimated. It is not conceivable that such as estimate could be usefully exported to an external population.

QUESTION 3

The best answer to this question is "it depends." These 2 provinces are far apart geographically, and the demographic features and culture of their populations also have differences. However, there are also similarities. If the differences between the provinces are not relevant to the association under consideration, an estimate could be generalized. If differences between these populations could alter the disease-exposure association, it would be unwise to generalize such estimates. External validity always needs to be considered on a case-by-case basis.

QUESTION 4

a. This is a problem. In epidemiology, adjustment for effect modifiers as if they were confounding variables is considered inappropriate. When there is effect measure modification, there is a different strength of association depending on the presence of the effect-modifying variable. Any type of adjusted estimate that pools across those strata produces a meaningless average of the differing associations. In stratified analysis, the heterogeneity or homogeneity of stratum-specific effects are readily apparent, but there is often a lack of clarity on this issue in model-based analyses, which is worrisome when it occurs.

b. The idea that significant variables should be retained in models is widespread, but it is not entirely central to the process of reasoning in epidemiological analysis. In epidemiology, the clearest justification for making an adjustment is that the variable in question acts as a confounder. In other words, the intent is to estimate the effect of an exposure, and the effect of that exposure is mixed with the effect of another variable, making adjustment necessary. Confounding is detected during modelling by determining whether a measure of effect—such as an odds ratio, risk ratio, risk difference, or hazard ratio—changes when an adjustment is made for a potential confounder (assuming that it has already been determined that the variable is not an effect modifier). The detection of confounding is not based on determining whether that particular confounder is significantly associated with the outcome.

QUESTION 5

Supplementary materials could include:

- Flowcharts: these can delineate inclusions, exclusions, attrition, and missing data—all factors related to participation that can assist with assessment of selection bias.

- Detailed information about the performance of measurement instruments (such as results of internal validation studies).

- Detailed tables: print editions often can't publish detailed tables. These could include more detailed modelling output, which would allow the presentation of tests for interaction—often not reported in published studies.

- Detailed stratified analysis: published studies often only include regression models.

- Archived versions of original study protocols: they can be useful because they lay out the analysis plan for a study as it stood before the data were examined. This helps with the assessment of type I error since it clarifies which analyses were planned ahead of time and which arose during exploratory phases of the analysis. Results of the latter type are vulnerable to type I error and therefore require replication.

- Study data set: some investigators believe that the study data set itself should be published along with the study. This would allow investigators to replicate the analysis, or conduct the analysis differently, as a means of assessing the robustness of the study's conclusions.

GLOSSARY

Adjusted estimate. An estimate of effect from which the confounding effects of an extraneous variable have been removed. Examples include stratified estimates, pooled estimates (e.g., the Mantel-Haenszel family of estimators), and estimates that have been adjusted using regression models.

Adjustment. A procedure to remove the effect of a confounding variable from an estimated parameter. Examples include direct and indirect standardization, as well as stratification or adjustments made using statistical models.

Analogy. A criterion employed in consideration of causation in epidemiology. It is rarely used because it is very subjective. It involves consideration of known causal pathways, and applying that information, by analogy, to a different health problem.

Analytical epidemiology. A branch of epidemiology that evaluates hypotheses, usually about disease etiology.

Attack rate. An incidence proportion usually calculated during an outbreak or epidemic, in which the risk interval for the incidence proportion consists of the duration of the outbreak or epidemic.

Attributable risk. The estimated amount (expressed either as a difference in incidence or as a percentage) by which the occurrence of disease could be reduced by removing a risk factor from a population or completely ameliorating its effects.

Attrition. This term usually applies to prospective studies, where it refers to loss of participants to a study (i.e., "drop outs").

Beneficence. An ethical principle that research should do good. Research should benefit people.

Bias. This term has many meanings in epidemiology. For example, judgement can be biased and testing procedures can also be biased. However, the most important meaning of this term in epidemiology relates to errors that studies make in their estimation of epidemiologic parameters. In this sense, bias is a systematic (as opposed to random) error in the estimation of a parameter that results from a defect in study design.

Biological gradient. A criterion that may be considered when weighing causal judgements. A biological gradient is a situation in which increasing levels of exposure lead to a stronger exposure-disease association. This is sometimes also called a dose-response relationship.

Biological plausibility. A criterion employed in consideration of causation in epidemiology. It refers to whether an association makes sense in view of biological data.

CANSIM. Statistics Canada's socioeconomic database. The name is an acronym for the Canadian Socioeconomic Information Management System. The CANSIM database is not limited to health. It comprises many categories of data. CANSIM has an online directory.[47] If you select health as a category in this directory, you can browse its extensive health data collections. CANSIM tables can be customized to flexibly provide output—e.g., for a specific province, age, or sex group.

Case-cohort study. A study, often considered a variant of the case-control design, in which the source population for the referent group includes all individuals in the population from which the cases derived, not just those without the disease.

Census. The enumeration, or counting, of all persons in a town, city, or country.

Coherence. This is a criterion employed in consideration of causation in epidemiology. It refers to whether an epidemiological observation is consistent with existing knowledge and theory.

Component cause. An exposure that causes a disease through its participation in causal mechanisms that typically include combinations of causes. Such combinations, together, comprise a causal mechanism.

Confidence interval (CI). An interval quantifying the degree of precision of an estimated epidemiologic parameter. A confidence interval provides a range of plausible parameters for a population parameter at a given level of confidence. Most commonly, a 95% level of confidence is used in the calculation.

Confidence limit. The number at the lower end of the range of a confidence interval (the lower limit) or at the upper end of the range (the upper limit).

Confounding. The intermixing (within a measure of association) of an effect of interest and the effect of an independent causal factor.

Consistency. This is a criterion employed in consideration of causation in epidemiology. It refers to the consistency with which an association has been reported in different studies conducted in different populations.

Coroner. An official involved in confirmation and certification of causes of death. Coroners also conduct investigations into causes of death.

Correlation coefficient. The most common measure of association seen in ecological studies. There are several types, but they all seek to quantify the extent of linear relationship between 2 variables. They assume values between -1 (representing a perfect negative correlation) and $+1$ (representing a perfect positive correlation). A value of 0 means no correlation. Most approaches (e.g., Pearson product moment coefficient, Spearman rank correlation) are based on pairs of observations, but the intraclass correlation coefficient (ICC) is based on groups of observations.

Correlational study. See *ecological study*.

Critical appraisal. Reading a study critically, with a view to identifying defects that could lead to inaccurate results.

Cross-product term. A term formed by multiplying 2 variables together. Such terms are useful in regression modelling because they provide an assessment of statistical interaction between those variables. This contributes to the assessment of effect measure modification, which must precede assessment and control of confounding in epidemiological analyses.

Cross-sectional study. A study in which all data are collected at a single point in time.

Crude parameter. A parameter that is not stratified (or otherwise adjusted) for the occurrence of other factors such as confounding variables. The term *crude* can be used for proportions (e.g., crude prevalence) or for measures of association (e.g., crude odds ratio).

Cumulative incidence. The incidence proportion expressed in terms of an accumulation of cases in an at-risk population over time intervals.

Death certificate. A form that provides official certification of death and records important information related to death.

Denominator. In a ratio (which is 1 number divided by another), the denominator is the number in the bottom of the fraction

Descriptive epidemiology. The study of the burden and distribution of diseases in populations. Describing these aspects of disease is essential for policy and planning purposes. Descriptive studies do not evaluate hypotheses about disease etiology, but sometimes generate such hypotheses.

Design effects. Complexities in the design of a study (usually this term is used when describing a survey that uses a complex sampling procedure) that must be accounted for in the way that the study data are analyzed.

Determinant. An exposure that determines the epidemiology of a disease, but not necessarily through a causal effect. Determinants can, for example, be exposures that alter mortality or prognosis, and therefore alter the connection between incidence and prevalence.

Differential misclassification bias. Systematic error that occurs due to misclassification of exposure or disease in a way that differs depending on exposure status (in classification of disease) or disease status (in classification of exposure). An example of such bias is recall bias in case-control studies.

Direct standardization. A procedure for increasing the comparability of 2 potentially confounded parameters by weighting them both by the same standardizing population. The weights are the proportion of the standardizing population within each stratum defined by the potential confounding variable (most commonly age and sex). Directly standardized rates are not real entities and have no meaning in themselves: their purpose is to facilitate comparisons between different populations.

Disability-adjusted life-year (DALY). A composite measure of disease burden composed of years lived with disability due to a disease (weighted by the extent of disability or health loss associated with the disease) and years of life lost.

Ecological fallacy. A methodological concern for studies assessing associations at the ecological (aggregate) level. The fallacy is assuming that an association at the aggregate level must also exist at the individual level.

Effect size. This term has different meanings in different disciplines. It is sometimes used to refer to a standardized measure of a treatment effect, but in epidemiology it usually refers to the strength of association of a health outcome with a risk factor.

Endemic disease. A disease that is maintained in a population at a relatively stable level, or steady state. Changes in the prevalence of endemic diseases, since they occur slowly, tend to be viewed as long-term trends, rather than as epidemics.

Epidemic. The occurrence of cases of disease in excess of what would normally be expected. Deciding what is expected may involve consideration of the history of the afflicted community, the geographical area in which it occurs or, sometimes, the season.

Epidemiology. The study of the distribution and determinants of disease in human populations. There are many variants of this definition. Veterinary epidemiology is closely related to human epidemiology, so *human* is often omitted. Also, some definitions refer to the study of the distribution and determinants of disease frequency, to emphasize that epidemiological research focuses on populations rather than individual people.

Equipoise. An ethical requirement for randomized controlled trials. It means there is neither enough evidence for or against a treatment to preclude its use as an intervention in research.

Extraneous variable. A variable whose effects fall outside of the exposure-disease association of primary interest.

False-negative rate (or proportion). The complement of sensitivity: the frequency with which people who have a disease are classified as not having it.

False-positive rate (or proportion). The complement of specificity: the frequency with which disease-free individuals are classified as having a disease.

Frequency weight. A type of sampling weight in which the value of the weight depicts the number of people in the general population represented by a survey participant.

Gold standard. A test or classification procedure that does not make errors.

Hazard ratio. A measure of association based on time-to-event data in survival analysis.

Health-adjusted life expectancy (HALE). An alternative approach to estimating disease burden. HALE is calculated in a way that resembles the estimation of life expectancy, but it accounts for years lived in a state of less-than-full health.

Healthy worker effect. The tendency of working people to be healthier, on average, than nonworking people. This creates an expectation that a standardized mortality ratio (SMR) calculated from an occupational cohort should be less than 1.

Incidence. The new occurrence of disease in those at risk of the disease. Incidence can be measured as a proportion, an odds, or an incidence rate. An incidence proportion is the proportion of an at-risk group that develops the disease in a defined risk interval. The incidence odds are the same thing, but quantified as an odds rather than a proportion. The incidence rate is an instantaneous rate of change in disease status within those at risk. Like all rates, the incidence rate has associated units, expressed in time^{-1} units, also called person-time units.

Incidence proportion. See *incidence.*

Incidence proportion ratio. A highly descriptive, but rarely used, term for a parameter consisting of a ratio of 2 incidence proportions. Also sometimes called a *cumulative incidence ratio, risk ratio,* or *relative risk.*

Incidence rate. See *incidence.*

Indirect standardization. An approach to standardization often encountered in the occupational health literature. The age and sex distribution of an occupational cohort, along with age- and sex-specific rates or frequencies from a standardizing population, is used to calculate an expected number of deaths (or cases), which is then compared to the observed number of deaths in a standardized mortality (or morbidity) ratio (SMR).

Induction period. The period of time between exposure to a risk factor and the establishment of a disease process. In the causal pie (or sufficient-component cause) model of etiology, the induction period is a period of time when exposure to other component causes is occurring. When a set of component causes forms a complete causal mechanism, disease onset occurs.

Infant mortality rate. The number of infant deaths (the death of a child under 1 year of age) divided by the number of live births in the same year.

Inference. The process of gaining information about a population by studying a sample drawn from that population.

Interaction. A situation in which the effects of 1 variable depend on the level of the another variable. Tests for interaction in statistical models are a way to detect effect measure modification.

International Classification of Disease. The international standard for classification of diseases and other health problems on death certificates and other administrative health records.

Interventional study. A study in which investigators assign an exposure to study participants, for example, through a random process (randomization).

Justice. An ethical principle stating (in the context of epidemiological research) that groups that endure the risks and harms of research should stand to benefit from the research.

Kappa coefficient. A coefficient used to quantify agreement between 2 ratings (e.g., in the assessment of interrater or test-rest reliability) that are categorical.

Late fetal deaths. A baby born with no signs of life but of 28 or more weeks gestation. In Canada, this typically excludes such births when they are of unknown gestational age.

Law of large numbers. A law of probability indicating that when an experiment is repeated many times, the result gets closer and closer to an expected value.

Life expectancy. A construct consisting of a projection of the age at which half of a hypothetical birth cohort would be dead.

Likelihood ratio. An alternative strategy for interpreting the results of a diagnostic test. This parameter allows posttest odds to be calculated from pretest odds using simple multiplication.

Live birth. A product of conception that, subsequent to birth, shows any signs of life such as breathing or movement.

Mantel-Haenszel estimators. A family of estimators that play a critical role in stratified analysis because they allow the pooling of stratum-specific estimates into a single, more precise, estimate of effect. This adjusts for confounding that arises from the variable on which the estimates were stratified.

Mantel-Haenszel test for homogeneity. A statistical test used in stratified analysis to determine whether 2 or more stratum-specific estimates differ from each other to a greater extent than could be explained by chance. The test provides a way of evaluating effect measure modification in stratified analysis.

Matching. Application of restriction rules to a referent group (e.g., controls in a case-control study or nonexposed participants in a prospective cohort study) to ensure that the distribution of a confounder, or confounders, is equal in the index (e.g., cases in a case-control study or exposed participants in a prospective cohort study) and referent groups, thereby controlling confounding.

Mean. A measure of the central tendency of a variable. It is calculated as the sum of values of the variable divided by the number of observations.

Median. The midpoint in a range of values taken by a variable. Half the observed values are greater than the median and half are less.

Medical examiner's office. This term is used in some Canadian jurisdictions in lieu of the term *coroner's office.*

Misclassification bias. Systematic error in the estimation of a parameter that is due to a study-design defect involving the classification of subjects into disease and exposure groups. Such bias can be differential or nondifferential.

Modelling. Statistical procedures used most often (in epidemiology) to produce estimates of the effect of an exposure that are unconfounded by the causal effects of other independent risk factors.

Modifiable determinant. A determinant of disease that can be changed, usually through public health action.

Morbidity. The diminishment from a healthy state caused by having a disease.

Mortality. Death. The rate of death in a population is the mortality rate. An unadjusted mortality rate is a crude mortality rate.

Necessary cause. A component cause that is a member of all causal mechanisms for a disease.

Negative predictive value. The probability that a disease is not present given a negative diagnostic test or a negative result on another type of classification procedure.

Neonatal mortality rate. Neonatal deaths occur in the first month of life. The neonatal mortality rate is expressed as a proportion of neonatal deaths among live births.

Nested case-control study. A case-control study nested within a prospective cohort study.

Nondifferential misclassification bias. Systematic error from misclassification that does not differ across the categories on the other axis of the classic 2 × 2 contingency table. For example, misclassification of exposure that does not depend on disease status is nondifferential.

Nonmaleficence. An ethical principle that states that research should not do harm.

Nonmodifiable determinant. A determinant of disease that cannot be changed. Such variables are usually treated as extraneous variables in epidemiological studies because, although they do not generally identify opportunities for prevention, they can confound or modify associations between modifiable risk factors and disease outcomes.

Normal distribution. A symmetrical bell-shaped distribution that arises often in nature and in statistical theory.

Numerator. In a ratio (which is 1 number divided by another), the numerator is the number in the top of a fraction, and the denominator is the number in the bottom.

Observational study. A study in which investigators do not assign exposure, as distinct from an interventional study (in which they do).

Observed survival proportion. This is the proportion of those with cancer who are alive after a specified period (usually 5 years). This parameter could be calculated for any condition, but the terminology is mostly used in the cancer literature.

Odds. A ratio in which the contents of the numerator are not counted in the denominator. For example, in a group of 10 people where 1 has a disease, you could say that the odds of disease are 1/9, which is equivalent to saying that the proportion with the disease is 1/10.

Odds ratio. A measure of association that is based on dividing the odds of disease in exposed study participants by the odds of disease in nonexposed study participants. Alternatively, the odds of exposure in diseased study participants could be divided by the odds of exposure in nondiseased study participants. This is the basic measure of association in case-control studies, but is widely used in other types of studies as well.

Outbreak. The occurrence of cases of a (usually) infectious disease in excess of expectation.

Pandemic. An epidemic that crosses international boundaries.

Parameter. A characteristic that defines an epidemiological feature or relationship, such as prevalence or relative risk.

Perinatal death. The death of a child under 1 week of age (0 to 6 days) or a stillbirth of 28 or more weeks gestation. The death of a child under 1 week of age is called an early neonatal death.

Perinatal mortality rate. The rate of occurrence of perinatal deaths (see above) during a year, usually expressed per 1000 births (where births include both live births and late fetal deaths) in that year.

Point estimate. A single estimate of a parameter calculated directly from the available data.

Population attributable risk. The extent to which the risk of disease could be diminished in an entire population by either removing a risk factor completely or completely ameliorating its effects.

Positive predictive value. The probability of disease given a positive diagnostic test or a positive result on another type of classification procedure.

Power calculation. A calculation that determines the power of an analysis to reject a null hypothesis, given parameters such as the sample size and an effect size.

Precision. The extent to which a study is free of vulnerability to random error. In epidemiology, precision is often quantified as the width of 95% CIs. Wide intervals indicate imprecision and narrow intervals indicate high precision.

Prevalence. There are 2 main types of prevalence. Point prevalence is the number or proportion of a population with a disease at a point in time. Period prevalence is the number or proportion of a population having a disease at any point during a defined interval of time—for example, annual prevalence is the number or proportion of a population having the disease at any point during a 1-year period.

Prevalence difference. A parameter quantifying the strength of association between an exposure and the prevalence of disease. It is calculated as the prevalence in exposed subjects minus the prevalence in nonexposed subjects.

Prevalence ratio. A parameter quantifying the strength of association between an exposure and the prevalence of disease. It is calculated as the prevalence in exposed subjects divided by the prevalence in nonexposed subjects.

Preventive fraction. The proportion or percentage of disease that could be prevented in a population through exposure to a protective factor (such as a preventive intervention).

Primary prevention. Prevention of the incidence of disease. Primary prevention intervenes at the level of risk-factor (or component-cause) exposures and thereby reduces the occurrence of disease.

Probability sample. A form of random sample in which the probability of any member of the population being selected into a sample is known.

Proportion. A proportion is a special type of ratio, in which the contents of the numerator are contained in the denominator. Descriptive epidemiology makes use of proportions a lot. For example, prevalence is usually expressed as a proportion and incidence can be expressed as a proportion.

Proportional mortality ratio. This ratio is calculated as the number of deaths due to a particular cause divided by the total number of deaths during an interval of time.

Public Health Agency of Canada. Usually known as PHAC. A federal government agency with a mission to promote and protect the health of Canadians through leadership, partnership, innovation, and action in public health.

Quasi-experiment. An intervention study in which the exposure is not assigned randomly.

Random error. Error introduced into an estimate as a result of sampling variability. Increasing the sample size of a study reduces its vulnerability to random error.

Random sample. A sample in which the selection of subjects is not predictable: it follows no rules (is random). Note this term is distinct from *random allocation* (as in a randomized trial).

Randomization. A procedure used in some interventional studies by which a random (unpredictable) procedure is used to assign exposure to a subset of study participants.

Randomized controlled trial. An interventional variant of the prospective cohort design in which the exposure is assigned randomly to study participants.

Recall bias. A type of bias that arises from recall errors. Recall bias due to misclassification of exposure in case-control studies is a type of differential misclassification bias.

Relative survival proportion. The ratio of survival in a group with a particular cancer to that of a comparable group free of the cancer. While relative survival proportions could be calculated for many conditions, this parameter has the highest profile in cancer research. It is recommended over the observed survival proportion by the Canadian Cancer Society.

Respect for persons principle. An ethical principle stating that people's autonomy must be respected. Potential participants decide, without coercion, whether to participate in a research study based on a thorough understanding of what participation would involve.

Restriction. A procedure to control confounding. Participants are selected such that they are always or never exposed to a confounder, eliminating the possibility that any effects of that confounder would be intermixed in parameters intended to reflect the causal impact of an exposure.

Retrospective. Looking back in time, into the past.

Retrospective cohort study. A cohort study having a forward logical direction but a backward (looking into the past) temporal direction.

Risk factor. An exposure that causes a disease.

Risk indicator. An exposure that is associated with a higher risk of disease, but is not necessarily the cause of that elevated risk.

Sample. A subset of a population. In epidemiology, this usually means a group of people sampled from a population.

Sample-size calculations. Calculations that determine the required sample size to achieve desired statistical power in the testing of a hypothesis or a desired level of precision in an estimate.

Sampling frame. A list of population elements that serves as the basis for the selection of a sample.

Screening. In its strictest sense, screening means the detection of latent disease (in a detectable preclinical stage), facilitating better outcomes through earlier intervention. Increasingly, the term is being used to describe any attempt to routinely or selectively assess any type of nonobvious health condition.

Secondary prevention. This term is synonymous with the less formal term, *screening.* It describes efforts to achieve better outcomes by earlier detection (in the latency phase) and earlier treatment of diseases.

Selection bias. A form of systematic error that results from study-design defects involving participation, or nonparticipation, in a study.

Sensitivity. The expected proportion of positive tests (or positive results on another type of classification procedure) among people who actually have the condition being tested for.

Sentinel indicators. Health statistics that reflect factors relevant to the health of entire populations, even if, on the surface, the statistics are based on a single age range. The classic examples are perinatal and infant mortality rates.

Simple random sample. A sample in which each individual in the population has the same probability of selection.

Source population. The population from which a study sample is drawn. Ideally, a source population should be directly representative of the population to which inference is directed (see *target population*). Otherwise, issues of generalizability arise.

Specific mortality rate. A rate calculated after stratification for a characteristic. Common examples include age- or sex-specific mortality rates.

Specificity. The expected proportion of negative tests (or negative results on another type of classification procedure) among those who actually do not have the condition being tested for.

Standard error. The standard deviation of the sampling distribution of a parameter, such as prevalence or an incidence proportion. It represents the amount of variability in estimates of such a parameter.

Standardized incidence ratio. This is the same as a standardized mortality ratio (see below), except that it is a standardization of incidence rather than mortality. This is most often found in the cancer epidemiology literature, due to the ability of cancer registries to support estimation of incidence.

Standardized mortality (or morbidity) ratio. The ratio of observed to expected deaths (mortality) or cases of disease (morbidity) in a population.

Statistical test. A procedure for evaluating the role of chance. A statistical test conducted at the 5% level of confidence determines whether observed results, or results that are more extreme, would occur by chance more than 5% of the time given a null hypothesis of no effect.

Stillbirth. A fetal death. In Canada, fetal deaths for which the product of conception has a birth weight of 500 grams or more, or the duration of pregnancy is 20 weeks or longer, are registered as stillbirths.

Stochastic error. This is another term for random error. Nonsystematic error in the estimation of study parameters. This form of error is reduced by increasing the sample size.

Strength of association. This is a criterion employed in consideration of causation in epidemiology. Stronger associations are generally viewed as more suggestive of causal effects.

Stratification. A procedure to detect and control confounding. At its most basic level, it involves estimating measures of association within strata defined by a potential confounding variable.

Stratify. Dividing a sample or population into groups based on some characteristic. When the groups are defined by the presence or level of a confounding characteristic, stratification is used as a method of adjustment for the confounding.

Stratum. A layer. In epidemiology, a stratum is usually a range of values for a characteristic in a sample. The plural of *stratum* is *strata*.

Study population. The population in a study. This term is confusing due to its use of the word *population* to describe a sample. Also, the term lacks consistent meaning in studies that use it.

Surveillance. Surveillance is a process of ongoing data collection, analysis, and communication of results (to those who need to know) for public health purposes.

Target population. A population to which inference is intended. This is the population that an epidemiologist is trying to learn about when conducting a research study.

Temporality. This is a criterion employed in consideration of causation in epidemiology. Since causes must precede effects, this criterion refers to the necessity of understanding the temporal relationship between exposure and disease before concluding that an association is causal.

Tertiary prevention. Efforts to diminish the negative impact of established diseases.

Type I error. A statistical error that results in rejection of a null hypothesis that is true.

Type II error. A statistical error that results in failure to reject a null hypothesis that is false.

Utilitarian principle. An ethical principle stating that the potential for research to harm may be allowable if offset by a suitable potential to do good. This is the idea that the potential harms of research can be weighed against the potential benefits.

Validity. This word has many different meanings in epidemiology. In every case, it refers to whether a result is accurate or correct. Where a diagnostic test is concerned, validity refers to the truthfulness of measurement. In critical appraisal, validity refers to the accuracy of an epidemiologic estimate.

Variable. A feature or factor that can assume different values.

REFERENCE LIST

1. Beck CA, Metz LM, Svenson LW, et al. Regional variation of multiple sclerosis prevalence in Canada. *Mult Scler*. 2005;11(5):516–9. http://dx.doi.org/10.1191/1352458505ms1192oa. Medline:16193887

2. Pappaioanou M, Spencer H. "One Health" initiative and ASPH. *Public Health Rep*. 2008;123(3):261. Medline:19006965

3. Johnson S. The ghost map. New York: The Penguin Group; 2006.

4. London School of Hygiene and Tropical Medicine. John Snow Bicentenary [Internet]. London (UK): London School of Hygiene and Tropical Medicine; 2013 [cited 2014 June 24]. Available from: http://johnsnowbicentenary.lshtm.ac.uk/.

5. Koch, R. Investigations into the etiology of traumatic infective diseases [Internet]. London (UK): New Sydenham Society: 1858 [cited 2014 September 19]. Available from: http://nrs.harvard.edu/urn-3:HMS.COUNT:1149035.

6. Howard-Jones N. Robert Koch and the cholera vibrio: a centenary. *Br Med J (Clin Res Ed)*. 1984;288(6414):379–81. http://dx.doi.org/10.1136/bmj.288.6414.379. Medline:6419937

7. Riley DL, Krepostman S, Stewart DE, et al. A mixed methods study of continuity of care from cardiac rehabilitation to primary care physicians. *Can J Cardiol*. 2009;25(6):e187–92. http://dx.doi.org/10.1016/S0828-282X(09)70096-0. Medline:19536388

8. Bernstein CN, Wajda A, Svenson LW, et al. The epidemiology of inflammatory bowel disease in Canada: a population-based study. *Am J Gastroenterol*. 2006;101(7):1559–68. http://dx.doi.org/10.1111/j.1572-0241.2006.00603.x. Medline:16863561

9. Maxwell CJ, Dalby DM, Slater M, et al. The prevalence and management of current daily pain among older home care clients. *Pain*. 2008;138(1):208–16. http://dx.doi.org/10.1016/j.pain.2008.04.007. Medline:18513871

10. Tyas SL, Manfreda J, Strain LA, et al. Risk factors for Alzheimer's disease: a population-based, longitudinal study in Manitoba, Canada. *Int J Epidemiol*. 2001;30(3):590–7. http://dx.doi.org/10.1093/ije/30.3.590. Medline:11416089

11. Vigen, T. Spurious Correlations [Internet]. [Cambridge (MA)]: Tyler Vigen; [cited 2014 June 24]. Available from: http://www.tylervigen.com.

12. Doll R, Hill AB. Smoking and carcinoma of the lung; preliminary report. *Br Med J*. 1950;2(4682):739–48. http://dx.doi.org/10.1136/bmj.2.4682.739. Medline:14772469

13. Statistics Canada. Smoking, 2013 [Internet]. Ottawa (ON): Government of Canada; 2014 June 13 [cited 2014 June 28]. Available from: http://www.statcan.gc.ca/pub/82-625-x/2014001/article/14025-eng.htm.

14. Statistics Canada. Table 103-0405 - Cancer incidence, by selected sites of cancer and sex, three-year average, census metropolitan areas, occasional (age-standardized rate per 100,000 population), in CANSIM [Internet]. Ottawa (ON): Government of Canada; 2013 December 12 [cited July 2014]. Available from: http://www5.statcan.gc.ca/cansim/a26?lang=eng&retrLang=eng&id=1030405&paSer=&pattern=&stByVal=1&p1=1&p2=-1&tabMode=dataTable&csid=

15. Health Canada. A National Strategy [Internet]. Ottawa (ON): Health Canada; 1999 [updated 2011 July 6; cited 2014 July 26]. Available from: http://www.hc-sc.gc.ca/hc-ps/pubs/tobac-tabac/ns-sn/index-eng.php#evidence.

16. Statistics Canada. Asthma, by sex, provinces and territories [Internet]. Ottawa (ON): Government of Canada; [updated 24 June 2012; cited 2014 July]. Available from: http://www.statcan.gc.ca/tables-tableaux/sum-som/l01/cst01/health50a-eng.htm.

17. Patten SB, Williams JV, Haynes L, et al. The incidence of delirium in psychiatric inpatient units. *Can J Psychiatry*. 1997;42(8):858–63. Medline:9356775

18. Tenenhouse A, Joseph L, Kreiger N, et al, and the CaMos Research Group. Canadian Multicentre Osteoporosis Study. Estimation of the prevalence of low bone density in Canadian women and men using a population-specific DXA reference standard: the Canadian Multicentre Osteoporosis Study (CaMos). *Osteoporos Int*. 2000;11(10):897–904. http://dx.doi.org/10.1007/s001980070050. Medline:11199195

19. Ebly EM, Parhad IM, Hogan DB, et al. Prevalence and types of dementia in the very old: results from the Canadian Study of Health and Aging. *Neurology.* 1994;44(9):1593–600. http://dx.doi.org/10.1212 /WNL.44.9.1593. Medline:7936280

20. Gravel R, Béland Y. The Canadian Community Health Survey: mental health and well-being. *Can J Psychiatry.* 2005;50(10):573–9. Medline:16276847

21. American Psychiatric Association. Diagnostic and statistical manual of mental disorders. 5th ed. Washington (DC): American Psychiatric Publishing; 2013.

22. Patten SB, Wang JL, Williams JV, et al. Descriptive epidemiology of major depression in Canada. *Can J Psychiatry.* 2006;51(2):84–90. Medline:16989107

23. Kessler RC, Andrews G, Mroczek D, Ustun B, Wittchen H. The World Health Organization Composite International Diagnostic Interview short-form (CIDI-SF). *Int J Methods Psychiatr Res.* 1998;7(4):171–85. http://dx.doi.org/10.1002/mpr.47.

24. Streiner DL, Patten SB, Anthony JC, et al. Has 'lifetime prevalence' reached the end of its life? An examination of the concept. *Int J Methods Psychiatr Res.* 2009;18(4):221–8. http://dx.doi.org/10.1002/mpr.296. Medline:20052690

25. Pringsheim T, Wiltshire K, Day L, et al. The incidence and prevalence of Huntington's disease: a systematic review and meta-analysis. *Mov Disord.* 2012;27(9):1083–91. http://dx.doi.org/10.1002/mds.25075. Medline:22692795

26. Bonaparte JP, Grant IA, Benstead TJ, et al. ALS incidence in Nova Scotia over a 20-year-period: a prospective study. *Can J Neurol Sci.* 2007;34(1):69–73. Medline:17352350

27. Wallington T, Berger L, Henry B, et al, and the SARS Investigation Team. Update: severe acute respiratory syndrome–Toronto, 2003. *Can Commun Dis Rep.* 2003;29(13):113–7. Medline:12861660

28. Gotay CC, Katzmarzyk PT, Janssen I, et al. Updating the Canadian obesity maps: an epidemic in progress. *Can J Public Health.* 2013;104(1):e64–8. Medline:23618109

29. Murray CJL, Lopez AC. Global burden of disease and injury. Boston: Harvard School of Public Health; 1996.

30. Murray CJ, Ezzati M, Flaxman AD, et al. GBD 2010: design, definitions, and metrics. *Lancet.* 2012;380(9859):2063–6. http://dx.doi.org/10.1016/S0140-6736(12)61899-6. Medline:23245602

31. Barendregt JJ, Van Oortmarssen GJ, Vos T, et al. A generic model for the assessment of disease epidemiology: the computational basis of DisMod II. *Popul Health Metr.* 2003;1(1):4. http://dx.doi .org/10.1186/1478-7954-1-4. Medline:12773212

32. United Nations. Handbook of vital statistical methods. Series F, No 7, Studies in methods. New York: United Nations; 1955.

33. Wellcome Library. Introduction to mortality statistics in England and Wales: 17th-20th century [Internet]. London (UK): Wellcome Library; [cited 2014 July 9]. Available from: http://wellcomelibrary.org /using-the-library/subject-guides/public-health/Mortality-statistics-in-England-and-Wales/.

34. Statistics Canada. Deaths and mortality rate, by selected grouped causes, sex and geography-Canada [Internet]. Ottawa (ON): Government of Canada; 2013 June 19 [cited 2014 July 9]. Available from: http://www.statcan.gc.ca/pub/84f0209x/2009000/tablesectlist-listetableauxsect-eng.htm.

35. Government of Ontario. Handbook on medical certification of death: prepared for registered nurses (extended class). Thunder Bay (ON): Office of the Registrar, Ontario Ministry of Consumer and Business Services; 2010.

36. World Health Organization. The International Classification of Diseases [Internet]. 10th rev. ed. Geneva (SU): World Health Organization: 1990 [cited 2014 July 9]. Available from: http://www.who.int /classifications/icd/revision/en/.

37. Statistics Canada. Leading causes of death in Canada [Internet]. Ottawa (ON): Government of Canada; 2012 July 25 [cited 2014 July 25]. Available from: http://www.statcan.gc.ca/pub/84-215-x/84-215 -x2012001-eng.htm.

38. Ashmore JP, Krewski D, Zielinski JM, et al. First analysis of mortality and occupational radiation exposure based on the National Dose Registry of Canada. *Am J Epidemiol.* 1998;148(6):564–74. http://dx.doi .org/10.1093/oxfordjournals.aje.a009682. Medline:9753011

39. Hwang SW. Mortality among men using homeless shelters in Toronto, Ontario. *JAMA.* 2000;283(16):2152–7. http://dx.doi.org/10.1001/jama.283.16.2152. Medline:10791509

40. Aronson H, Tough SC. Horse-related fatalities in the Province of Alberta, 1975-1990. *Am J Forensic Med Pathol.* 1993;14(1):28–30. http://dx.doi.org/10.1097/00000433-199303000-00006. Medline:8493964

41. Boyd J, Haegeli P, Abu-Laban RB, et al. Patterns of death among avalanche fatalities: a 21-year review. *CMAJ*. 2009;180(5):507–12. Medline:19213801

42. Service Nova Scotia and Municipal Relations. A handbook for physicians and medical examiners: medical certification of death and stillbirth [Internet]. Halifax (NS): Service Nova Scotia and Municipal Relations; 2002 [cited 2014 July]. Available from: https://www.novascotia.ca/snsmr/pdf/ans-vstat-physicians-handbook.pdf.

43. Choi BC. Perspectives on epidemiologic surveillance in the 21st century. *Chronic Dis Can*. 1998;19(4):145–51. Medline:10029510

44. Public Health Agency of Canada. Notifiable Disease Surveillance System [Internet]. Ottawa (ON): Government of Canada; 2014 March 31 [cited 2014 July 11]. Available from: http://dsol-smed.phac-aspc.gc.ca/dsol-smed/ndis/index-eng.php.

45. Public Health Agency of Canada. Public Health Agency of Canada Chronic Disease Infobase [Internet]. Ottawa (ON): Government of Canada; 2013 April 10 [cited 2014 July 11]. Available from: http://infobase.phac-aspc.gc.ca/.

46. Statistics Canada. CANSIM - Table directory [Internet]. Ottawa (ON): Government of Canada; 2014 July 26 [cited 2014 July 26]. Available from: http://www5.statcan.gc.ca/cansim/a29?lang=eng&p2=17.

47. Statistics Canada. CANSIM - Table directory [Internet]. Ottawa (ON): Government of Canada; [updated 2013 September 25; cited 1014 July]. Available from: http://www5.statcan.gc.ca/cansim/a05?lang=eng&id=1020030&pattern=1020030&searchTypeByValue=1&p2=35.

48. Maskalyk J, Hoey J. SARS update. *CMAJ*. 2003;168(10):1294–5. Medline:12743077

49. Canadian Medical Association. SARS: the struggle for containment. *CMAJ*. 2003;168(10):1229, 1231. Medline:12743047

50. Canadian Cancer Society's Advisory Committee in Cancer Statistics. Canadian cancer statistics 2014. Special topic: skin cancers. Toronto (ON): Canadian Cancer Society; 2014.

51. Statistics Canada. Potential years of life lost, by selected causes of death (ICD-9) and sex, population aged 0 to 74, Canada, provinces and territories [Internet]. Ottawa (ON): Government of Canada; 2002 May 2 [cited 2014 July 9]. Available from: http://www5.statcan.gc.ca/cansim/a26?lang=eng&retrLang=eng&id=1020010&paSer=&pattern=&stByVal=1&p1=1&p2=-1&tabMode=dataTable&csid=.

52. Statistics Canada. Life expectancy [Internet]. Ottawa (ON): Government of Canada; 2013 October 9 [cited 2014 July 13]. Available from: http://www.statcan.gc.ca/search-recherche/bb/info/life-vie-eng.htm.

53. World Health Organization. Life expectancy data by country [Internet]. Geneva (SU): World Health Organization; 2014 [cited 2014 July 24]. Available from: http://apps.who.int/gho/data/node.main.688?lang=en.

54. Ratnasingham S, Cairney J, Manson H, et al. The burden of mental illness and addiction in ontario. *Can J Psychiatry*. 2013;58(9):529–37. Medline:24099501

55. Public Health Agency of Canada. Health-Adjusted Life Expectancy (HALE) in Canada 2012 [Internet]. Ottawa (ON): Government of Canada; [updated 2012 September 25; cited 2014 July 13]. Available from: http://www.phac-aspc.gc.ca/cd-mc/hale-evas-eng.php.

56. Statistics Canada. Prevalence of migraine in the Canadian household population [Internet]. Ottawa (ON): Government of Canada; 2014 June 18 [cited 2014 July 9]. Available from: http://www.statcan.gc.ca/daily-quotidien/140618/dq140618c-eng.pdf.

57. Ellison LF, Wilkins K. Canadian trends in cancer prevalence. *Health Rep*. 2012;23(1):7–16. Medline:22590801

58. Oemar M, Janssen B. EQ-5D-5L user guide: basic information on how to use the EQ-5D-5L instrument. Rotterdam (NL): EuroQol Group; 2013.

59. Feng Y, Bernier J, McIntosh C, et al. Validation of disability categories derived from Health Utilities Index Mark 3 scores. *Health Rep*. 2009;20(2):43–50. Medline:19728585

60. Horsman J, Furlong W, Feeny D, et al. The Health Utilities Index (HUI): concepts, measurement properties and applications. *Health Qual Life Outcomes*. 2003;1(1):54. http://dx.doi.org/10.1186/1477-7525-1-54. Medline:14613568

61. Marra F, Cloutier K, Oteng B, et al. Effectiveness and cost effectiveness of human papillomavirus vaccine: a systematic review. *Pharmacoeconomics*. 2009;27(2):127–47. http://dx.doi.org/10.2165/00019053-200927020-00004. Medline:19254046

62. Vos T, Flaxman AD, Naghavi M, et al. Years lived with disability (YLDs) for 1160 sequelae of 289 diseases and injuries 1990-2010: a systematic analysis for the Global Burden of Disease Study 2010. *Lancet*. 2012;380(9859):2163–96. http://dx.doi.org/10.1016/S0140-6736(12)61729-2. Medline:23245607

63. Murray CJ, Vos T, Lozano R, et al. Disability-adjusted life years (DALYs) for 291 diseases and injuries in 21 regions, 1990-2010: a systematic analysis for the Global Burden of Disease Study 2010. *Lancet*. 2012;380(9859):2197–223. http://dx.doi.org/10.1016/S0140-6736(12)61689-4. Medline:23245608

64. Institute for Health Metrics and Evaluation. GBD 2010 Heat Map [Internet]. Seattle (WA): Institute for Health Metrics and Evaluation, University of Washington; 2013 [cited 2014 July]. Available from: http://vizhub.healthdata.org/irank/heat.php.

65. Sadovnick AD, Eisen K, Ebers GC, et al. Cause of death in patients attending multiple sclerosis clinics. *Neurology*. 1991;41(8):1193–6. http://dx.doi.org/10.1212/WNL.41.8.1193. Medline:1866003

66. Public Health Agency of Canada. Proportional Mortality by Major Causes, 2007: Canada [Internet]. Ottawa (ON): Government of Canada; 2013 July 29 [cited 2014 August 13]. Available from: http://www.cvdinfobase.ca/Proportions.aspx?l=eng&slng=eng&clng=f&DDListHR=00&Button1=Chart&DDListMethod=ByYear&DDListYr=2007.

67. Johansen HL, Wielgosz AT, Nguyen K, et al. Incidence, comorbidity, case fatality and readmission of hospitalized stroke patients in Canada. *Can J Cardiol*. 2006;22(1):65–71. http://dx.doi.org/10.1016/S0828-282X(06)70242-2. Medline:16450021

68. Shields M. Youth smoking. *Health Rep*. 2005;16(3):53–7. Medline:15971516

69. Fiest KM, Dykeman J, Patten SB, et al. Depression in epilepsy: a systematic review and meta-analysis. *Neurology*. 2013;80(6):590–9. http://dx.doi.org/10.1212/WNL.0b013e31827b1ae0. Medline:23175727

70. Thege BK, Colman I, El-guebaly N, Hodgins DC, Patten SB, Schopflocher D, Wolfe J, Wild TC. Substance-related and behavioural addiction problems: two surveys of Canadian adults. *Addict Res Theory*. Forthcoming 2014.

71. Kessler RC, Andrews G, Colpe LJ, et al. Short screening scales to monitor population prevalences and trends in non-specific psychological distress. *Psychol Med*. 2002;32(6):959–76. http://dx.doi.org/10.1017/S0033291702006074. Medline:12214795

72. Oremus M, Oremus C, Hall GB, et al, and the ECT & Cognition Systematic Review Team. Inter-rater and test-retest reliability of quality assessments by novice student raters using the Jadad and Newcastle-Ottawa Scales. *BMJ Open*. 2012;2(4):e001368. http://dx.doi.org/10.1136/bmjopen-2012-001368. Medline:22855629

73. Kassam A, Papish A, Modgill G, et al. The development and psychometric properties of a new scale to measure mental illness related stigma by health care providers: the Opening Minds Scale for Health Care Providers (OMS-HC). *BMC Psychiatry*. 2012;12(1):62. http://dx.doi.org/10.1186/1471-244X-12-62. Medline:22694771

74. Joseph L, Gyorkos TW, Coupal L. Bayesian estimation of disease prevalence and the parameters of diagnostic tests in the absence of a gold standard. *Am J Epidemiol*. 1995;141(3):263–72. Medline:7840100

75. Davidson BL, Elliott CG, Lensing AW, and the The RD Heparin Arthroplasty Group. Low accuracy of color Doppler ultrasound in the detection of proximal leg vein thrombosis in asymptomatic high-risk patients. *Ann Intern Med*. 1992;117(9):735–8. http://dx.doi.org/10.7326/0003-4819-117-9-735. Medline:1416575

76. Oremus M, Postuma R, Griffith L, et al, and the CLSA Algorithms Validation Group. Validating chronic disease ascertainment algorithms for use in the Canadian longitudinal study on aging. *Can J Aging*. 2013;32(3):232–9. http://dx.doi.org/10.1017/S0714980813000275. Medline:23924995

77. Foebel AD, Hirdes JP, Heckman GA, et al, and the ideas PNC research team. Diagnostic data for neurological conditions in interRAI assessments in home care, nursing home and mental health care settings: a validity study. *BMC Health Serv Res*. 2013;13(1):457. http://dx.doi.org/10.1186/1472-6963-13-457. Medline:24176093

78. Marrie RA, Yu BN, Leung S, et al, and the CIHR Team in the Epidemiology and Impact of Comorbidity on Multiple Sclerosis. The utility of administrative data for surveillance of comorbidity in multiple sclerosis: a validation study. *Neuroepidemiology*. 2013;40(2):85–92. http://dx.doi.org/10.1159/000343188. Medline:23095571

79. Statistics Canada. Canadian Community Health Survey - Annual Component [Internet]. Ottawa (ON): Government of Canada; 2013 September 30 [cited 2013 December 30]. Available from: http://www23.statcan.gc.ca/imdb/p2SV.pl?Function=getSurvey&SDDS=3226&lang=en&db=imdb&adm=8&dis=2.

80. Wells JE, Oakley Browne MA, Scott KM, et al, and the New Zealand Mental Health Survey Research Team. Te Rau Hinengaro: the New Zealand Mental Health Survey: overview of methods and findings. *Aust N Z J Psychiatry.* 2006;40(10):835–44. http://dx.doi.org/10.1111/j.1440-1614.2006.01902.x. Medline:16959009

81. Watson EK, Firman DW, Heywood A, et al. Conducting regional health surveys using a computer-assisted telephone interviewing method. *Aust J Public Health.* 1995;19(5):508–11. http://dx.doi.org/10.1111/j.1753-6405.1995.tb00419.x. Medline:8713202

82. Potthoff RF. Telephone sampling in epidemiologic research: to reap the benefits, avoid the pitfalls. *Am J Epidemiol.* 1994;139(10):967–78. Medline:8178785

83. Patten SB, Schopflocher D. Longitudinal epidemiology of major depression as assessed by the Brief Patient Health Questionnaire (PHQ-9). *Compr Psychiatry.* 2009;50(1):26–33. http://dx.doi.org/10.1016/j.comppsych.2008.05.012. Medline:19059510

84. Kish L. Survey sampling. New York: John Wiley & Sons Inc; 1995:1–34.

85. Jette N, Johnston M, Pringsheim T, et al. The case for neurological registry best practice guidelines in Canada. *Can J Neurol Sci.* 2013;40(4 Suppl 2):S1–3. Medline:23787261

86. Bladen CL, Rafferty K, Straub V, et al. The TREAT-NMD Duchenne muscular dystrophy registries: conception, design, and utilization by industry and academia. *Hum Mutat.* 2013;34(11):1449–57. http://dx.doi.org/10.1002/humu.22390. Medline:23913485

87. Furlan JC, Fehlings MG. The National Trauma Registry as a Canadian spine trauma database: a validation study using an institutional clinical database. *Neuroepidemiology.* 2011;37(2):96–101. http://dx.doi.org/10.1159/000330835. Medline:21921642

88. McLellan BA. A Canadian national trauma registry: the time is now. *J Trauma.* 1997;42(5):763–8. http://dx.doi.org/10.1097/00005373-199705000-00001. Medline:9191652

89. Shevell M, Dagenais L, Oskoui M. The epidemiology of cerebral palsy: new perspectives from a Canadian registry. *Semin Pediatr Neurol.* 2013;20(2):60–4. http://dx.doi.org/10.1016/j.spen.2013.06.008. Medline:23948680

90. Canadian Institutes of Health Research; Natural Sciences and Engineering Research Council of Canada; Social Sciences and Humanities Research Council of Canada. TCPS 2—2nd edition of Tri-Council Policy Statement: Ethical Conduct for Research Involving Humans [Internet]. Ottawa (ON): Government of Canada; 2010 [cited 2014 August 31]. Available from: http://www.pre.ethics.gc.ca/eng/policy-politique/initiatives/tcps2-eptc2/Default/.

91. Velasquez, J.C. MK-ULTRAViolence: or, how McGill pioneered psychological torture. *McGill Daily.* 2012;102(2):8–9.

92. Mosby I. Administering colonial science: nutrition research and human biomedical experimentation in aboriginal communities and residential schools, 1942–1952. *Soc Hist.* 2013;46(91):27.

93. Statistics Canada. Canadian Community Health Survey - Mental Health and Wellbeing [Internet]. Ottawa (ON): Government of Canada; 2013 December 18 [cited 2014 July]. Available from: http://www23.statcan.gc.ca:81/imdb/p2SV.pl?Function=getSurvey&SDDS=5015&lang=en&db=imdb&adm=8&dis=2.

94. Barnabe C, Joseph L, Bélisle P, et al. Prevalence of autoimmune inflammatory myopathy in the first nations population of Alberta, Canada. *Arthritis Care Res (Hoboken).* 2012;64(11):1715–9. http://dx.doi.org/10.1002/acr.21743. Medline:22623451

95. Supina AL, Patten SB. Self-reported diagnoses of schizophrenia and psychotic disorders may be valuable for monitoring and surveillance. *Can J Psychiatry.* 2006;51(4):256–9. Medline:16629350

96. Statistics Canada. Deaths and age-standardized mortality rate, by province and territory (deaths) [Internet]. Ottawa (ON): Government of Canada; 2013 September 25 [cited 2014 August 3]. Available from: http://www.statcan.gc.ca/tables-tableaux/sum-som/l01/cst01/hlth86a-eng.htm.

97. Statistics Canada. Table 051-0001. Estimates of population, by age group and sex for July 1, Canada, provinces and territories annual (persons unless otherwise noted) [Internet]. Ottawa (ON): Government of Canada; 2013 November 20 [cited 2014 August 3]. Available from: http://www5.statcan.gc.ca/cansim/a26?lang=eng&retrLang=eng&id=0510001&paSer=&pattern=&stByVal=1&p1=1&p2=37&tabMode=dataTable&csid=.

98. Statistics Canada. Table 102-05041. Deaths and mortality rates, by age group and sex, Canada, provinces and territories annual [Internet]. Ottawa (ON): Government of Canada; 2013 September 25 [cited 2014 August 3]. Available from: http://www5.statcan.gc.ca/cansim/a05?lang=eng&id=1020504&pattern=1020504&searchTypeByValue=1&p2=35.

99. Statistics Canada. Table 102-05631. Leading causes of death, total population, by sex, Canada, provinces and territories annual [Internet]. Ottawa (ON): Government of Canada; 2014 January 28 [cited 2014 August 3]. Available from: http://www5.statcan.gc.ca/cansim/a26.

100. Yergens DW, Dutton DJ, Patten SB. An overview of the statistical methods reported by studies using the Canadian community health survey. BMC Med Res Methodol. 2014;14(1):15. http://dx.doi.org/10.1186/1471-2288-14-15. Medline:24460595

101. Zablotska LB, Lane RS, Frost SE, et al. Leukemia, lymphoma and multiple myeloma mortality (1950-1999) and incidence (1969-1999) in the Eldorado uranium workers cohort. Environ Res. 2014;130: 43–50. http://dx.doi.org/10.1016/j.envres.2014.01.002. Medline:24583244

102. Spittal PM, Hogg RS, Li K, et al. Drastic elevations in mortality among female injection drug users in a Canadian setting. AIDS Care. 2006;18(2):101–8. http://dx.doi.org/10.1080/09540120500159292. Medline:16338767

103. Karamanis G, Skalkidou A, Tsakonas G, et al. Cancer incidence and mortality patterns in women with anorexia nervosa. Int J Cancer. 2014;134(7):1751–7. http://dx.doi.org/10.1002/ijc.28495. Medline:24114497

104. Callaghan RC, Gatley JM, Veldhuizen S, et al. Alcohol- or drug-use disorders and motor vehicle accident mortality: a retrospective cohort study. Accid Anal Prev. 2013;53:149–55. http://dx.doi.org/10.1016/j.aap.2013.01.008. Medline:23434842

105. Nijjar AP, Wang H, Quan H, et al. Ethnic and sex differences in the incidence of hospitalized acute myocardial infarction: British Columbia, Canada 1995-2002. BMC Cardiovasc Disord. 2010;10(1):38. http://dx.doi.org/10.1186/1471-2261-10-38. Medline:20723259

106. Afifi TO, MacMillan HL, Boyle M, et al. Child abuse and mental disorders in Canada. CMAJ. 2014;186(9):E324–32. http://dx.doi.org/10.1503/cmaj.131792. Medline:24756625

107. von Kries R, Koletzko B, Sauerwald T, et al. Breast feeding and obesity: cross sectional study. BMJ. 1999;319(7203):147–50. http://dx.doi.org/10.1136/bmj.319.7203.147. Medline:10406746

108. Weintraub D, Koester J, Potenza MN, et al. Impulse control disorders in Parkinson disease: a cross-sectional study of 3090 patients. Arch Neurol. 2010;67(5):589–95. http://dx.doi.org/10.1001/archneurol.2010.65. Medline:20457959

109. Hackam DG, Thiruchelvam D, Redelmeier DA. Angiotensin-converting enzyme inhibitors and aortic rupture: a population-based case-control study. Lancet. 2006;368(9536):659–65. http://dx.doi.org/10.1016/S0140-6736(06)69250-7. Medline:16920471

110. Friedenreich CM, Speidel TP, Neilson HK, et al. Case-control study of lifetime alcohol consumption and endometrial cancer risk. Cancer Causes Control. 2013;24(11):1995–2003. http://dx.doi.org/10.1007/s10552-013-0275-0. Medline:23929278

111. Rothwell DM, Bondy SJ, Williams JI. Chiropractic manipulation and stroke: a population-based case-control study. Stroke. 2001;32(5):1054–60. http://dx.doi.org/10.1161/01.STR.32.5.1054. Medline:11340209

112. Berkson J. Limitations of the application of fourfold table analysis to hospital data. Biometrics. 1946;2(3):47–53. Medline:21001024

113. Rothman KJ, Greenland S, Poole C, Lash TL. Causation and causal inference. In: Rothman KJ, Greenland S, Lash TL, editors. Modern epidemiology. Philadelphia: Lippincott Williams & Wilkins; 2008. p. 5–31.

114. Health Canada. Strong Foundation, Renewed Focus - An Overview of Canada's Federal Tobacco Control Strategy 2012-17 [Internet]. Ottawa (ON): Government of Canada; [updated 2014 January 23; cited 2014 August 4]. Available from: http://www.hc-sc.gc.ca/hc-ps/pubs/tobac-tabac/fs-sf/index-eng.php.

115. Walboomers JM, Jacobs MV, Manos MM, et al. Human papillomavirus is a necessary cause of invasive cervical cancer worldwide. J Pathol. 1999;189(1):12–9. http://dx.doi.org/10.1002/(SICI)1096-9896(199909)189:1<12::AID-PATH431>3.0.CO;2-F. Medline:10451482

116. Kleinbaum DG, Morgenstern H, Kupper LL. Selection bias in epidemiologic studies. Am J Epidemiol. 1981;113(4):452–63. Medline:6971055

117. Friedenreich CM, Biel RK, Lau DC, et al. Case-control study of the metabolic syndrome and metabolic risk factors for endometrial cancer. Cancer Epidemiol Biomarkers Prev. 2011;20(11):2384–95. http://dx.doi.org/10.1158/1055-9965.EPI-11-0715. Medline:21921255

118. Villeneuve PJ, Jerrett M, Brenner D, et al. A case-control study of long-term exposure to ambient volatile organic compounds and lung cancer in Toronto, Ontario, Canada. Am J Epidemiol. 2014;179(4):443–51. http://dx.doi.org/10.1093/aje/kwt289. Medline:24287467

119. Canadian Longitudinal Study on Aging/ Étude longitudinale canadienne sur le vieillissement. Canadian Longitudinal Study on Aging/ Étude longitudinale canadienne sur le vieillissement [Internet]. Hamilton (ON): Canadian Longitudinal Study on Aging/ Étude longitudinale canadienne sur le vieillissement; 2009 [cited 2014 August 5]. Available from: https://www.clsa-elcv.ca/.

120. Canadian Partnership Against Cancer/Partenariat canadien contre le cancer. Canadian Partnership for Tomorrow Project [Internet]. Toronto (ON): Canadian Partnership Against Cancer; [cited 2014 August 5]. Available from: http://www.partnershipagainstcancer.ca/about-this-site/.

121. Nurses' Health Study. The Nurses' Health Study [Internet]. Boston (MA): [publisher unknown]; [cited 2014 August 5]. Available from: http://www.channing.harvard.edu/nhs/.

122. Centers for Disease Control and Prevention. National Health and Nutrition Examination Survey [Internet]. Atlanta (GA): CDC; [updated 2014 July 30; cited 2014 August 5]. Available from: http://www.cdc.gov/nchs/nhanes.htm.

123. Sackett DL. Bias in analytic research. *J Chronic Dis.* 1979;32(1-2):51–63. http://dx.doi.org/10.1016/0021-9681(79)90012-2. Medline:447779

124. Moura C, Bernatsky S, Abrahamowicz M, et al. Antidepressant use and 10-year incident fracture risk: the population-based Canadian Multicentre Osteoporosis Study (CaMoS). *Osteoporos Int.* 2014;25(5):1473–81. http://dx.doi.org/10.1007/s00198-014-2649-x. Medline:24566587

125. Rothwell PM. External validity of randomised controlled trials: "to whom do the results of this trial apply?". *Lancet.* 2005;365(9453):82–93. http://dx.doi.org/10.1016/S0140-6736(04)17670-8. Medline:15639683

126. Modgill G, Jette N, Wang JL, et al. A population-based longitudinal community study of major depression and migraine. *Headache.* 2012;52(3):422–32. http://dx.doi.org/10.1111/j.1526-4610.2011.02036.x. Medline:22084834

127. Patten SB, Williams JV, Lavorato D, et al. Mortality associated with major depression in a Canadian community cohort. *Can J Psychiatry.* 2011;56(11):658–66. Medline:22114920

128. Vinceti M, Bonvicini F, Rothman KJ, et al. The relation between amyotrophic lateral sclerosis and inorganic selenium in drinking water: a population-based case-control study. *Environ Health.* 2010;9(1):77. http://dx.doi.org/10.1186/1476-069X-9-77. Medline:21134276

129. Stark CR, Mantel N. Effects of maternal age and birth order on the risk of mongolism and leukemia. *J Natl Cancer Inst.* 1966;37(5):687–98. Medline:4224604

130. Julious SA, Mullee MA. Confounding and Simpson's paradox. *BMJ.* 1994;309(6967):1480–1. http://dx.doi.org/10.1136/bmj.309.6967.1480. Medline:7804052

131. Tjepkema M, Wilkins R, Long A. Socio-economic inequalities in cause-specific mortality: a 16-year follow-up study. *Can J Public Health.* 2013;104(7):e472–8. Medline:24495823

132. Cheng I, Caberto CP, Lum-Jones A, et al. Type 2 diabetes risk variants and colorectal cancer risk: the Multiethnic Cohort and PAGE studies. *Gut.* 2011;60(12):1703–11. http://dx.doi.org/10.1136/gut.2011.237727. Medline:21602532

133. Frachon I, Etienne Y, Jobic Y, et al. Benfluorex and unexplained valvular heart disease: a case-control study. *PLoS One.* 2010;5(4):e10128. http://dx.doi.org/10.1371/journal.pone.0010128. Medline:20405030

134. Jadidi E, Mohammadi M, Moradi T. High risk of cardiovascular diseases after diagnosis of multiple sclerosis. *Mult Scler.* 2013;19(10):1336–40. http://dx.doi.org/10.1177/1352458513475833. Medline:23364857

135. Verhave JC, Tagalakis V, Suissa S, et al. The risk of thromboembolic events in kidney transplant patients. *Kidney Int.* 2014;85(6):1454–60. http://dx.doi.org/10.1038/ki.2013.536. Medline:24429408

136. Di Bartolomeo S, Valent F, Sbrojavacca R, et al. A case-crossover study of alcohol consumption, meals and the risk of road traffic crashes. *BMC Public Health.* 2009;9(1):316. http://dx.doi.org/10.1186/1471-2458-9-316. Medline:19723319

137. Redelmeier DA, Tibshirani RJ, Evans L. Traffic-law enforcement and risk of death from motor-vehicle crashes: case-crossover study. *Lancet.* 2003;361(9376):2177–82. http://dx.doi.org/10.1016/S0140-6736(03)13770-1. Medline:12842370

138. Band PR, Le ND, Fang R, et al. Cohort study of Air Canada pilots: mortality, cancer incidence, and leukemia risk. *Am J Epidemiol.* 1996;143(2):137–43. http://dx.doi.org/10.1093/oxfordjournals.aje.a008722. Medline:8546114

139. Dimich-Ward H, Lorenzi M, Teschke K, et al. Mortality and cancer incidence in a cohort of registered nurses from British Columbia, Canada. *Am J Ind Med.* 2007;50(12):892–900. http://dx.doi.org/10.1002/ajim.20505. Medline:17853402

140. Villeneuve PJ, Morrison HI. Coronary heart disease mortality among Newfoundland fluorspar miners. *Scand J Work Environ Health*. 1997;23(3):221–6. http://dx.doi.org/10.5271/sjweh.202. Medline:9243733

141. Villeneuve PJ, Lane RS, Morrison HI. Coronary heart disease mortality and radon exposure in the Newfoundland fluorspar miners' cohort, 1950-2001. *Radiat Environ Biophys*. 2007;46(3):291–6. http://dx.doi.org/10.1007/s00411-007-0108-1. Medline:17453229

142. Schulz KF, Altman DG, Moher D, and the CONSORT Group. CONSORT 2010 statement: updated guidelines for reporting parallel group randomised trials. *PLoS Med*. 2010;7(3):e1000251. http://dx.doi.org/10.1371/journal.pmed.1000251. Medline:20352064

143. Lam RW, Levitt AJ, Levitan RD, et al. The Can-SAD study: a randomized controlled trial of the effectiveness of light therapy and fluoxetine in patients with winter seasonal affective disorder. *Am J Psychiatry*. 2006;163(5):805–12. http://dx.doi.org/10.1176/appi.ajp.163.5.805. Medline:16648320

144. Rossouw JE, Anderson GL, Prentice RL, et al, and the Writing Group for the Women's Health Initiative Investigators. Risks and benefits of estrogen plus progestin in healthy postmenopausal women: principal results From the Women's Health Initiative randomized controlled trial. *JAMA*. 2002;288(3): 321–33. http://dx.doi.org/10.1001/jama.288.3.321. Medline:12117397

145. van Lonkhuijzen L, Kirsh VA, Kreiger N, et al. Endometrial cancer and meat consumption: a case-cohort study. *Eur J Cancer Prev*. 2011;20(4):334–9. http://dx.doi.org/10.1097/CEJ.0b013e328344747c. Medline:21422932

146. WHO Mortality Database [database]. Geneva (SU): World Health Organization; [updated 2104]. Available from: http://www.who.int/healthinfo/mortality_data/en/.

147. Cheng JJ, Schuster-Wallace CJ, Watt S, et al. An ecological quantification of the relationships between water, sanitation and infant, child, and maternal mortality. *Environ Health*. 2012;11(1):4. http://dx.doi.org/10.1186/1476-069X-11-4. Medline:22280473

148. Durbin A, Lin E, Taylor L, et al. First-generation immigrants and hospital admission rates for psychosis and affective disorders: an ecological study in Ontario. *Can J Psychiatry*. 2011;56(7):418–26. Medline:21835105

149. Auger N, Zang G, Daniel M. Community-level income inequality and mortality in Québec, Canada. *Public Health*. 2009;123(6):438–43. http://dx.doi.org/10.1016/j.puhe.2009.04.012. Medline:19482322

150. Reich KM, Chang HJ, Rezaie A, et al. The incidence rate of colectomy for medically refractory ulcerative colitis has declined in parallel with increasing anti-TNF use: a time-trend study. *Aliment Pharmacol Ther*. 2014;40(6):629–38. http://dx.doi.org/10.1111/apt.12873. Medline:25039715

151. Shiue I, Shiue M. Indoor temperature below 18°C accounts for 9% population attributable risk for high blood pressure in Scotland. *Int J Cardiol*. 2014;171(1):e1–2. http://dx.doi.org/10.1016/j.ijcard.2013.11.040. Medline:24315341

152. Kuendig H, Hasselberg M, Laflamme L, et al. Acute alcohol consumption and injury: risk associations and attributable fractions for different injury mechanisms. *J Stud Alcohol Drugs*. 2008;69(2):218–26. Medline:18299762

153. Yusuf S, Hawken S, Ounpuu S, et al, and the INTERHEART Study Investigators. Effect of potentially modifiable risk factors associated with myocardial infarction in 52 countries (the INTERHEART study): case-control study. *Lancet*. 2004;364(9438):937–52. http://dx.doi.org/10.1016/S0140-6736(04)17018-9. Medline:15364185

154. Patten SB, Williams JV, Love EJ. Depressive symptoms attributable to medication exposure in a medical inpatient population. *Can J Psychiatry*. 1996;41(10):651–4. Medline:8978945

155. Arseneault L, Cannon M, Witton J, et al. Causal association between cannabis and psychosis: examination of the evidence. *Br J Psychiatry*. 2004;184(2):110–7. http://dx.doi.org/10.1192/bjp.184.2.110. Medline:14754822

156. Hill AB. The environment and disease: association or causation? *Proc R Soc Med*. 1965;58:295–300. Medline:14283879

157. Surgeon General's Advisory Committee on Smoking and Health. Smoking and health: report of the advisory committee to the surgeon general of the public health service. Washington (DC): US Public Health Service, Office of the Surgeon General; 1964.

158. Bosch FX, Lorincz A, Muñoz N, et al. The causal relation between human papillomavirus and cervical cancer. *J Clin Pathol*. 2002;55(4):244–65. http://dx.doi.org/10.1136/jcp.55.4.244. Medline:11919208

159. VanderWeele TJ, Robins JM. The identification of synergism in the sufficient-component-cause framework. *Epidemiology*. 2007;18(3):329–39. http://dx.doi.org/10.1097/01.ede.0000260218.66432.88. Medline:17435441

160. Au B, Smith KJ, Gariépy G, Schmitz N. C-reactive protein, depressive symptoms, and risk of diabetes: results from the English Longitudinal Study of Ageing (ELSA). *J Pschosom Res*. 2014;77(3):180–6.

161. Mente A, de Koning L, Shannon HS, et al. A systematic review of the evidence supporting a causal link between dietary factors and coronary heart disease. *Arch Intern Med*. 2009;169(7):659–69. http://dx.doi.org/10.1001/archinternmed.2009.38. Medline:19364995

162. Hodgson C. What is the distribution of deaths due to cerebrovascular disease in Ontario? *CMAJ*. 1998;159(6 Suppl):s25–31.

163. Richards JB, Papaioannou A, Adachi JD, et al, and the Canadian Multicentre Osteoporosis Study Research Group. Effect of selective serotonin reuptake inhibitors on the risk of fracture. *Arch Intern Med*. 2007;167(2):188–94. http://dx.doi.org/10.1001/archinte.167.2.188. Medline:17242321

164. Agrawal S, Ebrahim S. Association between legume intake and self-reported diabetes among adult men and women in India. *BMC Public Health*. 2013;13(1):706. http://dx.doi.org/10.1186/1471-2458-13-706. Medline:23915141

165. Cedergren MI, Källén BA. Maternal obesity and infant heart defects. *Obes Res*. 2003;11(9):1065–71. http://dx.doi.org/10.1038/oby.2003.146. Medline:12972676

166. Petitti DB, Harlan SL, Chowell-Puente G, et al. Occupation and environmental heat-associated deaths in Maricopa county, Arizona: a case-control study. *PLoS One*. 2013;8(5):e62596. http://dx.doi.org/10.1371/journal.pone.0062596. Medline:23734174

167. O'Keefe JH, Lavie CJ. Run for your life ... at a comfortable speed and not too far. *Heart*. 2013;99(8):516–9. http://dx.doi.org/10.1136/heartjnl-2012-302886. Medline:23197444

168. O'Keefe JH, Schnohr P, Lavie CJ. The dose of running that best confers longevity. *Heart*. 2013;99(8):588–90. http://dx.doi.org/10.1136/heartjnl-2013-303683. Medline:23512971

169. Weber T. Response to 'Run for your life ... at a comfortable speed and not too far'. *Heart*. 2013;99(8):588. http://dx.doi.org/10.1136/heartjnl-2012-303556. Medline:23512970

170. Institute for Health Metrics and Evaluation. GBD profile: Canada [Internet]. Seattle (WA): Institute for Health Metrics and Evaluation, University of Washington; 2013 March 5 [cited 2014 July]. 4 p. Available from: http://www.healthdata.org/sites/default/files/files/country_profiles/GBD/ihme_gbd_country_report_canada.pdf.

171. MacLaren VV, Best LA. Multiple addictive behaviors in young adults: student norms for the Shorter PROMIS Questionnaire. *Addict Behav*. 2010;35(3):252–5. http://dx.doi.org/10.1016/j.addbeh.2009.09.023. Medline:19879058

172. Thombs BD, Coyne JC, Cuijpers P, et al. Rethinking recommendations for screening for depression in primary care. *CMAJ*. 2012;184(4):413–8. http://dx.doi.org/10.1503/cmaj.111035. Medline:21930744

INDEX

adjusted estimates, 170, 182
administrative data, 132–133
administrative record linkage, 146
age
   and confounding, 95, 96, 98–101,
     182–183
   and lifetime prevalence, 24
   and mortality rates, 41, 44–45, 98–101
age-specific mortality, 42
analogy, in causal judgement, 223
analysis stage, and confounding,
    169–171, 181
analytic studies, and descriptive
    studies, 113
analytical epidemiology, 2
area frame, 87
association
   case-control studies, 126–127
   and causality, 219–221
   concept and example, 11–12
   and confounding, 165–166, 170
   cross-sectional studies, 116–120
   measures, 162–163, 208–213
   prospective cohort studies, 155–157
   strength of, 219
attack rate, 27
attributable fraction/proportion,
    210, 212
attributable risk, 208–210
attributable risk among the exposed,
    209
attributable risk percent, 209, 212–213
attrition, 89–90, 158, 161, 202

base rate, 72
Bayes' theorem, 72–73, 75–76
beneficence, 91
Berkson's bias, 133
bias (systematic error)
   critical appraisal, 231
   and causality, 217
   characteristics, 144–145
   definition, 77
   direction and magnitude, 147, 235
   and measurement error, 65–66, 84

   and selection error, 84
   systematic error *vs.* random error, 16,
    52, 53, 80, 84
bias towards the null, 135, 147
binary outcomes, 15
biological gradient, 221
biological plausibility, 221–222
bivariate parameters, 162
blinding, 147
burden of disease, 30, 45, 47–48

Canadian Community Health Survey
    (CCHS), 114
Canadian Coroner and Medical
    Examiner Database, 38
Canadian Institute of Health
    Information (CIHI), 37
Canadian Mortality Registry, 37
cancer registries, 89, 132
CANSIM (Canadian Socio-Economic
    Information Management
    System), 28
cardinal data, 67
case-cohort studies, 203
case-control studies
   and association, 126–127
   cases and controls, 126, 127–129
   concept, 125–126
   design, 126–130
   differential misclassification bias,
    134–135, 145, 148–149
   direction, temporal and logical,
    151–152, 196
   efficiency, 129, 140
   and exposure, 126, 132–133,
    135–138, 140
   incidence and prevalence, 136–137
   misclassification bias, 133–135,
    140–141, 235–237
   nested case-control studies,
    195–197, 203
   nondifferential misclassification bias,
    135, 146, 148–149
   and odds ratios, 128–129, 130–132,
    133–134, 135–138

ABOUT THE AUTHOR

Dr. Scott Patten obtained an MD from the University of Alberta in 1986, and subsequently completed an FRCP(C) in psychiatry (1991) and a PhD in epidemiology (1994) at the University of Calgary. He is a professor in the department of Community Health Sciences at the University of Calgary and is a senior health scholar with Alberta Innovates, Health Solutions. He has over 20 years experience teaching epidemiology and supervising graduate students. As a researcher, he has published more than 400 scientific papers and is the editor-in-chief of the *Canadian Journal of Psychiatry*.